T0293620

OXFORD HANDBOOK OF
Pathology

Published and forthcoming Oxford Handbooks

OXFORD HANDBOOK OF
Pathology

THIRD EDITION

EDITED BY

James Carton

Consultant Histopathologist
North West London Pathology
Imperial College Healthcare NHS Trust
London, UK

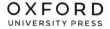

OXFORD
UNIVERSITY PRESS

Great Clarendon Street, Oxford, OX2 6DP,
United Kingdom

Oxford University Press is a department of the University of Oxford.
It furthers the University's objective of excellence in research, scholarship,
and education by publishing worldwide. Oxford is a registered trade mark of
Oxford University Press in the UK and in certain other countries

First Edition published in 2012
Second Edition published in 2017
Third Edition published in 2024

Published in the United States of America by Oxford University Press
198 Madison Avenue, New York, NY 10016, United States of America

British Library Cataloguing in Publication Data
Data available

Library of Congress Control Number: 2023951398

ISBN 978–0–19–289742–8

DOI: 10.1093/med/9780192897428.001.0001

Printed and bound in China by
C&C Offset Printing Co., Ltd.

To my husband for everything—Rob.
To my family for all the love—Mum, Dad, Keith, Betty, Anita,
Lorna, Kyle, Zack, Nicky, and Bella.
To my friends for all the laughs—Sheena, Allie, Tim, Emma, Jonny,
Jessie, Alastair, and Ian.

Contents

Preface to the third edition

I am thrilled to be able to present this third edition of the Oxford Handbook which I hope readers will find useful and informative.

Notable changes include a change in title to *Oxford Handbook of Pathology* rather than *Oxford Handbook of Clinical Pathology*. This revised title is thought to better reflect the content of the book which is predominantly anatomic/cellular pathology rather than the other pathology disciplines which are often collectively referred to as clinical pathology.

A new chapter on laboratory techniques has been added to explain the basics of commonly used ancillary techniques in pathology, particularly immunohistochemistry and molecular tests.

The cardiac and vascular chapters have been combined into a single cardiovascular pathology chapter, which reflects the very close relationship between these two organ systems.

A new entry on COVID-19 has been added to the infectious diseases chapter as one cannot possibly ignore the impact this novel coronavirus has had on the world since the previous edition.

All other chapters have also been updated, with particular focus on tumour pathology and new molecular diagnostic techniques.

I would like to take this opportunity to thank all the contributors who delivered their chapters whilst navigating the challenges of a pandemic and huge diagnostic reporting obligations. Thanks also to the team at Oxford University Press for their understanding and patience during the production of this new edition.

Dr James Carton, London, 2022

Contributors

Dr Scott Akker
Consultant Endocrinologist, Barts
Health NHS Trust, London, UK.

Professor Dan Berney
Professor of Genitourinary
Pathology, Barts Health NHS Trust,
London, UK.

Professor Robert Goldin
Professor of Liver and GI Pathology,
North West London Pathology,
London, UK.

Dr Monika Hofer
Consultant Neuropathologist,
Oxford University Hospitals NHS
Trust, Oxford, UK.

Dr Baljeet Kaur
Consultant Histopathologist,
North West London Pathology,
London, UK.

Dr Panagiota Mavrigiannaki
Consultant Histopathologist,
North West London Pathology,
London, UK.

Dr Rathi Ramakrishnan
Consultant Histopathologist,
North West London Pathology,
London, UK.

Dr Manuel Rodriguez-Justo
Consultant Histopathologist,
University College Hospitals NHS
Trust, London, UK.

Dr Candice Roufosse
Consultant Histopathologist,
North West London Pathology,
London, UK.

Dr James Sampson
Consultant Histopathologist,
Newcastle upon Tyne Hospitals
NHS Foundation Trust,
Newcastle, UK.

Dr Justin Weir
Consultant Histopathologist, Royal
Marsden NHS Foundation Trust,
London, UK.

Symbols and abbreviations

ABC	Aneurysmal bone cyst
ADH	Atypical ductal hyperplasia
ADTKD	Autosomal dominant tubulointerstitial kidney disease
AIDP	Acute inflammatory demyelinating polyneuropathy
AIDP	Atypical intraductal proliferation
AIN	Anal intraepithelial neoplasia
AITL	Angioimmunoblastic T-cell lymphoma
AKD	Acute kidney disease
AKI	Acute kidney injury
ALCL	Anaplastic large-cell lymphoma
ALH	Atypical lobular hyperplasia
ALL	Acute lymphoblastic leukaemia
AML	Acute myeloid leukaemia
AMSAN	Acute motor sensory axonal neuropathy
ANCA	Anti-neutrophil cytoplasm antibodies
APKD	Adult polycystic kidney disease
APP	Amyloid precursor protein
APTT	Activated partial thromboplastin time
ARDS	Acute respiratory distress syndrome
ARVD	Arrhythmogenic right ventricular dysplasia
ASD	Atrial septal defect
ATLL	Adult T-cell lymphoma
ATM	Ataxia-telangiectasia mutated
BCMA	B-cell maturation antigen
BL	Burkitt's lymphoma
BPH	Benign prostatic hyperplasia
CD	Cluster of differentiation
CD	Crohn's disease
CFTR	Cystic fibrosis transmembrane conductance regulator
CHD	Coronary heart disease
CIS	Carcinoma in situ
CKD	Chronic kidney disease
CLL	Chronic lymphocytic leukaemia

CML	Chronic myelogenous leukaemia
CNS	Central nervous system
COF	Cemento-ossifying fibroma
COPD	Chronic obstructive pulmonary disease
CRS	Cytokine-release syndrome
CS	Chondrosarcoma
CT	Computed tomography
DCIS	Ductal carcinoma in situ
DDD	Dense deposit disease
DIC	Disseminated intravascular coagulation
DLBCL	Diffuse large B-cell lymphoma
DPLD	Diffuse parenchymal lung disease
EATL	Enteropathy-associated T-cell lymphoma
ELISA	Enzyme-linked immunosorbent assay
ES	Epithelioid sarcoma
ESR	Erythrocyte sedimentation rate
ET	Essential thrombocythaemia
FAP	Familial adenomatous polyposis
FEA	Flat epithelial atypia
FESS	Functional endoscopic sinus surgery
FISH	Fluorescence in-situ hybridization
FISH	Fluorescent in-situ hybridization
FMTC	Familial medullary thyroid cancer
FNA	Fine-needle aspiration
FOB	Faecal occult blood
FSGS	Focal segmental glomerulosclerosis
FSH	Follicle-stimulating hormone
FVC	Forced vital capacity
GCNIS	Germ cell neoplasia in situ
GFR	Glomerular filtration rate
GvHD	Graft versus host disease
H&E	Haematoxylin & eosin
HAV	Hepatitis A virus

HBV	Hepatitis B virus
HCG	Human chorionic gonadotrophin
HCV	Hepatitis C virus
HDV	Hepatitis D virus
HEV	Hepatitis E virus
HIE	Hypoxic ischaemic encephalopathy
HIF	Hypoxia inducible factor
HIV	Human immunodeficiency virus
HLA	Human leucocyte antigen
HNPCC	Hereditary non-polyposis colorectal cancer
HPV	Human papilloma virus
HSCT	Haematopoietic stem cell transplant
HSV	Herpes simplex virus
IgAN	IgA nephropathy
IPF	Idiopathic pulmonary fibrosis
IPMN	Intraductal papillary neoplasms
ISLN	In situ lobular neoplasia
ISUP	International Society of Urologic Pathologists
ITP	Idiopathic thrombocytopenic purpura
JPOF	Juvenile psammomatoid ossifying fibroma
JTOF	Juvenile trabecular ossifying fibroma
LCIS	Lobular carcinoma in situ
LDL	Low-density lipoprotein
LFT	Liver function tests
LH	Luteinizing hormone
LP	Lymphocyte-predominant
MALT	Mucosa-associated lymphoid tissue
MASP	Mannose-binding lectin-associated serine protease
MCD	Minimal change disease
MCHC	Mean corpuscular haemoglobin concentration
MCV	Mean corpuscular volume
MEN	Multiple endocrine neoplasia
MFH	Malignant fibrous histiocytoma
MGUS	Monoclonal gammopathy of undetermined significance
MHC	Major histocompatibility complex
MoM	Metal-on-metal

MOMP	Mitochondrial outer membrane permeabilization
MPNST	Malignant peripheral nerve sheath tumour
NAFLD	Non-alcoholic fatty liver disease
NETS	Neuroendocrine tumours
NGS	Next generation sequencing
NK	Natural killer
NLPHL	Nodular lymphocyte-predominant Hodgkin's lymphoma
NOS	Not otherwise specified
NSAID	Non-steroidal anti-inflammatory drug
ONT	Oxford Nanopore Technologies
PBC	Primary biliary cholangitis
PCR	Polymerase chain reaction
PCV	Packed cell volume
PDA	Patent ductus arteriosus
PIN	Prostatic intraepithelial neoplasia
PPNAD	Primary pigmented nodular adrenocortical disease
PSA	Prostate-specific antigen
PT	Prothrombin time
PTH	Parathyroid hormone
PTLD	Post-transplant lymphoproliferative diseases
PV	Polycythaemia vera
RA	Rheumatoid arthritis
RAEB	Refractory anaemia with excess of blasts
RARA	Retinoic acid receptor alpha
RARS	Refractory anaemia with ring sideroblasts
RBC	Red blood cells
RCC	Renal cell carcinoma
RCU	Refractory cytopenia with unilineage
SCC	Squamous cell carcinoma
SCD	Sickle-cell disease
SIL	Squamous intraepithelial lesion
SLE	Systemic lupus erythematosus
SMA	Smooth muscle actin
TIA	Transient ischaemic attacks
TNBC	Triple negative breast cancer
TNM	Tumour, Node, Metastasis
TSH	Thyroid-stimulating hormone

TTP	Thrombotic thrombocytopenic purpura
UC	Ulcerative colitis
UEH	Usual epithelial hyperplasia
UIP	Usual interstitial pneumonia

UTI	Urinary tract infection
VSD	Ventricular septal defect
WCC	White cell count

Chapter 1

Basic pathology

Pathological terminology

Nomenclature of disease

- **Aetiology** refers to a disease's underlying cause. Diseases whose aetiology is unknown are described as **idiopathic**, **cryptogenic**, or **essential**.
- **Pathogenesis** refers to the mechanism by which the aetiological agent produces the manifestations of a disease.
- **Incidence** refers to the number of new cases of a disease diagnosed over a certain period of time.
- **Prevalence** refers to the total number of cases of a disease present in a population at a certain moment in time.
- **Prognosis** is a prediction of the likely course of a disease.
- **Morbidity** describes the extent to which a patient's overall health will be affected by a disease.
- **Mortality** reflects the likelihood of death from a particular disease.
- **Acute** and **chronic** refer to the time course of a pathological event. Acute illnesses are of rapid onset. Chronic conditions usually have a gradual onset and are more likely to have a prolonged course.
- **A syndrome** refers to a set of symptoms and clinical signs that, when occurring together, suggest a particular underlying cause(s).

Classification of disease

- **Genetic** diseases are inherited conditions in which a defective gene causes the disease (e.g. cystic fibrosis).
- **Infective** diseases are the result of invasion of the body by pathogenic microbes (e.g. malaria).
- **Inflammatory** diseases are due to excess inflammatory cell activity in an organ (e.g. rheumatoid arthritis).
- **Neoplastic** disease results from an uncontrolled proliferation of cells (e.g. breast carcinoma).
- **Vascular** diseases arise due to disorders of blood vessels (e.g. ischaemic heart disease).
- **Metabolic** disorders arise due to abnormalities within metabolic pathways (e.g. diabetes mellitus).
- **Degenerative** diseases occur as a consequence of damage and/or loss of specialized cells (e.g. loss of neurones from the cerebral cortex in Alzheimer's disease).
- **Iatrogenic** disease is the result of the effects of treatment (e.g. osteoporosis due to long-term glucocorticoid treatment).
- **Congenital** diseases are present at birth, whereas those occurring after birth are known as **acquired**.

Cellular adaptations

Atrophy

- A reduction in size of a tissue or organ.
- May occur through a reduction in cell number by deletion (apoptosis) or a reduction in cell size through shrinkage.
- Atrophy may occur as a normal physiological process (e.g. thymic atrophy during adolescence and post-menopausal ovarian atrophy).
- Examples of pathological atrophy include muscle atrophy following denervation and cerebral atrophy due to cerebrovascular disease.

Hypertrophy

- An increase in size of individual cells.
- Due to an increase in cell proteins and organelles.
- Seen in organs containing terminally differentiated cells that cannot multiply (e.g. cardiac and skeletal muscle).
- Examples of physiological hypertrophy include the myometrium of the uterus in pregnancy and muscles of a bodybuilder.
- Examples of pathological hypertrophy include left ventricular hypertrophy due to aortic stenosis (→ Calcific aortic stenosis, p. 42).

Hyperplasia

- An increase in cell number.
- Examples of physiological hyperplasia include endometrium and breast lobules in response to cyclical oestrogen exposure.
- Examples of pathological hyperplasia include benign prostatic hyperplasia (BPH) (→ Benign prostatic hyperplasia, p. 266) and parathyroid hyperplasia (→ Parathyroid hyperplasia, p. 393).

Metaplasia

- A change in which one cell type is switched for another.
- Thought to be the result of progenitor cells differentiating into a new type of cell, rather than a direct morphogenesis of cells from one type to another.
- Seen almost exclusively in epithelial cells, often in response to chronic injury.
- Metaplasia is named according to the new type of cell type (e.g. a change from non-squamous to squamous epithelium is called squamous metaplasia).
- Common sites of squamous metaplasia include the endocervix (creating the transformation zone where cervical neoplasia occurs) and the bronchi of smokers.
- Common sites of glandular metaplasia include the lower oesophagus in some people with reflux disease, creating a visible Barrett's oesophagus (→ Oesophagitis, p. 110).
- Metaplasia is a marker of long-term epithelial damage which, in **some** cases, may develop into epithelial **dysplasia** and eventually **carcinoma**.

Cellular death

Definitions
- **Cellular death** is the irreversible cessation of vital cellular functions culminating in the loss of cellular integrity.
- **Accidental cell death** is the virtually instantaneous and uncontrollable form of cell death corresponding to the physical disassembly of the plasma membrane caused by extreme physical, chemical, or mechanical cues.
- **Regulated cell death** is a controlled form of cell death in which superfluous, irreversibly damaged, or potentially harmful cells are targeted for elimination through activation of signalling pathways.
- **Programmed cell death** is a particular form of regulated cell death that occurs under physiological situations.

Morphological correlates of cell death
- Apoptosis: cell shrinkage, nuclear fragmentation, membrane blebbing, formation of small vesicles ('apoptotic bodies') taken up by neighbouring cells and degraded within lysosomes.
- Autophagy: degradation of unwanted cytoplasmic components within lysosomes.
- Necrosis: cellular breakdown with no phagocytic or lysosymal involvement.

Examples of regulated cell death
- **Extrinsic apoptosis** is propagated by CASP8 and precipitated by executioner caspases, mainly CASP3.
- **Intrinsic apoptosis** is demarcated by MOMP (mitochondrial outer membrane permeabilization), and precipitated by executioner caspases, mainly CASP3.
- **MPT-driven necrosis** is initiated by disturbances of the intracellular microenvironment such as severe oxidative stress and cytosolic calcium overload.
- **Necroptosis** depends on MLKL, RIPK3, and (in some settings) on the kinase activity of RIPK1.
- **Pyroptosis** depends on the formation of plasma membrane pores by members of the gasdermin protein family, often as a consequence of inflammatory caspase activation.
- Note that each type of regulated cell death can result in a range of immune reactions from anti-inflammatory/tolerogenic to pro-inflammatory/immunogenic.

Inflammation and healing

General concepts

- Inflammation is a response to cellular injury that aims to eliminate the cause and heal any damage that has been caused.
- Recognition of cellular injury triggers release of inflammatory mediators such as cytokines which stimulates recruitment of leukocytes and inflammatory proteins from the blood to the site of injury.
- Successful inflammatory response results in removal of the stimulus for inflammation and subsequent healing.
- Regulation of inflammation is critically important. Many diseases are the result of a misdirected or inadequately controlled inflammatory reaction.

Acute inflammation

- A rapid, non-specific response to cellular injury.
- Orchestrated by **cytokines** released from injured cells (e.g. histamine, serotonin, prostaglandins, leukotrienes, and platelet-activating factor).
- Cytokines activate endothelial cells, leading to the formation of an **acute inflammatory exudate** containing fluid, fibrin, and neutrophils.
- Severe acute inflammation may lead to a localized collection of pus within a necrotic cavity (**abscess**).
- Acute inflammation may resolve, heal with scarring, or progress to chronic inflammation.

Chronic inflammation

- Persistent form of inflammation in which there is simultaneous tissue damage and attempted repair.
- May arise from acute inflammation or occur from the outset.
- Characterized by the presence of chronic inflammatory cells, namely macrophages, lymphocytes, and plasma cells.
- More likely to heal with irreversible scarring than resolve.

Granulomatous inflammation

- A special type of chronic inflammation characterized by the presence of activated macrophages known as epithelioid histiocytes.
- Collections of epithelioid macrophages are known as **granulomas**.
- Granulomatous inflammation is associated with foreign bodies, persistent infections (e.g. mycobacteria), and diseases whose cause is unclear (e.g. sarcoidosis).

Healing

- Process of replacing dead and damaged tissue with healthy tissue.
- May occur through regeneration or repair.
- **Regeneration** (resolution) replaces damaged cells with the same type of cell and is the ideal outcome. This can only occur if the connective tissue framework of the tissue is not disrupted and if the tissue is capable of regeneration.
- **Repair** begins with the formation of granulation tissue which is then converted into a collagen-rich scar. Although the structural integrity is maintained, there is loss of function of the tissue that is scarred.

Innate immunity

Epithelial surfaces

- Epithelial surfaces form a physical barrier against infection.
- Low pH of skin and fatty acids in sebum inhibit microbial growth.
- The gut has gastric acid, pancreatic enzymes, mucosal immunoglobulin A (IgA), and normal colonic flora which act to prevent establishment of infection.
- The respiratory tract secretes mucus to trap organisms, and beating cilia transport them to the throat where they are swallowed.
- Continuous flushing of urine through the urinary tract prevents microbes from adhering to the urothelium.

Phagocytes

- Organisms breaching epithelial surfaces encounter tissue macrophages that recognize pathogens and attract neutrophils to the site.
- Macrophages and neutrophils are phagocytes that ingest microbes by phagocytosis into a phagosome.
- The phagosome is fused to cytoplasmic lysosomes that contain enzymes and reactive oxygen intermediates that kill the microbe.
- Phagocytes recognize organisms by pattern recognition receptors (e.g. mannose receptors, Toll-like receptors, and Nod-like receptors).

Acute phase proteins

- Cytokines produced by phagocytes stimulate the liver to rapidly synthesize and release acute phase proteins.
- **Mannose-binding lectin** recognizes microbial surface sugars and undergoes a conformational change, allowing it to bind a protein mannose-binding lectin-associated serine protease (MASP) and form a complex which activates complement.
- **C-reactive protein** binds to the phosphorylcholine portions of microbial lipopolysaccharide and targets them for phagocytosis by macrophages.

Complement

- A collection of circulating proteins that assist the immune system in killing microbes.
- May be activated by antibodies bound to a microbe (**classical pathway**), triggered automatically on microbes lacking a regulatory protein present on host cells (**alternative pathway**), or by mannose-binding protein (**lectin pathway**).
- A sequential cascade leads to the generation of C3 convertase, an enzyme that splits many molecules of C3 into C3b.
- Microbes coated in C3b are destroyed either by phagocytosis or the **membrane attack complex**, a polymer of the terminal complement components which forms holes in the cell membrane of the microbe.
- The complement system is tightly regulated to prevent uncontrolled activation. **Decay accelerating factor** disrupts binding to C3b to cell surfaces and **membrane co-factor** protein breaks down C3b.

Adaptive immunity

Antibody-mediated immunity

- Mediated by proteins called **antibodies** or **immunoglobulins**.
- Binding of antigen to the Fab antigen-binding region unmasks the binding sites on the Fc portion which mediates the functions of the antibody.
- Antibodies work in four main ways:
  - Neutralize the biological activity of a vital microbial molecule (e.g. a binding protein or toxin).
  - Target microbes for phagocytosis.
  - Activate complement.
  - Activate cytotoxic immune cells.
- Antibody production is initiated following binding of an antigen to its specific B-cell receptor on the surface of naïve B-lymphocytes in the presence of an additional signal from CD4+ helper T-lymphocytes.

Cell-mediated immunity

- Predominantly mediated by T-lymphocytes.
- CD4+ helper T-cells are activated by foreign peptides presented by class II major histocompatibility complex (MHC) molecules expressed by specialized antigen-presenting cells such as dendritic cells and macrophages.
- Activated CD4+ helper T-cells proliferate and secrete cytokines that mediate a variety of immune responses.
- Many subtypes of helper T-cells are recognized, depending on the cytokines they produce when activated, including Th1, Th2, Th3, and Th17.
- CD8+ cytotoxic T-cells are activated by foreign peptides presented by class I MHC expressed by all nucleated cells.
- Activated CD8+ cytotoxic T-cells destroy the presenting host cell either by stimulating apoptosis through the **Fas ligand** or by inserting a membrane pore called **perforin** through which the T-cell pours in proteolytic enzymes.

Hypersensitivity reactions

Definition

- A group of diseases caused by an abnormal immune-mediated reaction.
- May be directed at an exogenous antigen from the environment or a self-antigen (in which case the reaction is a form of autoimmunity).

Immediate (type 1) hypersensitivity

- Characterized by the production of immunoglobulin E (IgE) antibodies in response to an antigen.
- Cross-linkage of surface IgE receptors on mast cells releases mediators, such as histamine, which stimulate acute inflammation.
- Typical of people with **atopy**, a genetic disposition to produce large quantities of IgE in response to environmental antigens such as pollen and house dust mites.
- **Anaphylaxis** represents a systemic form of immediate hypersensitivity caused by the widespread release of histamine. In its most severe form, it can lead to **anaphylactic shock**.
- Immediate hypersensitivity diseases affect >20% of people and the incidence is rising.

Antibody-mediated (type 2) hypersensitivity

- Caused by immunoglobulin G (IgG) or immunoglobulin M (IgM) antibodies binding to a fixed antigen in a tissue.
- Binding of the antibody may activate complement and lead to cellular injury (e.g. bullous pemphigoid; ➲ Bullous pemphigoid, p. 486), or cause a change in cellular function (e.g. thyroid-stimulating hormone [TSH] receptor-stimulating antibody in Graves' disease; ➲ Graves' disease, p. 378).

Immune complex-mediated (type 3) hypersensitivity

- Caused by circulating IgG or IgM antibodies forming immune complexes with antigen in the blood and depositing in tissues where they activate complement.
- Sites of predilection for the deposition of immune complexes include small blood vessels, kidneys, and joints.
- Immune complex-mediated hypersensitivity reactions tend to be multisystem diseases in which vasculitis, arthritis, and glomerulonephritis feature (e.g. systemic lupus erythematosus; ➲ Systemic lupus erythematosus, p. 620).

T-cell-mediated (type 4) hypersensitivity

- Caused by activated T-lymphocytes that injure cells by direct cell killing or releasing cytokines that activate macrophages.
- Because T-cell responses take 1–2 days to occur, this type is also known as delayed-type hypersensitivity.
- Examples include contact dermatitis (➲ Eczema, p. 478), Hashimoto's thyroiditis (➲ Hashimoto's thyroiditis, p. 376), primary biliary cholangitis (➲ Primary biliary cholangitis, p. 158), and TB (➲ Tuberculosis, p. 24).

Neoplasia

Definitions

- **A neoplasm** is an abnormal mass of tissue which shows uncoordinated growth and serves no useful purpose. The word is often used synonymously with the word **tumour** which simply means a swelling.
- **Benign** neoplasms usually have a slow rate of growth and remain confined to their site of origin. Benign neoplasms usually run an innocuous course but can be dangerous if they compress vital nearby structures or if the neoplasm secretes hormones uncontrollably.
- **Malignant** neoplasms have capacity to spread or metastasize to distant sites and produce secondary tumours called metastases which can grow independently from the primary tumour.
- **Cancer** is a broad term for any malignant neoplasm.

Nomenclature of neoplasms

Epithelial neoplasms

- Benign neoplasms of squamous epithelium are called **acanthomas** if they are flat or **papillomas** if they grow in branching fronds.
- Benign neoplasms of glandular epithelium are called **adenomas**.
- Epithelial malignancies are called **carcinomas**. Carcinomas showing squamous differentiation are called **squamous cell carcinomas**. Carcinomas showing glandular differentiation are called **adenocarcinomas**.
- Carcinomas are often preceded by a phase of epithelial **dysplasia**, in which the epithelium contains neoplastic cells but invasion beyond the confines of the epithelium has not yet occurred.

Connective tissue neoplasms

- Lipoma is a benign adipocytic tumour.
- Leiomyoma is a benign smooth muscle tumour.
- Rhabdomyoma is a benign skeletal muscle tumour.
- Angioma is a benign vascular tumour.
- Osteoma is a benign bony tumour.
- Liposarcoma is a malignant adipocytic tumour.
- Leiomyosarcoma is a malignant smooth muscle tumour.
- Rhabdomyosarcoma is a malignant skeletal muscle tumour.
- Angiosarcoma is a malignant vascular tumour.
- Osteosarcoma is a malignant bony tumour.

Other types of neoplasms

- Lymphomas, leukaemias, and myeloma are haematological malignancies derived from cells of blood or the bone marrow.
- Malignant melanoma is a malignant melanocytic neoplasm.
- Malignant mesothelioma is a malignant mesothelial tumour.
- Germ cell tumours usually arise in the testes or ovaries.
- Embryonal tumours are a group of malignant tumours seen predominantly in children and composed of very primitive cells (e.g. neuroblastoma; ➔ Neuroblastoma, p. 402) and nephroblastoma (➔ Childhood renal tumours, p. 262).

Carcinogenesis

General concepts

- Malignant tumours arise through the accumulation of mutations in multiple genes which allow tumour cells to proliferative uncontrollably, evade cell death, invade locally, and spread to distant sites (**metastasize**).
- Many malignant tumours show characteristic **initiating mutations** that are acquired early in carcinogenesis.
- Over time further critical **driver mutations** are acquired by tumour cells.

Common mutations in cancers

- Activating mutations in genes stimulating cell growth (e.g. *EGFR*, *HER*, *RET*, *PDGFB*, *KIT*, *ALK*, *RAS*, *BRAF*, *JAK2*, *MYC*, *CCND1*, *CDK4*).
- Loss of function mutations in genes inhibiting cell growth (e.g. *RB*, *CDKN2A*, *NF1*, *PTCH*, *PTEN*).
- Loss of function mutations in genes controlling genomic stability (e.g. TP53). The protein product of TP53, the p53 protein, is known as the 'guardian of the genome' as it is upregulated in cells with DNA damage stimulating them to either repair the DNA damage, become senescent, or undergo apoptosis. Mutation of p53 is a critical step in carcinogenesis as it allows cells with DNA damage to continue to proliferate and acquire further driver mutations.

Common carcinogens

- Chemical carcinogens (e.g. cigarette smoke).
- Ultraviolet radiation (e.g. sunlight).
- Ionizing radiation (e.g. CT scans).
- Oncogenic viruses (e.g. human papillomavirus, Epstein–Barr virus, HTLV-1, hepatitis B and C viruses).
- Chronic inflammatory diseases which stimulate proliferation of cells (e.g. ulcerative colitis).
- Hormones which stimulate proliferation of hormonally responsive tissues (e.g. oestrogens).

Laboratory techniques

Histopathology

Introduction

- Histopathology is the microscopic study of tissue samples from patients.
- Samples for histopathology require chemical processing that ends with the tissue sample embedded in a **paraffin wax block**.
- This allows very thin sections of the tissue to be cut and stained for microscopic examination by a histopathologist.

Tissue processing

- Tissue samples for histopathology require a number of steps to produce a paraffin block.
- Fixation: this preserves the cells and prevents autolysis. The most common fixative is formalin.
- Dehydration: water needs to be removed from the tissue. This is achieved by immersing the tissue in increasing concentrations of alcohol such that water is gradually replaced by alcohol.
- Clearing: a clearing agent is then used to remove the alcohol in the tissue and allow the tissue to be infiltrated by molten wax.
- Embedding: the wax-infiltrated tissue is now formed into a paraffin block at an embedding station where a mould is filled with molten wax and the tissue placed into it. Once solidified, the paraffin block is ready for cutting (microtomy) and staining.

Stains

- Cells are colourless and transparent, so histology sections need to be stained with dyes to make them visible.
- Basic dyes react with acidic components in cells, such as nuclei acids in nuclei.
- Acidic dyes react with basic components in cells, such as proteins and other cytoplasmic elements.
- **Haematoxylin & eosin (H&E)** is the most commonly used stain in histopathology. Haematoxylin is a basic stain that stains the nucleus of cells purple, whilst eosin is an acidic dye which stains the cytoplasm of cells pink (Fig. 2.1).

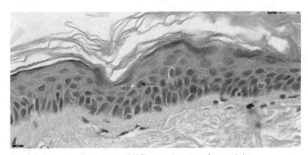

Fig. 2.1 Haematoxylin and eosin (H&E) stained section of normal skin. Haematoxylin stains the nucleus of cells purple (red arrow). Eosin stains the cytoplasm of cells pink (green arrow) (see Plate 1).

- Examination of H&E-stained sections alone may be enough to make a diagnosis on a tissue sample, but often ancillary tests are required to make a diagnosis (e.g. immunohistochemistry or molecular testing).

Cytopathology

Introduction

- Cytopathology, or cytology, is the microscopic study of individual cells from patients (as opposed to intact tissue samples in histopathology).
- Cytology is mostly used in tumour pathology to diagnose an array of benign and malignant tumours as well as for the detection of pre-cancerous changes.
- Cytology is often divided into **gynaecological cytology** (assessment of pre-cancerous changes of the cervix—predominantly in the context of cervical screening programmes) and **non-gynaecological** or **diagnostic cytology** (the assessment of other tissues of the body).

Cytology samples

- Cytology samples may be obtained by brushing the areas of interest with a sampling device (e.g. cervical cytology, bronchial cytology or by inserting a fine needle into an abnormal area; i.e. fine needle aspiration [FNA] cytology). Fluids may also be sent (e.g. urine or effusions).

Cytology sample preparation

- Cytology samples require fixation and then staining—common cytology stains include Papanicolaou, Diff Quick.
- Rinsing of needles and syringes from FNA samples and fluid samples can also be centrifuged with the resulting deposit processed into a paraffin cell block similar to a histopathology sample from which sections can be cut for H&E staining and immunohistochemical analysis.

Immunohistochemistry

Introduction

- Immunohistochemistry (IHC) is a special technique that allows visualization of antigens in cells by using labelled antibodies that bind specifically to the antigen of interest. This is a very commonly used ancillary technique used in histopathological diagnosis.
- Hundreds of antibodies are now available for use in diagnostic histopathology.
- Examples of some common antibodies used in diagnostic practice include:
  - Cytokeratins (e.g. MNF116 or AE1/AE3)—epithelial markers
  - Desmin—muscle marker
  - ERG—endothelial marker
  - CD45—leukocyte marker
  - MelanA—melanocyte marker

Laboratory method

- IHC is typically performed on sections taken from formalin-fixed paraffin-embedded tissue.
- Thin sections are cut with a microtome and mounted onto glass slides coated with an adhesive.
- The sections are then dried in an oven or microwave.
- The paraffin is then removed using xylene or a xylene-free alternative.
- Epitope/antigen retrieval may be required for some antigens, which is achieved by either heating the tissue or digesting the tissue using a proteolytic enzyme.
- The labelled antibody of interest is applied to the tissue section.
- Any antigen-bound antibody can then be detected by adding a conjugate which generates a coloured signal which is usually brown or red (Fig. 2.2).

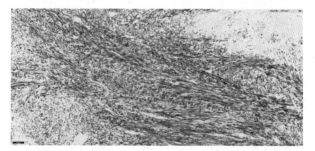

Fig. 2.2 An example of a leiomyosarcoma demonstrating positive brown staining for desmin by immunohistochemistry, indicating muscle phenotype (see Plate 2).

Molecular pathology

Introduction

- Molecular techniques in pathology are used to evaluate the genetics of tissue samples (i.e. DNA or RNA analysis).
- Molecular pathology is employed mostly in tumour pathology and may be used to help diagnose a specific tumour, predict the behaviour of a tumour and/or predict the response of a tumour to therapy.
- Some common cancers in which molecular genetic testing is frequently performed include:
  - Lung cancer: *EGFR, ALK, ROS-1, PDL-1*
  - Melanoma: *BRAF*
  - Colon cancer: *K-RAS*, mismatch repair genes
  - Breast cancer: *HER2*
  - Chronic myelogenous leukaemia: *BCR/ABL1*
  - Sarcomas with characteristic molecular aberrations (e.g. well-differentiated liposarcoma)
- Reliable molecular results are critically dependent on the quality of the specimen being analysed. The sample needs to have sufficient tumour cells present and have had adequate formalin fixation to ensure optimum DNA/RNA quality.
- Common techniques include **polymerase chain reaction** (PCR) to detect short DNA sequence abnormalities and hybridization techniques (e.g. **fluorescent in-situ hybridization** to detect larger abnormalities such as deletions, duplications, or translocations).

Polymerase chain reaction

- PCR techniques use DNA polymerases to amplify a segment of target DNA lying between two primer sites. Subsequent analysis can be performed using different techniques including **next-generation sequencing (NGS)** or **real-time PCR**.
- NGS uses primers for many genetic regions with a mixture of PCR products then enriched for specific areas of interest. NGS is a sensitive test as it can detect mutations even if only a small proportion of the examined products are abnormal.
- Real-time PCR uses fluorescent indicators to detect particular genetic sequences during DNA amplification (e.g. detection of *BRAF* V600E codon mutation in melanoma; Fig. 2.3).

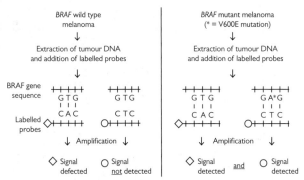

Fig. 2.3 Example of real-time polymerase chain reaction technique for the detection of *BRAF* codon 600 mutation in melanoma.

Fluorescent in-situ hybridization (FISH)

- FISH uses large segments of fluorescently labelled DNA to target chromosomal areas of interest, which can then be visualized under a fluorescent microscope. *FISH* can be used to detect gene amplifications (e.g. *HER2* in breast cancer, *MDM2* in well-differentiated liposarcoma) or translocations (e.g. *PDGFB-COL1A1* in dermatofibrosarcoma protuberans).

Chapter 3

Infectious diseases

Microbes

Bacteria

- Single-celled organisms with their double-stranded DNA lying free in the cytoplasm surrounded by a cell membrane and cell wall.
- Most grow in air (aerobes) but can grow without it (facultative anaerobes). Some only grow in the absence of oxygen (strict anaerobes).
- Gram-positive bacteria have a thick cell wall composed of peptidoglycan and a second polymer, often teichoic acid.
- Gram-negative bacteria have a thinner peptidoglycan wall overlaid by an outer lipid membrane composed of lipopolysaccharide.
- Mycobacteria are a type of bacteria with a thick waxy cell wall which can be stained with the Ziehl–Neelsen stain.

Viruses

- Smallest and simplest microbes composed of genetic material in the form of deoxyribonucleic acid (DNA) or ribonucleic acid (RNA) enclosed in a protein shell (capsid). Some viruses also have an outer lipid membrane acquired from the host cell in which they formed.
- Obligate intracellular organisms that can only replicate by infecting a host cell and hijacking its metabolic apparatus.
- Cause disease by destroying host cells (direct cytopathic effect) or due to the immune reaction against the infection.
- Some viruses are able to establish latent infection (e.g. herpes simplex).
- Some viruses are oncogenic and implicated in the transformation of the host cell and development of malignancy (e.g. human papillomavirus in cervical carcinoma; ➲ Cervical carcinoma, p. 300 and Epstein–Barr virus in nasopharyngeal carcinoma (➲ Nasopharyngeal diseases, p. 100).

Fungi

- Contain DNA within a nucleus and have a cell membrane containing ergosterol and an outer cell wall composed of chitin.
- Yeasts are unicellular fungi that reproduce by budding (e.g. *Candida*).
- Moulds grow as branching filaments called hyphae that interlace to form a tangled mass known as a mycelium. Mycelia produce spores.
- Some fungi can exist in yeast and mould forms (e.g. *Histoplasma*).

Protozoa

- Single-celled organisms which may live inside host cells or in the extracellular environment.
- Intracellular protozoa derive nutrients from the host cell (e.g. *Plasmodium, Leishmania, Toxoplasma*).
- Extracellular protozoa feed by direct nutrient uptake and/or ingestion of shed epithelial cells (e.g. *Giardia, Trichomonas*).

Helminths

- Complex multicellular parasitic worms, ranging in size from microscopic organisms to giant organisms several metres in length.
- Many have complex life cycles involving more than one host.
- Divided into nematodes (roundworms), cestodes (tapeworms), and trematodes (flukes).

Human immunodeficiency virus (HIV)

Pathogen
- Single-stranded, positive-sense, enveloped RNA virus.
- Member of lentivirus genus, part of the retrovirus family.

Epidemiology
- Very common worldwide, most notably in sub-Saharan Africa.

Transmission
- Major routes of transmission are unprotected sex, contaminated needles, breast milk, and transmission from mother to baby at birth.
- Transmission via transfused blood products now virtually eliminated by stringent donor screening.

Immunopathogenesis
- Infects CD4+ helper T-lymphocytes, macrophages, and dendritic cells.
- Widespread seeding of lymphoid tissue occurs following infection.
- HIV-specific CD8+ cytotoxic T-cells initially control the disease.
- Eventually, HIV escapes immune control through antigenic mutation.
- Viral load rapidly rises and CD4+ counts fall precipitously.

Presentation
- Acute seroconversion causes a flu-like illness with fever, lymphadenopathy, sore throat, myalgia, rash, and mouth ulcers.
- Latency phase then follows, which is usually asymptomatic.
- Final phase presents with opportunistic infections and/or neoplasms (Fig. 3.1).
- Common opportunistic infections include pulmonary tuberculosis, *Pneumocystis* pneumonia, oesophageal candidiasis, intestinal cryptosporidiosis, and *Mycobacterium avium*, cryptococcal meningitis, cerebral toxoplasmosis.
- Common neoplasms include cervical/anal warts and carcinoma, non-Hodgkin's B-cell lymphomas, and Kaposi's sarcoma.

Histopathology
- Lymph nodes show florid follicular hyperplasia with follicle lysis. Lymphomas are usually of diffuse large B-cell type (➲ Diffuse large B-cell lymphoma, p. 452).
- Bone marrow appears dysplastic with jumbling of haematopoietic lineages and increased numbers of plasma cells.
- Skin may show eosinophilic folliculitis (infiltration of hair follicles by eosinophils). Cutaneous Kaposi's sarcoma shows an irregular proliferation of human herpesvirus (HHV)-8-positive spindle cells in the dermis which form slit-like vascular spaces.
- *Pneumocystis* pneumonia shows a lymphocytic alveolitis with silver-positive organisms in the alveolar spaces.

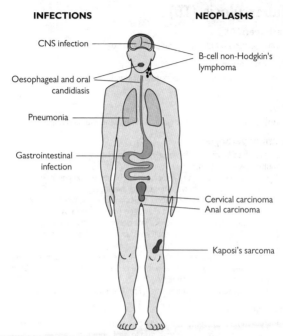

INFECTIONS

NEOPLASMS

CNS infection

B-cell non-Hodgkin's lymphoma

Oesophageal and oral candidiasis

Pneumonia

Gastrointestinal infection

Cervical carcinoma
Anal carcinoma

Kaposi's sarcoma

Fig. 3.1 Manifestations of advanced HIV infection.

Reproduced with permission from *Clinical Pathology* (Oxford Core Texts), Carton, James, Daly, Richard, and Ramani, Pramila, Oxford University Press (2006), p. 50, Figure 4.8.

Prognosis

- With modern anti-HIV therapy, many patients can expect to have a near normal lifespan such that they die with HIV rather than from it.
- Importantly it is now well established that patients with undetectable viral loads do not transmit the virus.

Tuberculosis (TB)

Pathogen
- *Mycobacterium tuberculosis*, an acid-fast rod-shaped bacillus.

Epidemiology
- Most common infectious disease worldwide.
- Kills 2 million people per year.

Transmission
- Respiratory spread from an infectious patient with active pulmonary TB.

Immunopathogenesis
- Inhaled bacilli are engulfed by alveolar macrophages but survive and multiply within them.
- Mycobacteria spread in macrophages in blood to oxygen-rich sites such as the lung apices, kidneys, bones, and meninges.
- After a few weeks, mycobacteria-specific CD4+ helper T-cells are activated following MHC class II antigen presentation by macrophages.
- Th1 subset helper T-cells secrete interferon-γ, activating macrophages into which aggregate into granulomas and wall off the mycobacteria in an anoxic and acidic environment.
- Most immunocompetent hosts contain the infection, leading to scarring.
- Active disease tends to be seen in the elderly, malnourished, diabetic, immunosuppressed, alcoholic.
- Active disease may be pulmonary (75%) or extrapulmonary (25%).

Presentation
- Pulmonary TB presents as a chronic pneumonia with persistent cough, fever, night sweats, weight loss, and loss of appetite.
- Extrapulmonary TB may present with meningitis, lymphadenopathy, genitourinary symptoms, and bone or joint pain.

Diagnosis
- Acid-fast bacilli may be seen in sputum, pleural fluid, or bronchoalveolar lavage fluid.
- Culture is the definitive investigation but takes up to 12 weeks.
- Polymerase chain reaction can be used for diagnosis and identification of drug-resistant strains.

Histopathology
- Necrotizing granulomatous inflammation.

Prognosis
- With antituberculous treatment, most people make a full recovery.
- Untreated, about half of people will eventually die of the infection.
- Prognosis is worse with coexisting HIV or organisms with multidrug resistance.

Infectious mononucleosis

Pathogen
- Epstein–Barr virus (EBV), a DNA herpesvirus.

Epidemiology
- Most patients are teenagers or young adults.
- No gender or racial predilection.

Transmission
- Saliva or droplet spread from an EBV-infected person.
- Incubation period of 4–5 weeks.

Pathogenesis
- EBV infects oropharyngeal epithelial cells via the C3d receptor and replicates within them.
- EBV also infects B-lymphocytes where the linear genome circularizes and persists as an episome.
- Viral persistence allows ongoing replication in oropharyngeal epithelial cells and the release of infectious particles into the saliva.

Presentation
- Sore throat, fever, malaise.
- Clinical examination may reveal lymphadenopathy, palatal petechiae, and splenomegaly.

Diagnosis
- Lymphocytosis.
- Peripheral blood film shows large, atypical lymphocytes (these are not specific for EBV).
- 90% have heterophil antibodies (Paul–Bunnell; Monospot test).
- EBV-specific IgM antibodies imply current infection.

Histopathology
- Lymph nodes and tonsils show marked paracortical expansion by large lymphoid blasts which are a mixture of B- and T-cells.
- EBV-LMP1 antigen can be detected in some of the B-blasts immunohistochemically.

Prognosis
- In most cases, the illness is self-limiting.
- Rare complications include meningitis, encephalitis, cranial nerve lesions, Guillain–Barré syndrome, depression, and fatigue.

COVID-19

Pathogen

- SARS-CoV-2, a single-stranded, positive-sense RNA coronavirus.
- Significant variants of the virus with increased transmissibility have arisen, most notably Delta (first identified in India) and Omicron (first identified in South Africa).

Epidemiology

- Emerged in December 2019 leading to a global pandemic.
- Mostly a disease of adults with symptomatic infection being rare in children.

Transmission

- Primary mechanism is through infected respiratory droplets.
- Target host receptors are found mainly in respiratory tract epithelium.
- Most transmission occurs through close contact (15 minutes face to face within 2 metres).
- Spread is especially efficient indoors with poor ventilation.

Pathogenesis

- Virus spike protein binds to host angiotensin converting enzyme 2 (ACE 2) receptor.
- After viral entry, virus-specific T-cells are recruited to the site of infection, eliminating the virus and leading to recovery in most patients.
- Patients who develop severe disease elicit an aberrant immune response.

Presentation

- Fever (90%), cough (60–70%), breathlessness (30–50%).
- Temporary loss of smell and/or taste is also commonly reported.
- Severe disease occurs on average 8 days from onset of symptoms with patients showing evidence of acute respiratory distress syndrome (ARDS).
- Other critical manifestations include acute cardiac injury, shock, coagulopathy, and multiple organ failure.

Diagnosis

- Identification of viral RNA through reverse transcription polymerase chain reaction or viral antigens through lateral flow testing.

Histopathology

- Lungs: diffuse alveolar damage with hyaline membranes, oedema, pneumocyte hyperplasia.
- Cardiovascular: lymphocytic myocarditis reported.
- Gastrointestinal: steatosis, mild hepatitis.
- Renal: acute tubular injury.
- Skin: perniosis-like changes in digits with microthrombi ('COVID toe').

Prognosis

- One large study in mainland China early in the pandemic found 14% of patients presented with severe respiratory compromise and 5% to be

critically unwell with respiratory failure, shock, or multiorgan failure. A fatality rate of 2% was reported in the same study.
• Increasing age and co-morbidities including obesity and other cardiorespiratory diseases are associated with risk of fatality.

Malaria

Pathogen
- Plasmodia protozoa: *Plasmodium falciparum, P. vivax, P. ovale, P. malariae.*

Epidemiology
- Endemic in tropical Africa, Asia, and South America.
- ~10 million new infections each year.
- ~1 million deaths each year (mostly *P. falciparum*).

Transmission
- *Plasmodium* sporozoites are injected by the female *Anopheles* mosquito during a blood meal.

Pathogenesis
- Sporozoites infect hepatocytes and proliferate into merozoites.
- Merozoites infect and multiply in red cells, causing haemolytic anaemia.
- Sequestration of red cells heavily parasitized by *P. falciparum* causes acute renal failure and cerebral malaria (Fig. 3.2).

Presentation
- Non-specific flu-like illness initially with headache, malaise, and myalgia.
- Fevers and chills then follow.
- Cerebral malaria presents with confusion, seizures, and coma.

Diagnosis
- Parasitized red cells may be seen on examination of blood films.

Prognosis
- Non-falciparum malaria has a very low mortality.
- Severe falciparum malaria can kill. Poor prognostic signs include high levels of parasitaemia, hypoglycaemia, disseminated intravascular coagulation, and renal impairment.

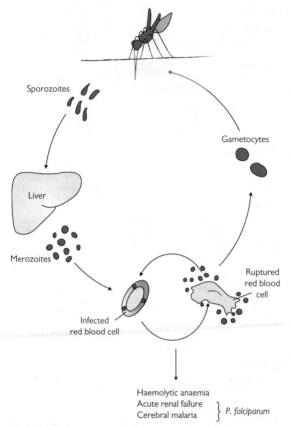

Fig. 3.2 Malaria life cycle. An infected mosquito injects sporozoites into blood which home to the liver and multiply in hepatocytes, forming merozoites. Merozoites released into blood infect red blood cells and multiply again, rupturing the red cells and infecting more red cells. Some merozoites mature into gametocytes which newly infect a mosquito, completing the life cycle.

Reproduced with permission from *Clinical Pathology* (Oxford Core Texts), Carton, James, Daly, Richard, and Ramani, Pramila, Oxford University Press (2006), p. 26, Figure 3.5.

Syphilis

Pathogen
- *Treponema pallidum*, a coiled spirochaete.

Epidemiology
- Worldwide distribution.
- Incidence increasing since the 1990s.

Transmission
- Almost always through sexual contact with an infected person.
- Can pass from mother to baby and cause congenital syphilis.

Pathogenesis
- Organisms enter the body via minor abrasions in epithelial surfaces.
- The organism produces a non-antigenic mucin coat which facilitates rapid spread throughout the body via blood and lymphatics.

Presentation
- Primary syphilis causes a firm, painless skin ulcer ('chancre') which appears about 3 weeks following exposure. The chancre occurs at the point of contact and is usually genital or perianal. There may be mild regional lymph node enlargement.
- Secondary syphilis presents 1–2 months after the chancre with rash, malaise, lymphadenopathy, and fever.
- Tertiary syphilis present years after exposure with so-called gummas in the skin, mucosa, bone, joints, lung, and testis. Gummas are inflammatory masses caused by a granulomatous reaction to the organism.
- Quaternary syphilis causes ascending aortic aneurysms, cranial nerve palsies, dementia, and tabes dorsalis.

Diagnosis
- In primary syphilis, the organisms may be visualized by microscopy of chancre fluid. Serology is often negative at this stage.
- In secondary syphilis, the organisms may be seen in the lesions and serology is usually positive.
- Organisms are usually not seen in later stages of syphilis, but serology usually remains positive.

Prognosis
- Antibiotic treatment during primary or secondary stages is usually curative and prevents risk of longer-term complications related to later-stage disease.

Lyme disease

Pathogen
- *Borrelia burgdorferi*, a spirochaete.

Epidemiology
- Found in temperate zones of Europe, North America, and Asia.

Transmission
- Arthropod-borne infection transmitted via ticks of the genus *Ixodes*.

Pathogenesis
- *Borrelia* organisms are injected into the skin via the tick bite where they establish infection and proliferate.
- Days to weeks later, *Borrelia* spreads via the bloodstream to distant sites, notably the joints, heart, and nervous system.
- *Borrelia* evades the immune system through antigenic variation of its surface proteins and inactivating complement components.

Presentation
- The earliest sign is an outwardly expanding erythematous rash at the site of the tick bite, known as **erythema migrans**. Many patients do not present with, or recall, the rash.
- Later signs include arthralgia, myalgia, neuropathies, changes in cognition, and palpitations.
- ➔ The presence of non-specific features across multiple body systems can make the diagnosis extremely challenging.

Diagnosis
- Western blot, enzyme linked immunosorbent assay (ELISA), or PCR analysis on blood or cerebrospinal fluid (CSF).

Prognosis
- Most people diagnosed and treated recover fully with no complications.

Leishmaniasis

Pathogen

- *Leishmania* protozoa.

Epidemiology

- 1–2 million new cases each year worldwide.
- Seen in Africa, India, South America, the Middle East, and the Mediterranean.

Transmission

- Inoculation from the bite of an infected sandfly.

Pathogenesis

- The parasite is inoculated into the dermis and phagocytosed by dermal macrophages.
- The ability of each species to survive within macrophages and evade host immunity dictates the clinical outcome.

Presentation

- **Cutaneous leishmaniasis**, caused by *Leishmania tropica* and *L. mexicana*, usually present with a single nodule which ulcerates and heals with scarring.
- **Mucocutaneous leishmaniasis**, caused by *L. braziliensis*, presents with skin lesions resembling the cutaneous form which may spread to the mucosa of the nose, mouth, and pharynx.
- **Visceral leishmaniasis** (kala-azar), caused by *L. donovani*, presents with fever, anaemia, lymphadenopathy, and hepatosplenomegaly due to widespread dissemination of the organism via macrophages through the reticuloendothelial system.

Diagnosis

- Microscopy, culture, fluorescence *in situ* hybridization, or polymerase chain reaction.

Histopathology

- Skin biopsies show a heavy dermal inflammatory infiltrate composed of lymphocytes, plasma cells, and many parasitized macrophages.
- The organisms are round to oval, 2–4 micrometres in size, with an eccentric kinetoplast.

Prognosis

- Cutaneous disease usually resolves spontaneously over a period of months.
- Mucocutaneous disease should be treated early as outcome is less satisfactory once mucosal sites are involved.
- Visceral disease is fatal without treatment due to liver failure and bone marrow failure.

Cardiovascular pathology

Congenital heart disease

Ventricular septal defect (VSD)

- Most common type of congenital heart disease.
- An abnormal hole in the interventricular septum.
- May occur anywhere in the septum, but most occur in the upper part.
- A small VSD may have little functional significance and may close spontaneously as the child ages. There remains, however, a risk of infective endocarditis.
- A larger VSD causes a left-to-right shunt and increased volume load on the right ventricle, with symptoms of cardiac failure.

Patent ductus arteriosus (PDA)

- Persistence of the ductus arteriosus after 10 days of life.
- Systemic blood flows from the aorta to the pulmonary artery, causing a left-to-right shunt.
- Blood flow to the lungs is increased two-fold, as is the volume return to the left side of the heart, causing left ventricular hypertrophy.
- Infective endocarditis is a frequent complication.

Atrial septal defect (ASD)

- An abnormal hole in the atrial septum.
- Most common site is in the middle of the septum away from the atrioventricular valves.
- Blood flows from the left-to-right atrium, causing an increase in circulation through the lungs.
- May be asymptomatic or cause easy fatiguability in childhood.
- Many present in adulthood due to atrial arrhythmias.

Atrioventricular septal defect (AVSD)

- A defect at the junction of the atrial and ventricular septae.
- In a complete AVSD, there is a combination of a low ASD and high VSD (creating essentially a hole in the centre of the heart).
- Most function like a VSD with a volume overload to the right ventricle.
- Most common form of coronary heart disease (CHD) seen in children with Down's syndrome.

Tetralogy of Fallot

- Comprises pulmonary stenosis, VSD, overriding aorta, and right ventricular hypertrophy.
- Pulmonary stenosis causes a right-to-left shunt and reduced blood flow to the lungs, resulting in cyanosis.

Transposition of the great arteries

- Incorrect placement of the aorta to the right ventricle and the pulmonary artery to the left ventricle.
- Always an associated defect to allow mixing of blood from both circulations (e.g. VSD or PDA) or the abnormality is incompatible with life.

Coarctation of the aorta

- A localized narrowing of the lumen of the aortic arch, distal to the origin of the left subclavian artery.
- In the infantile form, a PDA distal to the coarctation allows cardiac output to the lower body, but most of this is deoxygenated blood from the right side of the heart, so there is cyanosis of the lower half of the body.
- In the adult form, there is no PDA. Increased blood flow to the upper half of the body is increased and most patients develop upper extremity hypertension. This form is often not recognized until adult life.

Bicuspid aortic valves

- Tend to function well at birth and go undetected.
- Most bicuspid valves eventually develop calcific aortic stenosis (at an earlier age than typical 'senile' aortic stenosis) or aortic regurgitation.
- Increased risk of aortic dissection in adult life (➲ Aortic dissection, p. 50).

Ischaemic heart disease

Definition
- Myocardial damage as a result of impaired perfusion.

Epidemiology
- Very common disease seen mostly in older adults.
- Men are affected more than women, largely as a result of the protective effects of oestrogen.

Aetiology
- **Coronary artery atherosclerosis** (CAD) is the major underlying cause.
- CAD is a progressive inflammatory disease in which plaques of lipid, inflammatory cells and collagen develop in the media of coronary arteries leading to obstruction of the lumen and weakening of the vessel wall.
- Risk factors for CAD include smoking, diabetes, elevated low-density lipoprotein (LDL) cholesterol, hypertension.

Pathogenesis
- Stable atheromatous plaques narrow the lumen of the coronary artery leading to symptoms of cardiac ischaemia on exertion – this presents as **stable angina**.
- Unstable or 'vulnerable' plaques which rupture lead to thrombosis over the plaque and sudden, complete occlusion of the coronary artery – this presents as an **acute coronary syndrome** (unstable angina, acute myocardial infarction, or sudden death).

Presentation
- Stable angina: chest pain on exertion which is relieved by rest or use of nitroglycerin.
- Unstable angina: chest pain at rest or minimal exertion.
- Acute myocardial infarction: chest pain at rest radiating to left arm with ST segment elevation and raised serum troponin levels.
- Sudden death: usually due to a fatal arrhythmia such as ventricular
- Chronic left ventricular failure.

Macroscopy
- Coronary arteries with atherosclerosis show variable stenosis by white yellow plaques. Ruptured plaques show complete occlusion of the lumen by red thrombus overlying the plaque.
- Myocardium infarcted by an occluded coronary artery initially shows mottling (12–24 hours) then a yellow centre with a red border (3-10 days) then grey edges (10–14 days) before white scar tissue is laid down (3–8 weeks).

Histopathology
- Coronary artery atheromatous plaques are composed of variable proportion of smooth muscle, macrophages, lymphocytes, lipid, and extracellular matrix including collagen and elastic fibres. Plaques

that have ruptured show a fibrin-rich thrombus overlying the plaque occluding the lumen.
• Myocardium infarcted by an occluded coronary artery initially shows myocyte contraction bands, neutrophil infiltration and interstitial oedema (first 24 hours) then infiltration of macrophages with granulation tissue (7–14 days) before a dense fibrous scar is laid down.

Arrhythmogenic right ventricular cardiomyopathy

Definition
- Rare inheritable disorder of myocardium characterized by replacement of right ventricle myocardium by fibrofatty tissue.

Synonyms
- Arrhythmogenic right ventricular dysplasia (ARVD).
- Arrhythmogenic cardiomyopathy.

Epidemiology
- 1 in 1000 to 1 in 5000 people.
- Male:female ratio of 3:1.
- Accounts for 5% of sudden death in people aged under 65.

Aetiology
- Mutations in genes encoding desmosomal proteins (e.g. desmoplakin, plakophilin-2, and plakoglobin).
- Inheritance is predominantly autosomal dominant with incomplete penetrance.

Pathogenesis
- Mutations in desmosomal proteins cause disruption of connections between cardiac myocytes leading to myocardial cell death, apoptosis, and fibrofatty replacement.

Presentation
- Palpitations, syncope, fatigue.
- Cardiac arrest following physical exertion.
- Family history of sudden death.

Histopathology
- Loss of myocardial fibres with replacement by fibrous tissue, fat, and some inflammation.
- No granulomas or giant cells are seen.

Prognosis
- Patients have an increased risk of arrythmias and sudden death.
- Treatments aim to reduce this risk with options including drug treatment, ablation, implantable defibrillator.

Hypertrophic cardiomyopathy

Definition
- Inherited cardiac disorder characterized by ventricular hypertrophy, usually asymmetric, involving the interventricular septum.

Synonyms
- Hypertrophic obstructive cardiomyopathy (HOCM).

Epidemiology
- Common, involving about 0.5% of the population.

Aetiology
- Most cases are linked to mutations in sarcomeric proteins (e.g. beta-myosin heavy chain and myosin binding protein C).
- Autosomal dominant pattern of inheritance.

Presentation
- Syncope, palpitations, chest pain, breathlessness on exertion.
- First presentation may be sudden cardiac death.

Macroscopy
- Asymmetric hypertrophy of the interventricular septum is the classical finding.
- Symmetric hypertrophy seen in about 40% of cases.
- Dilated end stage form present in about 10% of cases.

Microscopy
- Myocyte hypertrophy with bizarre myocyte nuclei.
- Interstitial fibrosis.

Prognosis
- Most patients are asymptomatic.
- First presentation may be sudden cardiac death related to ventricular fibrillation.

Idiopathic dilated cardiomyopathy

Definition
- Left ventricular failure where the exact cause is initially unknown.

Epidemiology
- Patients are generally young adults aged 20–60 years who are therefore still in the prime of their life.

Aetiology
- May be a consequence of a wide variety of causes.
- This includes alcohol, chemotherapeutic drugs, viral myocarditis, immune dysregulation, and inherited mutations in genes encoding cytoskeletal or sarcomeric proteins.

Presentation
- Symptoms of left ventricular failure (i.e. fatigue and breathlessness).

Macroscopy
- Hearts are enlarged with dilated chambers, particularly the ventricles.
- Cardiac weight is increased (up to 3× normal).
- Mural thrombi may be present related to stasis of blood.

Microscopic
- Histological changes are non-specific.
- Myocytes may have hypertrophic features.
- Myocardial fibrosis present to a variable degree.

Prognosis
- DCM is generally a progressive disease with gradually worsening left ventricular function.
- Treatment aims to slow disease progression and improve survival.

Calcific aortic stenosis

Definition
- Degenerative condition causing calcification and narrowing of a trileaflet aortic valve.

Epidemiology
- Most common acquired cardiac valve abnormality.
- Affects about 3% of people aged over 65 years.
- Males affected slightly more frequently affected than females.

Pathogenesis
- Mechanical injury to the endothelium of the valve surface causes an inflammatory reaction with subendothelial accumulation of lipids and inflammatory cells.
- Quiescent interstitial cells become activated and acquire an osteoblastic phenotype leading to laying down of calcium and bone.

Presentation
- Breathlessness, angina, syncope, and reduced exercise tolerance.

Macroscopy
- Firm calcified nodules present on valve leaflets, located predominantly near the base of the cusps on aortic side of leaflets with sparing of free margins (Fig. 4.1).
- Accompanying fibrosis and retraction of cusps.

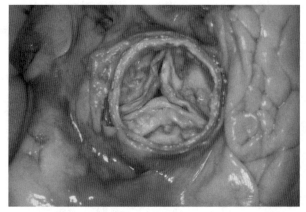

Fig. 4.1 Calcific aortic stenosis. This aortic valve is studded with nodules of calcium causing significant narrowing of the valve orifice (see Plate 3).

Reproduced with permission from *Clinical Pathology* (Oxford Core Texts), Carton, James, Daly, Richard, and Ramani, Pramila, Oxford University Press (2006), p.96, Figure 6.18.

Histopathology

- Calcium and bone deposits in the valve leaflets associated with inflammation, lipid deposition, and fibrosis.

Prognosis

- Treatment is important in patients with symptomatic disease as about half will die within 3 years without intervention.
- Surgical valve replacement is the gold standard.

Myxomatous mitral valve disease

Definition
- Myxoid degeneration of the mitral valve leading to weakening.
- Most common cause of primary mitral valve regurgitation.

Epidemiology
- Common cardiac valve abnormality affecting up to 3% of the population.
- Equal incidence in men and women.

Aetiology
- Likely to be a genetic disorder with highly variable penetrance.

Pathogenesis
- Precise molecular pathways are yet to be elucidated but the end result is the accumulation of glycosaminoglycans in valve leaflets with collagen fragmentation and weakening of the valve.

Presentation
- Wide spectrum of clinical features.
- Many patients have stable disease with no symptoms or complications.
- Patients with symptoms present with palpitations and chest pain.

Macroscopy
- Excised valve leaflets appear enlarged, thickened, and rubbery in consistency.
- Cut surface appears gelatinous and glistening.

Histopathology
- Increase in myxomatous tissue in the spongiosa layer of the valve leaflet.
- Extension of myxomatous tissue into the fibrous later causes collagen disruption and fragmentation of elastin fibres.

Prognosis
- Complications of progressive disease include left ventricular failure, atrial fibrillation, and infective endocarditis.

Rheumatic mitral valve disease

Definition
- Mitral valve scarring and deformity as a complication of acute rheumatic fever.

Epidemiology
- Incidence varies among countries depending on availability of antibiotics for treatment streptococcal pharyngitis.
- Low level of incidence remains even in developed countries due to cases of untreated asymptomatic group A streptococcal infection.

Pathogenesis
- Antibodies to *Streptococcus* M protein cross react with myosin, laminin, and vimentin proteins in the heart.
- Antibody binding to host tissue in the mitral valve leads to tissue injury and scarring of the mitral valve.

Presentation
- Most patients present in adulthood many years after initial episode of acute rheumatic fever.
- Symptoms include those of left ventricular failure and atrial fibrillation.

Macroscopy
- Surgically excised valves show leaflet fibrosis with thickening of the cords.
- If the sample includes the commissures then commissural fusion is present.
- Calcification may be present.

Histopathology
- Fibrous and fibroelastin thickening with loss of the normal valve layers.
- Neovascularisation, lymphocyte rich inflammation, and calcification.

Prognosis
- Patients with mild disease usually do not progress and can be observed.
- Patients with more severe disease require surgical intervention with either balloon valvulotomy or valve replacement and usually do well.

Infective endocarditis

Definition
- Infection of the interior surface of the heart, usually a heart valve.

Classification
- Acute endocarditis is caused by pathogenic organisms infecting a structurally normal heart.
- Subacute endocarditis is a more insidious illness caused by weakly pathogenic organisms infecting a structurally abnormal heart.

Epidemiology
- Uncommon, but important to recognize.

Microbiology
- Acute endocarditis is usually due to *Staphylococcus aureus*.
- Subacute endocarditis is most commonly due to *Streptococcus viridans* or enterococci.

Pathogenesis
- *S. aureus* usually gains access to the blood from the skin via indwelling vascular lines or via intravenous drug abuse.
- *S. viridans* gains access to the blood from the oropharynx after tooth brushing or dentistry.
- Enterococci gain access to the blood following instrumentation of the bowel or bladder.

Presentation
- Left-sided acute endocarditis presents acutely with fever and signs of valve damage. Major systemic embolic events are also common with septic emboli travelling to multiple organs.
- Right-sided acute endocarditis presents with fevers, chills, and prominent pulmonary symptoms due to numerous septic emboli in the lungs.
- Subacute endocarditis causes low-grade fever and constitutional symptoms. The diagnosis may be difficult and easily overlooked.

Macroscopy
- The involved endocardial surface is covered with friable vegetations (Fig. 4.2).
- Acute cases may show extensive underlying tissue destruction and abscess formation.

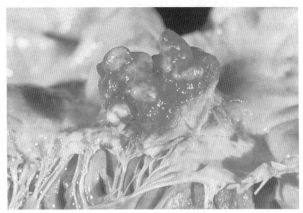

Fig. 4.2 Close-up of a vegetation of infective endocarditis. This is on the mitral valve; you can see the chordae tendinae attached to the valve leaflets (see Plate 4).

Reproduced with permission from *Clinical Pathology* (Oxford Core Texts), Carton, James, Daly, Richard, and Ramani, Pramila, Oxford University Press (2006), p.97, Figure 6.19.

Histopathology
- Vegetations are composed of a mixture of fibrin, inflammatory cells, and bacterial colonies which are usually Gram-positive cocci.

Prognosis
- Acute endocarditis has a high mortality due to rapid valve destruction and the development of acute cardiac failure.
- Subacute endocarditis has a more protracted course but remains a serious disease if undiagnosed and untreated.

Myocarditis

Definition
- Inflammation of the myocardium unrelated to ischaemia.

Epidemiology
- Rare.

Aetiology
- Most cases are infective in origin.
- Drugs and toxins have also been implicated.
- Some cases are idiopathic.

Microbiology
- Coxsackie virus is the most commonly implicated organism.
- Other organisms include HIV, *Clostridia*, *Meningococcus*, *Mycoplasma*, *Borrelia*, leptospirosis, and Chagas' disease.

Pathogenesis
- Myocyte injury causes a variable degree of necrosis and inflammation.

Presentation
- Depends on the extent of myocardial necrosis.
- Mild cases may cause a flu-like illness without obvious localizing symptoms to the heart and go undiagnosed.
- More severe cases cause breathlessness, chest pain, and palpitations.
- Very severe cases present as a medical emergency with acute cardiac failure and cardiogenic shock, mimicking a massive acute myocardial infarction.

Macroscopy
- Macroscopic changes vary widely, depending on severity.
- Importantly, many cases of myocarditis produce no gross pathology and the heart appears macroscopically normal.
- Very severe cases of myocarditis producing extensive necrosis may give a macroscopic abnormality similar to myocardial infarction.

Histopathology
- All forms of myocarditis show an inflammatory cell infiltrate together with myocardial necrosis or degeneration. The infiltrate is usually a mixture of lymphocytes and histiocytes.

Prognosis
- In most cases, recovery is complete without complications.

Pericarditis

Definition
- Inflammation of the pericardium.

Epidemiology
- Uncommon.

Aetiology
- Infection is a common cause and may be viral (Coxsackie, EBV, HIV), bacterial (extension from lung pneumonia, acute rheumatic fever, tuberculosis), or fungal.
- Full-thickness acute myocardial infarction causes pericarditis overlying the infarct.
- Other miscellaneous causes include severe renal failure ('uraemic' pericarditis), hypothyroidism, multisystem autoimmune diseases (e.g. RA, SLE), cardiac surgery, radiotherapy, malignant infiltration, and some drugs.

Pathogenesis
- Injury to the pericardium causes an inflammatory response.

Presentation
- Central chest pain which is worse on inspiration or lying flat and relieved by sitting forward.
- A superimposed large pericardial effusion may cause breathlessness.

Macroscopy
- The pericardial surface of the heart is roughened due to the presence of an inflammatory exudate
- Strands of fibrinous material may be present between the two pericardial surfaces.
- The exudate may be purulent if associated with bacterial infection.
- An associated pericardial effusion may be present.

Histopathology
- The pericardium is infiltrated by inflammatory cells, often with fibrin deposition.
- Malignant cells may be seen in cases due to malignant infiltration.

Prognosis
- Infective pericarditis often resolves with appropriate treatment.
- Pericarditis associated with an acute myocardial infarction is governed by the outcome of the infarction.
- Uraemic pericarditis implies severe renal failure with attendant risk of mortality.
- Malignant pericarditis usually implies significant metastatic disease and poor prognosis.
- Any cause of pericarditis may lead to a reactive pericardial effusion which, if large, requires urgent drainage to prevent cardiac tamponade.

Aortic dissection

Definition
- A tear in the aortic wall through which blood tracks.

Classification
- Type A (75%) involve the ascending aorta or aortic arch.
- Type B (25%) involve the descending aorta without involvement of the ascending aorta or arch.

Epidemiology
- Most cases occur in adults aged 50–70 years old.
- Male-to-female ratio is 2:1.

Aetiology
- Most cases are related to hypertension.
- Other associations include connective tissue disorders (e.g. Marfan's syndrome).

Pathogenesis
- Degenerative changes in the media weaken the aortic wall and predispose to dissection.
- Hypertension is thought to act through pressure and ischaemic related injury.
- Connective tissue disorders are associated with upregulation of TGF-β and remodelling of the aortic wall.

Presentation
- Acute severe 'tearing' chest pain which may closely mimic acute myocardial infarction.
- External rupture causes massive internal haemorrhage and shock.

Macroscopy
- A tear is usually visible in the intima of the aorta where the dissection starts and ends.
- If the dissection ruptures externally, large quantities of blood clot will be found around the site of rupture.

Histopathology
- Cystic medial degeneration of variably severity is seen with loss of elastic fibres and excess myxoid ground substance.
- Haematoma is present in a plane between the inner two-thirds and the outer third of the media.

Prognosis
- Untreated cases have a high mortality rate (50% within the first week).
- Treated cases have good initial survival but remain at risk of death from rupture of the dissection or development of a new dissection.

Abdominal aortic aneurysm

Definition
- A localized permanent dilation of the abdominal aorta >3 cm in diameter.

Epidemiology
- Incidence is reported to be 5–10%.

Aetiology
- Almost all are caused by aortic atherosclerosis.

Pathogenesis
- Proteolytic enzymes weaken the media of the aorta, leading to aneurysmal change.
- Increased levels of matrix metalloproteinases have been found in aneurysmal aortas. These enzymes are known to degrade elastin.

Presentation
- Unruptured aneurysms are often asymptomatic and most are discovered incidentally on abdominal examination or imaging.
- Ruptured abdominal aortic aneurysms present as a surgical emergency with abdominal pain and shock.

Macroscopy
- The aorta is dilated, usually below the level of the renal arteries.
- Extensive atherosclerosis is invariably present, often with secondary thrombosis and calcification.

Histopathology
- Aortic atherosclerosis shows intimal collections of lipid, inflammatory cells, and fibrosis. Complicated lesions may show haemorrhage in the plaque or overlying thrombus.
- Aortic aneurysms show severe atherosclerosis with marked loss of the media layer.

Prognosis
- The natural history is that of gradual enlargement.
- Risk of rupture is exponentially related to the diameter.
- Mortality after rupture exceeds 80%.
- Elective surgical repair should be considered for aneurysms with a maximum diameter of 5.5 cm or more.

Giant cell (temporal) arteritis

Definition
- Large vessel vasculitis with predilection for extracranial carotid artery branches.

Epidemiology
- Disease of older adults aged 70–80.
- Women affected 2–3 times more frequently than men.

Aetiology
- Unknown.

Presentation
- Headache, scalp tenderness, jaw claudication.
- Partial or complete visual loss.
- Polymyalgia rheumatica present in one-third of cases.

Histopathology
- Diagnosis is usually made on temporal artery biopsy.
- Inflammatory infiltrate present in all layers of the artery with lymphocytes and macrophages predominating.
- Giant cells may be seen but are not necessary to make the diagnosis.

Prognosis
- Condition is responsive to steroids.
- Visual loss is the most important complication to prevent.

Varicose veins

Definition
- Dilation and tortuosity of saphenous leg veins.

Epidemiology
- Affect up to 20% of the population.
- Marked female predilection (female: male ratio 9:1).

Aetiology
- Risk factors include family history, age, female gender, prolonged standing, obesity, pregnancy.

Pathogenesis
- Incompetence of the vein valves leads to venous hypertension and remodelling of the vein wall

Presentation
- Palpably dilated superficial leg veins.
- Associated skin and soft tissue changes such as oedema, stasis dermatitis, lipodermatosclerosis, and ulceration.

Histopathology
- Intimal hyperplasia with neovascularization and fibrosis of the media.
- Thrombus formation may be seen.

Peripheral vascular diseases

Definition

- Diseases relating to obstruction to blood flow to the extremities, most commonly the lower limb.

Epidemiology

- Incidence increases with increasing age, with up to 15% of over 70s affected.
- Male predilection (up to 3:1).

Aetiology

- Vast majority related to atherosclerotic disease.
- In younger patients, unusual causes should be considered such as vasculitis or clotting disorder.

Pathogenesis

- Atherosclerosis of arteries supplying the extremities narrows the lumen and results in ischaemia.
- Thrombosis or embolization can completely occlude the artery.

Presentation

- Obstruction of flow to the lower limbs results in pain in the calf on exercise known as intermittent claudication. Severe disease causes pain at rest and ischaemic ulceration.
- Complete blockage of an artery by thrombus results in an acutely ischaemic leg.

Histopathology

- Tissue from affected arteries show atherosclerosis +/− overlying thrombus.
- Tissue from amputation specimens show necrotic tissue +/− secondary infection.

Lung pathology

Respiratory tract malformations

Congenital diaphragmatic hernia

- A defect in the diaphragm caused by failure of the pleuroperitoneal canals to close during 8–10 weeks of gestation.
- Bowel loops and the liver can pass into the thorax and compress the developing lung, causing lung hypoplasia.
- Infants usually present with respiratory failure and 50% die within 24h of birth.

Congenital (cystic) adenomatoid malformation

- A lung mass composed of terminal bronchioles. There are no normal alveoli.
- Usually, a single lobe is involved.
- Many cases diagnosed by antenatal ultrasound at 20 weeks' gestation.
- Most cause a degree of respiratory distress and so are surgically removed.

Pulmonary sequestration

- A discrete mass of lung tissue that has no normal connection with the respiratory tract.
- Sequestrations have a systemic blood supply.
- Most are intrapulmonary and found in the left lower lobe.
- Up to half of extrapulmonary sequestrations may be associated with other anomalies.
- Pulmonary sequestrations may become infected or cause massive haemoptysis.

Acute respiratory distress syndrome (ARDS)

Definition
- A very severe form of acute lung injury defined as a ratio of $PaO_2:FiO_2$ <200mmHg in the presence of bilateral alveolar infiltrates on chest X-ray and in the absence of let ventricular failure.

Epidemiology
- Incidence rates range from 17 to 34 per 100 000 people years.
- 10–15% of all intensive care patients meet criteria for ARDS.

Aetiology
- Any severe injury to the lung may lead to ARDS.
- Common causes include severe pneumonia, shock, trauma, multiple transfusions.
- In many cases, multiple factors act together.

Pathogenesis
- Severe damage to the lung causes widespread alveolar necrosis with severe impairment of normal gas exchange.

Presentation
- Severe breathlessness, in addition to signs of the underlying cause.

Macroscopy
- Both lungs are typically markedly heavy and fluid-filled, often weighing >1000 g each (a normal lung weighs 300–400 g).

Histopathology
- The histopathological hallmark is **diffuse alveolar damage**, characterized by the presence of hyaline membranes lining alveolar spaces.
- Hyaline membranes are composed of a mixture of fibrin and necrotic alveolar epithelial cells.

Prognosis
- Severe condition with high mortality rates averaging between 30% and 50%, depending on the cause.
- Survivors usually demonstrate residual pulmonary functional abnormalities.

Bronchiectasis

Definition
- An abnormal permanent dilation of bronchi, accompanied by inflammation in their walls and in adjacent lung parenchyma.

Epidemiology
- Incidence rates between 20 and 35 per 100 000 people years.
- More common in underdeveloped countries due to higher incidence of severe childhood pulmonary infections.

Aetiology
- A structural condition resulting from a number of different causes.
- In developed countries, bronchiectasis is usually related to obstruction to an area of the lung (e.g. tumour or foreign body) or in association with cystic fibrosis (CF). Many cases prove to be idiopathic.
- In less developed countries, severe pulmonary infections are a major cause.

Pathogenesis
- Thought to be the result of weakening in bronchial walls caused by recurrent inflammation.
- Scarring in the adjacent lung parenchyma places traction on the weakened bronchi, causing them to permanently dilate.

Presentation
- Persistent productive cough and haemoptysis (which may be massive).

Macroscopy
- Affected areas of the lung contain visibly dilated airways filled with mucopurulent material which extend right up to the pleural surface.
- In obstructive cases, the cause may be seen proximally (e.g. a tumour).

Histopathology
- Bronchial dilation with marked chronic inflammation in the wall, often with lymphoid aggregates and germinal centres.
- Adjacent alveoli may show an acute and organizing pneumonia.

Complications
- Pulmonary hypertension and right ventricular failure (RVF).
- Deposition of serum amyloid A protein in β-pleated sheets in multiple organs (AA amyloidosis).

Cystic fibrosis

Definition
- An inherited disorder caused by a mutation in the **cystic fibrosis transmembrane conductance regulator** (*CFTR*) gene.

Epidemiology
- The most common lethal genetic disease in Caucasian populations.
- About 1 in 2500 live births in Caucasian populations.

Genetics
- Inherited in an autosomal recessive manner.
- *CFTR* is on chromosome 7q and codes for an anion channel that regulates multiple cellular ion channels.
- Over 1400 mutations have been described, though the most common is a deletion at position 508 that leads to loss of a phenylalanine amino acid (the ΔF508 mutation).

Pathogenesis
- The ΔF508 mutation is a processing mutation that causes abnormal folding of the CFTR protein and its subsequent degradation in the cell.
- In sweat ducts, abnormal CFTR function causes reduced absorption of sodium chloride with production of salty sweat.
- In the lungs and gut, abnormal CFTR function result in reduced chloride secretion and increased sodium absorption. As a result, passive water reabsorption increases lowering surface water content of epithelial cells.
- In the lungs, this causes viscid secretions that obstruct the airways and predispose to recurrent infections.

Presentation
- Most patients present with pulmonary disease due to recurrent infections. Initially, common bacteria colonize the lungs, but eventually *Pseudomonas aeruginosa* often becomes the dominant organism.
- Pancreatic insufficiency is also common.
- Bowel obstruction may occur in the neonatal period due to thick meconium (meconium ileus) or develop later in childhood.
- Liver disease develops late.
- Some cases may be diagnosed when a raised serum immunoreactive trypsin is picked up on neonatal screening.

Macroscopy
- Lungs from older children usually show widespread bronchiectasis.
- The liver may appear fatty and, in severe cases, may be cirrhotic.

Histopathology
- Lungs show bronchiectatic airways containing thick mucus. Acute inflammation may be seen if there is active infection.
- The liver shows inspissated bile in intrahepatic bile ducts. There may be periportal fibrosis and, in more severe cases, cirrhosis.

Prognosis

- Major improvements in management have extended average life expectancy to 50 years.
- Most patients die as a result of pulmonary disease.
- Novel genetic treatments for restoring CFTR function are being investigated in clinical trials.

Pulmonary thromboembolism

Definition
- Occlusion of a pulmonary artery by an embolic thrombus.

Epidemiology
- Common condition with incidence rates of 100 per 100 000 people years.

Aetiology
- As pulmonary emboli originate from deep vein thromboses, the risk factors are the same as for that condition, i.e. immobility, acute medical illness, recent surgery, malignancy, pregnancy, and congenital and acquired thrombotic disorders.

Pathogenesis
- A fragment of a detached thrombus from a deep vein thrombosis embolizes via the right side of the heart into the pulmonary arterial circulation and lodges in a pulmonary artery.

Presentation
- Blockage of a major pulmonary artery usually may cause instant death due to a sudden huge rise in pulmonary arterial pressure, acute RVF, and cardiac arrest.
- Blockage of medium-sized arteries causes an area of ventilation/ perfusion mismatch in the lungs with breathlessness.
- Smaller pulmonary emboli may lead to subtle symptoms of breathlessness, chest pain, and dizziness; these can easily go undiagnosed.

Macroscopy
- Emboli are visible as fragments of thrombi within pulmonary arteries.
- Thrombi are firm and brown and the cut surface may show visible bands (lines of Zahn).

Histopathology
- Fresh thromboemboli are composed of a mixture of fibrin and enmeshed blood cells, often arranged in alternating linear bands that correspond to the macroscopic lines of Zahn.
- Thromboemboli organize after 2–3 days with ingrowth of granulation tissue composed of fibroblasts and capillaries from the vessel wall.
- Old thromboemboli may be evident as fibrous nodules projecting from the vessel wall or fibrous bands crossing the lumen of a pulmonary artery.

Prognosis
- Mortality rates range from 3% to 25%.
- Risk of death is higher for larger emboli or if the diagnosis is made late.

Pulmonary hypertension

Definition
- A mean pulmonary artery pressure >25 mmHg at rest or >30 mmHg during exercise.

Subtypes
- Secondary pulmonary hypertension is a complication of chronic lung or cardiac disease.
- Primary pulmonary hypertension occurs in the absence of chronic lung or heart disease.

Epidemiology
- Secondary pulmonary hypertension is quite common.
- Primary pulmonary hypertension is rare.

Aetiology
- Common causes of secondary hypertension include COPD, interstitial lung disease, left ventricular failure (LVF), and chronic pulmonary thromboemboli.
- Primary pulmonary hypertension may be idiopathic or associated with certain drugs, HIV infection, collagen vascular disease, and congenital systemic-to-pulmonary shunts.

Pathogenesis
- Chronic hypoxia and obliterative pulmonary fibrosis both lead to the development of raised pressure in the pulmonary arterial circulation.

Presentation
- Secondary pulmonary hypertension causes worsening of the symptoms of the pre-existing condition with increasing breathlessness.
- Primary pulmonary hypertension presents with exertional dyspnoea and fatigue. Dizziness and syncope are also common.

Macroscopy
- The presence of atherosclerosis in large pulmonary arteries is a clue to underlying pulmonary hypertension.
- Right ventricular hypertrophy may also be present.

Histopathology
- Muscular hypertrophy and intimal proliferation of small pulmonary arteries and muscularization of pulmonary arterioles.
- Severe cases show plexiform lesions, characterized by a proliferation of slit-like vascular spaces from the arterial wall.
- Very severe cases may display fibrinoid necrosis of the arterial wall.

Prognosis
- Secondary pulmonary hypertension generally implies significant underlying cardiac or lung disease with poor prognosis.
- Prognosis of primary pulmonary hypertension is also very poor with 5-year survival rates of only 25–50%.

Asthma

Definition
- A chronic inflammatory disorder of large airways characterized by recurrent episodes of reversible airway narrowing.

Epidemiology
- Very common, affecting >10% of children and 5% of adults.

Aetiology
- Atopic asthma typically begins in childhood and is triggered by environmental allergens such as pollen, dust, and food. These patients are more likely to have a positive family history of asthma and atopy.
- Non-atopic asthma is more often triggered by upper respiratory tract viral infection, inhaled air pollutants, exercise, or cold air.

Pathogenesis
- Atopic asthma is caused by an exaggerated Th2 immune response to environmental allergens.
- B-cells are stimulated to produce large amounts of IgE which binds to mast cells and cause them to degranulate.
- Degranulated mast cells stimulate airway inflammation and bronchospasm.

Presentation
- Intermittent episodes of breathlessness, wheeze, and chest tightness.
- Cough, particularly at night, is also common.

Macroscopy
- Lungs of most asthmatics may be macroscopically normal.
- Thick mucus plugs in airways may be seen in severe disease.

Histopathology
- Airways show evidence of inflammatory activity with eosinophils which are not usually seen in normal airways.
- There may also be basement membrane thickening, goblet cell hyperplasia, and prominent smooth muscle.

Prognosis
- Generally good with appropriate treatment.
- There is a small mortality rate associated with severe acute asthma.

Chronic obstructive pulmonary disease (COPD)

Definition
- A chronic lung condition characterized by breathlessness due to poorly reversible and progressive airflow obstruction.

Epidemiology
- Very common disease with a prevalence of 1–4% of the population.
- Mostly a disease of middle-aged to elderly adult smokers.

Aetiology
- 85% of cases are caused by smoking.
- Most of the remainder are attributable to previous workplace exposure to dusts and fumes.
- A very small number are related to α1-antitrypsin deficiency.

Pathogenesis
- Inflammation and scarring of small bronchioles are thought to be the main source of airflow obstruction.
- Imbalance of proteases and antiproteases causes destruction of the lung parenchyma with dilation of terminal airspaces (emphysema) and air trapping.
- Mucous gland hyperplasia and irritant effects of smoke causes productive cough (chronic bronchitis).

Presentation
- Sudden onset of exertional breathlessness on a background of prolonged cough and sputum production.
- Spirometry shows ↓ forced expiratory volume in 1 s (FEV_1) and ↓ FEV_1/forced vital capacity (FVC) ratio (Fig. 5.1).

Macroscopy
- The lungs are hyperinflated with thick mucus in the airways and dilated terminal airspaces.
- Bullae may be present.

Histopathology
- Chronic inflammation and fibrosis of small bronchioles (chronic obstructive bronchiolitis).
- Finely pigmented macrophages in respiratory bronchioles (respiratory bronchiolitis).
- Dilated terminal airspaces (emphysema).

Prognosis
- Gradual decline in lung function with episodes of acute exacerbation due to infection, pneumothorax, or pulmonary embolism.
- Pulmonary hypertension and right ventricular failure then occur.
- Left ventricular failure often coexists due to ischaemic heart disease.
- Death is often related to both respiratory and cardiac failure.

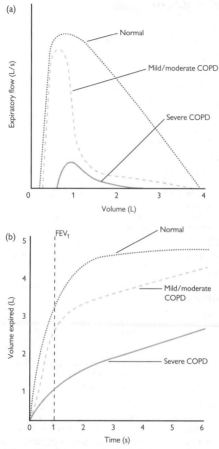

Fig. 5.1 (a) Flow–volume loops in a normal individual, compared with patients with COPD. In mild to moderate COPD, the immediate flow is relatively normal (this is why peak flow can be normal in patients with early COPD), but then the airflow rapidly decreases. In severe COPD, the airflow is very poor with prominent air trapping (note how at the start of expiration, there is already nearly 1 L of air in the lungs). (b) Spirometry in a normal individual, compared with patients with COPD. Note how in COPD, the forced expiratory volume in 1 s (FEV_1) is reduced, but the final volume expired is relatively normal (they just take longer to get there!), hence the FEV_1-to-FVC ratio is lowered.

Reproduced with permission from *Clinical Pathology* (Oxford Core Texts), Carton, James, Daly, Richard, and Ramani, Pramila, Oxford University Press (2006), p. 115, Figure 7.7.

Bacterial pneumonia

Definition
- An infection of the lung parenchyma caused by bacterial organisms.

Classification
- Community-acquired.
- Hospital-acquired.
- Aspiration.
- Immunosuppression.

Epidemiology
- Very common.

Microbiology
- Community-acquired: *Streptococcus pneumoniae, Mycoplasma pneumoniae, Haemophilus influenzae, Legionella pneumophila*.
- Hospital-acquired: Gram-negative bacteria, e.g. *Klebsiella, Escherichia coli, Pseudomonas*.
- Aspiration: mixed aerobic and anaerobic bacteria.
- Immunosuppression: all the previously mentioned possible (as well as viral, mycobacterial, and *Pneumocystis*).

▶ Multiple coexisting infections are common in the immunosuppressed.

Pathogenesis
- Bacterial organisms overcome the defences of the lung and establish infection in alveoli.

Presentation
- Productive cough, breathlessness, chest pain, and fever.

Macroscopy
- The infected lung parenchyma feels firm and appears yellowish.
- Purulent material may be expressed from small airways.
- The overlying pleura may show evidence of pleuritis.

Histopathology
- The alveolar spaces are filled with an inflammatory infiltrate rich in neutrophils. Bacterial colonies are often visible within the exudate.
- In cases of aspiration pneumonia, food material may be present within the lung parenchyma.
- Severe cases complicated by abscess formation show destruction of the lung tissue and replacement by confluent sheets of neutrophils.

Prognosis
- Recovery is usually expected with appropriate antimicrobial therapy in an otherwise healthy individual.
- Complications include respiratory failure, septicaemia, pleural effusion, empyema, and lung abscess. These are more likely with virulent organisms or in patients with coexisting heart and lung disease.

Idiopathic pulmonary fibrosis (IPF)

Definition
- An idiopathic interstitial pneumonia limited to the lung and associated with a histological appearance of usual interstitial pneumonia (UIP).

Epidemiology
- The majority of patients are between 50 and 70y.
- Men are affected about twice as often as women.
- Cigarette smoking increases the risk by several fold.

Aetiology
- Unknown but currently thought that recurrent exposure to environmental irritants leads to repetitive episodes of alveolar injury and an abnormal repair mechanism.

Pathogenesis
- Injured alveolar epithelial cells in susceptible individuals react by overexpressing profibrotic cytokines, such as transforming growth factor-beta and interleukin-10, which stimulate irreversible lung scarring (Fig. 5.2).

Presentation
- Progressive breathlessness and non-productive cough.

Macroscopy
- Marked lung fibrosis with honeycomb change.
- Disease most marked at the peripheries of the lower lobes.

Histopathology
- Heterogeneous, non-uniform fibrotic process, characterized by markedly scarred areas of the lung juxtaposed to islands of relatively normal lung ('spatial variability').
- Evidence of active ongoing fibrosis in the form of numerous fibroblastic foci ('temporal variability').

▶ This histopathological picture, known as **UIP**, is always seen in IPF but is not specific for it.

Prognosis
- Very poor, with average survival of only 2–3 years from diagnosis.
- A common terminal event is an acute exacerbation of IPF, characterized histologically by diffuse alveolar damage on a background of the UIP histological pattern.

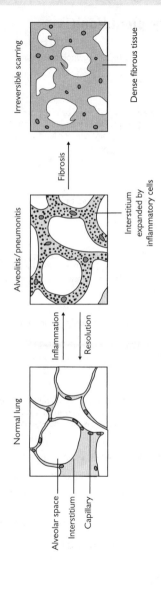

Fig. 5.2 Evolution of diffuse parenchymal lung disease (DPLD). The normal interstitium is thin and contains pulmonary artery capillaries. In DPLD, the interstitium becomes expanded by an inflammatory cell infiltrate ('pneumonitis' or 'alveolitis'), impairing gas exchange. Complete resolution can occur, but the danger is the development of fibrosis which permanently destroys the lung parenchyma.

Reproduced with permission from *Clinical Pathology* (Oxford Core Texts), Carton, James, Daly, Richard, and Ramani, Pramila, Oxford University Press (2006), p. 126, Figure 7.10.

Hypersensitivity pneumonitis

Definition
- An interstitial lung disease caused by an immunologic reaction to inhaled antigens.

Synonyms
- Extrinsic allergic alveolitis.
- Individual forms of the disease are also known by many other names (farmer's lung, humidifier lung, maple bark stripper's lung, mushroom worker's lung, pigeon breeder's lung, bird fancier's lung, etc.).

Epidemiology
- Uncommon.

Aetiology
- Thermophilic bacteria (mouldy hay, compost, air conditioner ducts).
- Fungi (mouldy maple bark, barley, or wood dust).
- Avian proteins (bird droppings and feathers).

Pathogenesis
- Inhaled antigens lead to an abnormal immune reaction in the lungs.
- Involves a combination of antibody (type 2), immune complex (type 3), and cell-mediated (type 4) hypersensitivity reactions (◓ Hypersensitivity reactions, p. 8).

Presentation
- Acute disease follows exposure to large amounts of antigen and causes severe breathlessness, cough, and fever 4–6 h after exposure. Resolution occurs within 12–18h after exposure ceases.
- Chronic disease results from prolonged exposure to small amounts of antigen with gradual onset of breathlessness, dry cough, and fatigue.

Radiology
- High-resolution computed tomography (CT) shows middle to upper lobe-predominant linear interstitial opacities and small nodules.
- Often associated with traction bronchiectasis and honeycomb areas.

Histopathology
- Cellular chronic interstitial pneumonia with peribronchiolar accentuation.
- Foci of organizing pneumonia and poorly formed granulomas may also be present.

Prognosis
- Generally good if the causative antigen is identified and exposure is avoided.
- Persistent exposure can lead to irreversible lung fibrosis and respiratory failure.

Lung carcinoma

Definition
- A malignant epithelial tumour arising in the lung.

Epidemiology
- One of the most common and deadly cancers with nearly 2 million deaths annually.
- Most present in patients aged over 60 years.

Aetiology
- About 80% of cases are directly attributable to smoking.

Classification
- Adenocarcinoma (40%).
- Squamous cell carcinoma (20%).
- Small cell carcinoma (15%).
- A number of rare subtypes make up the remainder.

Carcinogenesis
- Similar to other carcinomas, lung carcinomas are likely to arise from a precursor phase of epithelial dysplasia, representing neoplastic transformation of lung epithelium without invasion.
- Adenomatous dysplasia/adenocarcinoma *in situ* precedes adenocarcinoma.
- Squamous dysplasia/squamous carcinoma *in situ* precedes squamous cell carcinoma.

Genetic mutations
- Adenocarcinoma: Gain of function mutations in receptor tyrosine kinase genes such as *EGFR*, *ALK*, *ROS*, and *MET*.
- Squamous cell carcinoma: Loss of function mutations in tumour suppressor genes such as *TP53* and *CDKN2A*.
- Small cell carcinoma: Inactivation of *TP53* and *RB*; amplification of MYC family.

Presentation
- Symptoms related to local growth of the tumour include progressive breathlessness, cough, chest pain, hoarseness, or loss of voice, haemoptysis, weight loss, and recurrent pneumonia.
- Abdominal pain, bony pain, and neurological symptoms may occur from metastases.
- A small proportion of small cell carcinomas present with paraneoplastic syndromes or the superior vena cava syndrome.

Macroscopy
- A firm white/grey tumour mass within the lung.
- Yellow consolidation may be seen in the lung parenchyma distal to large proximal tumours due to an obstructive pneumonia (Fig. 5.3).
- Pleural puckering may be seen overlying peripheral tumours that have infiltrated the pleura.
- Metastatic tumour deposits may be seen in hilar lymph nodes.

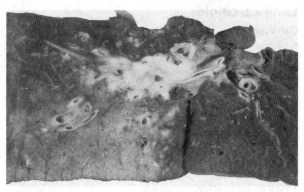

Fig. 5.3 A central lung carcinoma. Note how the lung tissue distal to the tumour shows flecks of yellow consolidation due to an obstructive pneumonia. The tumour was found to be a squamous cell carcinoma when examined microscopically (see Plate 5).

Reproduced with permission from *Clinical Pathology* (Oxford Core Texts), Carton, James, Daly, Richard, and Ramani, Pramila, Oxford University Press (2006), p.131, Figure 7.13.

Histopathology

- Adenocarcinoma: malignant epithelial tumour showing glandular differentiation and/or mucin production.
- Squamous cell carcinoma: malignant epithelial tumour showing keratinization and/or intercellular bridges.
- Small cell carcinoma: high grade neuroendocrine carcinoma composed of small cells with scant cytoplasm, ill-defined cell borders, finely granular chromatin, and absent nucleoli. Mitotic activity is high and necrosis is often extensive.

Immunohistochemistry

- The main histological types of lung carcinomas show differing patterns of immunohistochemistry which can aid in diagnosis.
- Adenocarcinoma: p63/p40 negative; TTF1 positive.
- Squamous cell carcinoma: p63/p40 positive; TTF1 negative.
- Small cell carcinoma: neuroendocrine marker (CD56, chromogranin, synaptophysin) positive; TTF1 positive.

Prognosis

- Poor with 5-year survival rates of ~10% in most countries.

Lung carcinoids

Definition
- Neuroendocrine epithelial tumours of the lung with low to intermediate grade malignant behaviour.

Classification
- Divided into **typical carcinoids** (90%) and **atypical carcinoids** (10%).

Epidemiology
- Rare tumours comprising <5% of all lung malignancies.
- Most present in patients aged under 60 years—than younger lung carcinomas.

Aetiology
- Most are not associated with smoking.

Presentation
- About 25% are diagnosed incidentally during investigation for another reason.
- Symptoms include coughing, wheezing, haemoptysis, pneumonia.
- Most cases are endocrinologically silent clinically.

Histopathology
- Epithelial tumours growing in organoid nests, rosettes, and trabeculae.
- Cells are relatively small with stippled 'salt and pepper' chromatin.
- TC have <2 mitoses per square millimetre and absence of necrosis.
- AC have 2–10 mitoses per square millimetre and may have necrosis.

Immunohistochemistry
- Positive for neuroendocrine markers such as CD56, chromogranin, and synaptophysin.
- TTF1 is also usually positive.

Prognosis
- Typical carcinomas are low grade malignancies with about 15% showing regional lymph node metastasis and <5% showing distant metastasis. 5-year survival rate is 90%.
- Atypical carcinoids are intermediate grade malignancies with up to 20% showing metastatic behaviour and 5-year survival rate of 60%.

Pleural effusion

Definition

- An accumulation of excess fluid within the pleural space.

Epidemiology

- Common.

Aetiology

- LVF.
- Pneumonia.
- Pulmonary embolism.
- Malignancy.
- Multisystem autoimmune diseases (e.g. lupus, RA).

Pathogenesis

- Increased pulmonary venous congestion (LVF), inflammation of the pleura (pneumonia, pulmonary embolism, autoimmune disease), infiltration of the pleura (malignancy).

Presentation

- Small effusions may be asymptomatic (though visible on imaging).
- Large effusions cause breathlessness.

Macroscopy

- Fluid is seen within the pleural space.
- Fluid may be straw-coloured, haemorrhagic, or purulent.

Cytopathology

- Cytological examination of pleural fluid in benign conditions shows mesothelial cells and variable numbers of inflammatory cells, depending on the cause.
- Pleural fluid due to malignancy may contain malignant cells with enlarged pleomorphic nuclei.

Prognosis

- Parapneumonic effusions and those due to pulmonary emboli resolve upon treatment.
- Pleural effusion due to LVF usually implies advanced disease and poor prognosis.
- Pleural effusion due to malignancy is invariably due to metastatic disease and so has a very poor prognosis.

Pneumothorax

Definition
- The presence of air in the pleural space.

Epidemiology
- Common.
- Men are affected more than women.

Aetiology
- Spontaneous pneumothorax typically occurs in thin, tall young men. It is thought to be due to the rupture of small delicate apical blebs of lung tissue which result from stretching of the lungs.
- Underlying lung disease (e.g. COPD, asthma, pneumonia, TB, CF, sarcoidosis, lung carcinoma, IPF. Rare conditions often associated with pneumothorax include pulmonary Langerhans cell histiocytosis, pulmonary lymphangioleiomyomatosis, and thoracic endometriosis).
- Trauma (e.g. penetrating chest wound, rib fractures).
- Iatrogenic, e.g. subclavian vein cannulation, lung biopsy.

Pathogenesis
- Air leaks out of the damaged lung into the pleural space until the pressures equalize.
- The lung collapses to a variable degree, depending on the size of the pneumothorax.
- Rarely, the tissues near the lung defect act as a one-way valve, preventing the equalization of pressure. The continuous build-up of pressure and volume in the pleural space displaces mediastinal structures, causing cardiorespiratory arrest (**tension pneumothorax**).

Presentation
- Sudden onset of unilateral pleuritic chest pain.
- There may be breathlessness, depending on the size of the pneumothorax. Patients with an underlying lung disease will usually notice a worsening in their symptoms.

Radiology
- Air is present within the pleural space, together with varying amounts of lung collapse.

Histopathology
- Apical lung tissue excised from patients with spontaneous pneumothoraces shows one or more bullae associated with subpleural alveolar collapse and fibrosis.
- The overlying visceral pleura shows reactive mesothelial hyperplasia and inflammation which is often rich in eosinophils.

Prognosis
- About one-third of patients with spontaneous pneumothorax suffer from recurrent episodes, usually on the same side.

Pleural mesothelioma

Definition
- An aggressive malignant tumour arising in pleural mesothelium.

Epidemiology
- Most cases are seen in males aged over 60 years old.
- Nearly 7000 cases were diagnosed in the UK between 2016 and 2018.
- An expected downward trend in incidence is still yet to be seen.

Aetiology
- >90% of cases are directly attributable to asbestos exposure.
- Amphibole asbestos is the most potent type, followed by chrysotile, and then amosite.
- Rarer causes include exposure to non-asbestos mineral fibres and therapeutic radiation.

Pathogenesis
- Inhaled asbestos fibres become permanently entrapped in the lung.
- Most do not cause a tissue reaction and these are probably the ones responsible for the carcinogenic effects.
- A minority become coated with iron, forming asbestos bodies.

Genetic mutations
- A relatively low tumour mutation burden is seen in comparison with lung carcinomas.
- Involved genes are mostly tumour suppressor genes, the most common being *CDKN2A*, *BAP1*, and *NF2*.

Presentation
- Breathlessness, often due to a large pleural effusion, and chest pain.
- Weight loss and malaise are often profound.

Macroscopy
- Initially, multiple small nodules stud the parietal pleura.
- As the tumour grows, the nodules become confluent and form a tumour mass that encases the entire lung and fuses to the chest wall (Fig. 5.4).

Cytopathology
- Cytological examination of pleural fluid from a pleural effusion may reveal the presence of malignant mesothelial cells forming sheets, clusters, and papillae.

Histopathology
- **Epithelioid mesothelioma** (representing the majority of cases) is composed of round malignant cells forming tubules and papillae. Grading of epithelioid mesothelioma can predict behaviour with high grade tumours showing shorter survival than low grade tumours.
- **Sarcomatoid mesothelioma** is composed of elongated spindled malignant cells.
- **Biphasic mesothelioma** contains a mixture of epithelioid and sarcomatoid types.

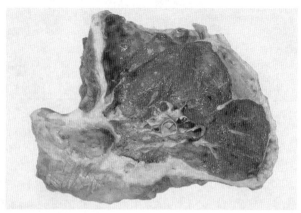

Fig. 5.4 Typical macroscopic appearance of malignant mesothelioma. Note how the tumour encases and compresses the lung (see Plate 6).

Reproduced with permission from *Clinical Pathology* (Oxford Core Texts), Carton, James, Daly, Richard, and Ramani, Pramila, Oxford University Press (2006), p. 136, Figure 7.15.

Ancillary tests

- Immunohistochemistry shows positive staining for mesothelial markers such as cytokeratin 5/6, WT1, D2-40, and calretinin.
- Loss of BAP1 expression by immunohistochemistry and deletion of *CDKN2A* by fluorescence in situ hybridization (FISH) analysis supports a diagnosis of mesothelioma.

Prognosis

- Very poor, with half of patients dying within a year of diagnosis.
- Few survive >2 years from diagnosis.

Head and neck pathology

Inflammatory oral cavity diseases

Oral ulceration

Recurrent aphthous stomatitis (RAS)

- Common and painful condition.
- Typically begins in childhood or adolescence, F>M.
- No single causative agent has been identified (food allergy, stress, trauma, hormone).
- Clinically 3 types: major, minor, and herpetiform.
  - Minor aphthous ulcerations range from 3 to 10 mm and generally heal within 1–2 weeks.
  - Major form measures more than 1 cm and can take up to 6 weeks to heal, and may scar. Typically on buccal and labial mucosa.
  - Herpetiform aphthae are named because of their clinical appearance and not necessarily related to herpes virus. They are less common and consist of small individual lesions which can combine to form larger lesions. Usually heal within 7–10 days, but are often more frequent.

Traumatic ulcer

- Localized ulcer found on the buccal mucosa, tongue, and lips.
- Appear as areas of erythema and a rolled hyperkeratotic border may develop adjacent to the ulcer.
- Caused by mechanical damage from food, self-inflicted injury (such as biting), malocclusion, sharp teeth, thermal, chemical, or electrical burns.
- Prognosis is excellent if source identified.
- If non-healing after 2–3 weeks, a biopsy must be performed.

Geographic tongue (benign migratory glossitis)/erythema migrans

- Common benign lesion affects the tongue and other oral mucosal surfaces (erythema migrans). Inflammatory in nature with multiple erythematous areas representing loss of filiform papillae.
- Geographical areas of red and white, usually resolve within a few days, but may quickly develop in another area.
- Aetiology unknown, though some histological similarity to psoriasis.
- Typically, it is a chronic condition with periods of exacerbation and remission.

Oral candidiasis

- Fungal infection which is more common in the immunosuppressed.
- Clinically, erythema with pseudo-membrane formation.
- **Central papillary atrophy/median rhomboid glossitis.** Midline with variably sized areas of papillary atrophy and erythema caused by chronic fungal infection.
- About 1% of the population—men between the ages of 30–50 years of age.
- **Histology.** A yeast (*Candida albicans*) that develops pseudo-hyphae and resides in the stratum corneum.

Oral actinomycosis

- **Definition.** Gram-positive anaerobic bacteria—normal oral flora that colonizes tonsillar crypts, dental plaque, and the gums.
- Pathological infection occurs if it enters deeper tissue through trauma (e.g. tooth extraction).

Oral herpes simplex

- Usually caused by herpex simplex type 1, less frequently herpes simplex type 2.
- Primary herpes simplex: Symptomatic and occur during childhood. Orally—painful gingivostomatitis. Occasionally, the infection occurs later in life and in an adult may manifest as a pharyngotonsillitis. Patients are typically symptomatic for 1–2 weeks.
- Secondary or recurrent herpes simplex: A small number of patients and the vermillion zone of the lip affected as well as the keratinized oral mucosa.
- May occur spontaneously or be triggered by sunlight, trauma, or systemic infection. Lesions heal within a week to 10 days. Frequency is highly variable from patient to patient—some have regular recurrences.
- Histology shows typical herpetic changes in keratinocytes.

Oral lichen planus

- Seen mostly in middle-aged females and shows fine lace-like pattern of lines known as Wickham's striae.
- Two main forms recognized: reticular and erosive.
- Reticular form is more common—multiple lesions with a bilateral symmetrical pattern.
- Erosive form is usually symptomatic—atrophic, erythematous lesions with central ulceration.
- Cause is unknown, multifactorial, and characterized by a T-cell mediated chronic immune response and abnormal epithelial keratinization.
- There is still controversy whether oral lichen planus is associated with an increased risk of malignancy but excessive tobacco and alcohol use should be discouraged.

Mucous membrane pemphigoid

- Also known as cicatricial pemphigoid.
- Autoimmune blistering disease predominantly affecting mucosal sites.
- Presents between ages 50–70 years with oral blistering.
- The conjunctiva, upper airways, and skin are also often involved.
- Histology shows separation of the squamous epithelium from the underlying connective tissue with a variable inflammatory infiltrate.
- Direct immunofluorescence shows linear deposition of IgG and C3 along the basement membrane zone.

Benign oral cavity neoplasms

Squamous papilloma

- Benign exophytic proliferation of squamous epithelium.
- Most occur in adults aged 30–50 y.
- The exact aetiology is unknown but the role of human papilloma virus strains 6 and 11 has been implicated in its causation.
- Predilection for hard and soft palates and the uvula.
- Histology shows papillary fronds lined by squamous epithelium.
- Prognosis is excellent. Do not undergo malignant transformation.

Fibroepithelial polyp

- Benign proliferation of fibrous tissue in response to irritation/trauma.
- Presents as a painless oral lump in an adult aged 30–50 y.
- Histology shows a subepithelial mass of dense collagenous tissue.
- Prognosis is excellent with no inherent tendency to recur.

Peripheral ossifying fibroma

- Asymptomatic, slow-growing, pale-pink firm growth of the gingiva.
- Seen mostly in young adult females.
- Probably arises from the periodontal ligament due to chronic irritation.
- Histology shows randomly dispersed foci of bone, cementum-like material, and dystrophic calcification in a fibroblastic stroma.
- Prognosis is excellent. Recurrence rate of ~15% if incomplete removal.

Peripheral giant cell granuloma

- Painless, well circumscribed, reddish-purple mass on the gingiva, anterior to the molar teeth (mandible > maxilla). Female 30–50 years of age.
- Thought to arise from the periodontal ligament space and the giant cells are of odontoclastic origin.
- Histology shows multiple multinucleated giant cells in a vascularized fibroblastic stroma with haemorrhage and haemosiderin.
- Prognosis is excellent. Recurrence rate of ~15% if incomplete removal.

Pyogenic granuloma

- Benign vascular lesion, also known as 'lobular capillary haemangioma'.
- Presents as a dark red polypoid mass which often ulcerates.
- Histology shows a lobulated proliferation of small blood vessels.

Mucocele

- Caused by blockage or rupture of a salivary gland duct.
- Presents as a fluctuant lesion, most commonly on the lower lip.
- Histology shows a cystic space filled with mucin and lined by inflammatory tissue.

Amalgam tattoo

- An exogenous pigment associated discoloration of the oral mucosa, composed of granules of silver amalgam used in the filling of dental cavities.
- Appears as a grey-black macule of few millimetres in size.

- Commonly located on the alveolar ridge, interdental papillae, alveolar mucosa, floor of the mouth, and the vestibule.
- Histology shows large amounts of dark metal or brown pigment often coursing along reticulin fibres in the connective tissue especially around blood vessels.
- Prognosis is excellent. There is little to no response by the host tissue to the embedded silver amalgam.

Oral carcinoma

Definition

- Malignant epithelial neoplasm arising from the mucosal epithelium of the oral cavity.

Epidemiology

- Most frequent in the fifth and sixth decades.
- Incidence of 4/100 000 globally and mortality rate of 1.9 deaths/ 100 000.
- High incidence in Asia, Europe, and Latin America.
- Males > females.
- As smoking rates decline there is decrease in intraoral cancer.

Aetiology

- Smoking and high alcohol intake are the dominant risk factors for oral carcinoma. These two factors are strongly synergistic.
- Smokeless tobacco, betel quid also increases risk.
- Smoking-related cancers commonly show *TP53* mutations.
- *P16 only seen in 3% of OSCC.*

Presentation

- Early oral carcinomas appear as small red/white/ulcerated plaques and may be picked up during routine oral examination, often by dentists.
- Advanced oral carcinomas present with problems with talking and eating due to tumour obstruction. Most frequent sites are tongue, floor of mouth, gingiva. In betel quid and tobacco chewing cultures it is the buccal mucosa.
- There may be coexisting neck swelling due to cervical lymph node metastasis.

Macroscopy

- Early tumours appear as red/white plaques (Fig. 6.1).
- Advanced tumours appear as ulcerated exophytic masses.

Histopathology

- >90% are **squamous cell carcinomas**, characterized by invasive growth of epithelial cells showing variable squamous differentiation.
- Tumours are graded into well, moderate, or poorly differentiated.
- Special subtypes include verrucous, papillary (good prognosis), spindle cell, adenosquamous (worse prognosis).
- Tumour growth at the invasive front is divided into cohesive or non-cohesive.
- Thickness >4 mm and bone invasion are poor prognostic factors.

Prognosis

- Conventional OSCC is aggressive—the 5-year survival is 80% for early disease and 20% for advanced tumours. These patients are also at high risk of developing multiple tumours due to a field change effect throughout the upper aerodigestive tract, particularly if there is high-grade dysplasia at the margins.

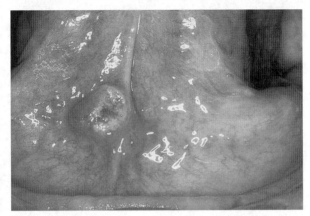

Fig. 6.1 Early squamous cell carcinoma of the oral cavity, presenting as a persistent ulcerated lesion on the undersurface of the tongue (see Plate 7).

Reproduced with permission from *Clinical Pathology* (Oxford Core Texts), Carton, James, Daly, Richard, and Ramani, Pramila, Oxford University Press (2006), p.452, Figure 19.4.

Oropharyngeal carcinoma

Definition
- Malignant epithelial neoplasm arising in the oropharynx.
- The majority are squamous cell carcinomas associated with high-risk human papilloma virus (HPV) (OPSCC-HPV).
- A small subset are non-HPV-associated and more frequently found in older patients on the soft palate.

Epidemiology
- OPSCC-HPV incidence has risen over the last three decades.
- Typically male, white, non-smoking, and 50–56 years old.

Aetiology
- HPV infection (typically type 16) is implicated in a high proportion (~90%) of oropharyngeal carcinomas.
- Oral sex is an established risk factor.
- Localization—base of tongue and palatine tonsils.

Carcinogenesis
- HPV-related cancers show overexpression of the cell cycle protein *p16*.

Presentation
- Typically present at an advanced clinical stage, often as a small primary with nodal involvement, which may be cystic.

Histopathology
- Distinctive non-keratinizing morphology, grading is **not** used.
- Unlike oral carcinoma, associated dysplasia is rarely seen.
- The tumour arises from the crypt epithelium and surrounded by lymphoid cells. It is composed of lobules and nests with central necrosis.
- HPV can be detected by in-situ hybridization and PCR-based assays.
- Diffuse immunoreactivity for p16 is a reliable surrogate marker for high-risk HPV.

Prognosis
- HPV-associated carcinomas show a much more favourable prognosis, with overall 5-year survival rates of 85%.

Salivary gland tumours

A diverse array of epithelial tumours have been described in the salivary glands (11 benign and 21 malignant types in the current WHO classification). Only the more common ones will be mentioned here.

Pleomorphic adenoma

- Most common salivary gland neoplasm.
- Majority occur in the parotid gland as a painless, slowly growing lump.
- Cytology is cellular with abundant epithelial and myoepithelial cells and fibrillary stromal fragments.
- Histology shows a circumscribed tumour composed of a mixture of ductal epithelium, myoepithelial cells, and a myxochondroid stroma. (Fig. 6.2).
- Benign tumour but may recur following incomplete excision. If left untreated, there is a small risk (6%) of malignant transformation ('carcinoma ex pleomorphic adenoma').
- Metastasizing Pleomorphic adenoma is histologically indistinguishable from PA but produces secondary tumours in distant sites (bone, lung, lymph nodes). More common if after multiple local recurrences.

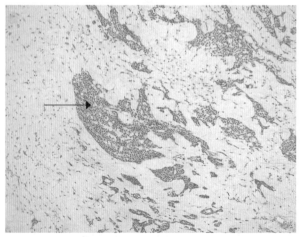

Fig 6.2 Pleomorphic adenoma. Typical microscopic appearance of a pleomorphic adenoma with an intermingling of epithelial elements (arrow) set within a mesenchymal component (see Plate 8).

Reproduced with permission from *Clinical Pathology* (Oxford Core Texts), Carton, James, Daly, Richard, and Ramani, Pramila, Oxford University Press (2006), p.456, Figure 19.7.

Warthin tumour
- Second most common salivary gland neoplasm.
- Almost all occur in the parotid gland as a painless, slowly growing lump. May be bilateral and linked with smoking.
- Cytology shows sheets of oncocytic epithelial cells with abundant lymphoid cells in the background.
- Histology shows a circumscribed tumour composed of papillary-cystic structures lined by a double layer of oncocytic epithelium with an underlying dense lymphoid stroma.
- Benign tumour but may recur following incomplete excision.

Mucoepidermoid carcinoma
- Most common malignant salivary gland neoplasm.
- Wide age range and the commonest malignancy in children and young adults.
- Presents with a tender mass related to a major salivary gland, but can occur in minor glands.
- Cytology shows mucus, intermediate cells, and mucus cells.
- Histology shows an infiltrative tumour composed of a mixture of intermediate, squamoid, and mucous cells. Cystic change may be seen.
- Most are characterized by *CRTC1-MAML2* gene fusion.
- Most tumours are low-grade and behave well, with survival >95%.
- High-grade tumours are aggressive, with 10-year survival ~25%.

Acinic cell carcinoma
- Malignant salivary gland tumour, mostly arising in the parotid (90%).
- Presents with a mass which may be painful.
- Histology shows a tumour composed of serous acinar cells with granular cytoplasm which may grow in a variety of architectural patterns (solid, microcystic, follicular).
- 20-year survival ~90%.

Adenoid cystic carcinoma
- Malignant salivary gland tumour, mostly arising in major salivary glands, but >1/3rd occur in minor glands.
- Presents with a slowly growing mass which may be painful and mean age 50 years.
- Histology shows an infiltrative tumour composed of basaloid epithelial and myoepithelial cells, classically forming cribriform sheets, tubules, or solid sheets surrounded by a hyalinized basement membrane. Perineural invasion is very frequently seen.
- Fusion of the *MYB/MYBL1* oncogene and the transcription factor *NFIB*.
- The tumour shows a relentless clinical course, with a 10-year survival rate of 50–70%. Distant metastases reported in >50%.

Polymorphous adenocarcinoma
- Second commonest intraoral malignant salivary neoplasm. Average age 50–70 years.
- Most involve the palate and present as painless mass.

- Submucosal and composed of cytologically uniform cells with a diverse morphology (lobular, trabecular., microcystic, solid, cribriform with perineural invasion).
- Good overall survival, but local recurrence can occur in 10–33%.

Salivary duct carcinoma
- Aggressive malignancy resembling mammary ductal carcinoma.
- 10% of all salivary gland malignancies, usually male and elderly.
- Most occur in parotid and often rapidly growing with facial nerve palsy, pain, and metastatic disease.
- Histology shows high-grade ductal carcinoma with comedonecrosis, lymphovascular, and perineural invasion.
- Often express androgen receptor and 25–30% express Her2.
- 35–45% 5-year survival.

Secretory carcinoma
- Low-grade salivary carcinoma, arising predominantly in the parotid gland with a morphological resemblance to mammary secretory carcinoma.
- Mean age 46 years, most commonly presents with a painless mass in the parotid.
- Histology shows an epithelial tumour with solid, cystic, or papillary growth and eosinophilic secretions.
- Harbours a t(12;15) translocation, leading to an *ETV6-NTRK3* fusion oncogene.
- Indolent tumour, rarely distant metastases with 85% 5-year survival.

Benign sinonasal diseases

Sinonasal polyps

- Benign polypoid lesions of the sinonasal tract.
- Usually related to repeated episodes of inflammation from infection or allergic rhinitis.
- Occur predominantly in adults. Presence in children should raise the possibility of cystic fibrosis.
- Present with nasal obstruction.
- Histologically, the polyps comprise an oedematous, inflamed stromal core, covered by a sinonasal-type epithelium with a mixed eosinophilic and chronic inflammatory infiltrate.

Sinonasal papillomas

- EXOPHYTIC TYPE/SCHNEIDERIAN TYPE arises from the lower anterior nasal septum and is composed of papillary fronds covered by a bland multilayered squamous epithelium.
- Age 20–50 and more common in men.
- Aetiologically related to HPV, and malignant change extremely rare.
- ENDOPHYTIC/INVERTED TYPE arises from the lateral nasal wall and is composed of inverted lobules of non-keratinizing epithelium covered by a layer of ciliated columnar epithelium with many intraepithelial microcysts and neutrophils.
- Premalignant and malignant features can be seen arising in inverted papillomas.
- Aetiologically related to HPV (low-risk > high-risk subtypes).
- Higher rate of local recurrence.
- ONCOCYTIC/CYLINDRICAL TYPE arises from the lateral nasal wall and is composed of exophytic and endophytic proliferation of a columnar oncocytic epithelium with many intraepithelial microcysts.

Fungal rhinosinusitis

- INVASIVE. Acute—is aggressive with 50% mortality. Invasion of submucosa, bone, vascular, and neural structures by *Aspergillus* or *Mucor*. Occurs in immunosuppressed and diabetics.
- Managed by surgical debridement and systemic antifungals.
- NON-INVASIVE. Often a fungal ball of *Aspergillus* in the maxillary sinus associated with previous dental treatment. Managed by functional endoscopic sinus surgery (FESS).

Allergic fungal sinusitis

- Allergic reaction to ubiquitous fungal antigens.
- Presents with nasal itching and discharge.
- Severe cases can give rise to a large destructive inflammatory mass.
- Histology shows a layered arrangement of mucoid material with abundant eosinophils and eosinophilic cellular debris. Fungal hyphae can be highlighted within the material with special stains.

Sinonasal malignancies

Sinonasal squamous cell carcinoma

KERATINIZING SQUAMOUS CELL CARCINOMA (KSCC)

- These are rare and typically occur in elderly males. Can originate from inverted papillomas.
- Exhibit same histological features as conventional squamous cell carcinoma (SCC).
- 5-year survival is 50–60%.

NON-KERATINIZING SQUAMOUS CELL CARCINOMA (NKSCC)

- These also typically occur in elderly males.
- 30–50% harbour high-risk HPV.
- Most common sites are the maxillary sinus, lateral nasal wall, and nasal septum.
- Histologically expanding nests or ribbons of non-keratinizing squamous epithelium sometimes with papillae.
- 5-year survival is 50–60%. Not yet known if HPV confers a better survival.

Sinonasal adenocarcinomas

INTESTINAL-TYPE ADENOCARCINOMA (ITAC)

- Marked male predilection and usually arise in the ethmoid sinus and nasal cavity. There is a well-recognized association with occupational exposure, particularly in wood workers.
- Most occur in ethmoid sinus>nasal cavity>maxillary sinus.
- Histologically similar to adenocarcinomas of the gastrointestinal (GI) tract.
- Prognosis depends on grade and stage. 68% 5-year survival.

NON-INTESTINAL-TYPE ADENOCARCINOMA (non-ITAC)

- No sex predilection and wide age range. No known aetiology.
- Tend to involve the ethmoid sinus and maxillary sinus.
- Histologically low-grade tumours have a papillary/tubular pattern. 'Back-to-back' appearance of single layer of uniform cuboidal/columnar cells.
- High-grade tumours are more diverse with solid growth pattern.

SALIVARY-TYPE ADENOCARCINOMA

- Have an equal gender incidence and mostly arise in the maxillary sinuses. The most common histological type is adenoid cystic carcinoma.

Sinonasal undifferentiated carcinoma

- A rare, but highly aggressive, malignancy arising in the sinonasal tract.
- Presents with a large mass with bone destruction.
- Histology shows sheets of undifferentiated epithelial cells with high mitotic activity and necrosis. There are no glandular or squamous features.
- Prognosis is poor (35% 5-year survival).

NUT carcinoma

- Poorly differentiated carcinoma with squamous differentiation defined by presence of nuclear protein in testis (NUT) gene rearrangement.
- Median age 21 years and occurs in midline structures such as the nasal cavity and paranasal sinuses.
- 50% cases present with lymph node or distant metastases.
- Poor prognosis—median survival <1 year.

Olfactory neuroblastoma

- Rare sinonasal malignancy or neuroectodermal origin arising from the olfactory epithelium.
- Even distribution across all ages.
- Presents with nasal obstruction, anosmia, and headaches.
- Histology shows lobules/nests of closely packed, small, round, blue cells which may form pseudorosettes or true rosettes, which are surrounded by sustentacular cells.
- A histological grading system from 1 (low) to 4 (high) is used (after Hyams).
- The 5-year survival ranges from 40% to 90%, depending on the stage and grade.

Malignant melanoma

- Very rare sinonasal malignancy which presents with symptoms of nasal obstruction, discharge, and pain.
- Histology shows malignant melanocytes which can grow in a multitude of different patterns.
- More likely to have a *KIT* mutation or amplification and less likely to have a *BRAF* mutation than cutaneous melanoma.
- Prognosis is generally poor.

Nasopharyngeal diseases

Nasopharyngeal angiofibroma

- Rare, locally aggressive, benign soft tissue tumour which arises exclusively in the nasopharynx of young males (peak age of onset 15 y).
- Histology shows a highly vascular neoplasm, in which variably sized vessels are surrounded by a cellular fibroblastic stroma. The lesion is covered by an intact sinonasal epithelium.
- Local recurrence occurs in about 5–25% of cases following surgery.

Nasopharyngeal carcinoma

- A carcinoma arising in the nasopharynx with evidence of squamous differentiation.
- Presents in adults (M>F) with nasal obstruction, hearing loss, and tinnitus.
- Marked geographical variation in incidence, being particularly common in southern China, Thailand, and the Philippines.
- Strong association with Epstein–Barr virus (EBV) and diet (salted and fermented foods).
- Histology recognizes three subtypes: non-keratinizing, keratinizing, and basaloid.
- Most cases are treated with radical radiotherapy.
- 5-year survival rates are 75–98% depending on stage.

Benign laryngeal diseases

Vocal cord nodules

- Benign growths of the laryngeal mucosa.
- Nodules are seen mostly in young women associated with vocal abuse.
- Present with vocal changes.
- Small lesions arising in the middle third of both vocal cords.
- Histology shows a nodule with an oedematous stroma which then becomes fibrotic.

Vocal cord polyp

- Benign growth of the laryngeal mucosa.
- Occurs at any age and with equal gender incidence.
- Presents with vocal changes.
- Involves the ventricular space, or Reinke's space, of one vocal cord.
- Histology shows a polyp with a stroma that may be variably oedematous, myxoid, hyaline, or fibrous.

Laryngeal amyloidosis

- A localized form of amyloidosis.
- Usually arises in the false vocal cord.
- Presents with vocal changes.
- Histology shows deposition of amorphous eosinophilic material beneath the epithelium. Amyloid stains with Congo red and demonstrates chromatic changes under polarized light.
- The amyloid is usually derived from light-chain immunoglobulin.

Squamous papillomas

- Most common benign laryngeal neoplasms.
- Associated with HPV types 6 and 11.
- Bimodal age of incidence <5 y and 20–40 y.
- Present with vocal changes.
- Histology shows branching exophytic papillary fronds covered by a bland squamous epithelium.
- Children tend to develop a more aggressive disease with early recurrences and a higher change of spread beyond the larynx.
- Adults tend to show a more favourable course with less frequent recurrences.

Laryngeal carcinoma

Definition
- Malignant epithelial neoplasm arising in the larynx.

Epidemiology
- 1% of all cancers.
- Men affected more frequently than women, though the incidence in women is increasing.
- Patients usually present in sixth and seventh decades.
- Geographic variation in topographical site affected (Supraglottic SCC commoner in France, Italy, Spain; Glottic in UK, USA, Canada).

Aetiology
- Strong association with heavy smoking and alcohol consumption.

Carcinogenesis
- *TP53* and *CDKN2A* mutations frequently observed.

Presentation
- Glottic tumours: hoarseness.
- Supraglottic tumours: dysphagia, foreign body sensation in the throat.
- Subglottic tumours: dyspnoea, stridor.

Histopathology
- >90% are squamous cell carcinomas, characterized by invasive growth of epithelial cells showing variable squamous differentiation.
- Tumours are graded into well, moderate, or poorly differentiated.
- Tumour growth at the invasive front is divided into cohesive or non-cohesive.

Prognosis
- Tumour, Node, Metastasis (TNM) stage correlates well with survival.
- The 5-year survival approaches 90% for stage 1 tumours, but <50% for stage 4.

Odontogenic cysts

General points

- Odontogenic cysts are a group of epithelial-lined cysts that originate from tooth-forming (odontogenic) tissue and therefore arise in tooth-bearing regions of the maxilla and mandible.
- May be developmental or inflammatory in origin.
- Usually diagnosed when dental radiographs are taken in dentistry practice.
- Cyst removal is advised to prevent destructive effects on the surrounding jaw and teeth.

Radicular (periapical) cyst

- Most common type of odontogenic cyst.
- Inflammatory in origin.
- Arises around the apex of a non-vital tooth, usually due to deep caries or trauma.
- Tends to be asymptomatic, unless it becomes inflamed.
- Radiologically appears as a well-defined, round radiolucency.
- Histologically shows an inflamed fibrous wall lined by a non-keratinizing stratified squamous epithelium.

Dentigerous cyst

- Second most common type of odontogenic cyst.
- Developmental in origin. Wide age range with peal incidence 10–40.
- Arises around the crown of an unerupted tooth, most commonly an impacted wisdom tooth.
- Radiologically appears as a radiolucent lesion.
- Histologically lined by a thin layer of stratified epithelium, most likely of dental follicular origin.
- Complete removal is curative.

Odontogenic keratocyst

- Third most common type of odontogenic cyst.
- Developmental in origin.
- Wide age range with peak incidence 10–30 and second peak 50–70.
- Radiologically presents as a well-demarcated radiolucency, often with scalloped margins; 25% are multiloculated.
- 80% occur in the mandible.
- Histology is distinctive with an uninflamed fibrous wall lined by a thin, parakeratinized stratified squamous epithelium with a corrugated surface. The basal epithelial layer is well-defined and palisaded.

▶ Multiple lesions should prompt consideration of Gorlin's syndrome (naevoid basal cell carcinoma syndrome) caused by mutations in the *PTCH* gene.

Calcifying odontogenic cyst

- Rare, <1% of all odontogenic cysts.
- Mean age of 30.
- Developmental and part of the group of ghost cell lesions of the jaws.
- Radiolucent swelling anterior jaw.
- Histology shows a unicystic variably thickened epithelium with palisading basal layer and focal accumulations of ghost cells and small sheets of dentinoid.

Jawbone neoplasms

Ossifying fibroma

- Benign fibro-osseous neoplasm, arising most commonly in the mandible.
- Three subtypes; Cemento-ossifying fibroma (COF); and two juvenile types: juvenile trabecular ossifying fibroma (JTOF) and juvenile psammomatoid ossifying fibroma (JPOF).
- COF is rare—patients in the third and fourth decades. F > M. Tooth-bearing area of the mandible and maxilla.
- JTOF is rare—patients 8–12 years. F=M. Maxilla > mandible.
- JPOF is rare—patients 16–33 years. F=M. Mostly extragnathic craniofacial bones.
- More common in females.
- Radiologically appear as well-demarcated, radiolucent lesions with varying degrees of radio-opacity.
- Histologically COF contains cementum-like material or bone in a fibroblastic stroma. JTOF consists of cellular osteoid trabeculae in spindle cell rich stroma. JPOF consists of small uniform psammommatoid bodies in a fibroblastic stroma.

Ameloblastoma

- Rare, slowly growing, locally aggressive odontogenic tumour.
- Most arise in the posterior mandible.
- Occurs mostly from 30 to 60 y, with no gender predilection.
- Follicular/plexiform type (80%) shows islands of odontogenic epithelium with columnar epithelial cells and inner cells resemble stellate reticulum.
- Unicystic type (5–20%) shows a cyst lined by ameloblastomatous epithelium. Usually second decade.
- Ameloblastomas commonly show a *BRAF* V600E mutation.
- Treated by excision, though recurrences are common if surgery is conservative.

Melanotic neuroectodermal tumour of infancy

- Rare, locally aggressive, rapidly growing tumour composed of a biphasic population of small neuroblast-like cells and larger melanin producing epithelioid cells.
- 90% occur in the craniofacial region, commonly the maxilla.
- 90% are infants.

Central giant cell lesion

- Uncommon lesion of the jawbones.
- Presents in young adults 20–30 y, with a predilection for the mandible.
- Radiologically appears as a radiolucent defect with scalloped borders.
- Histologically composed of osteoclastic giant cells and spindled fibroblasts in a vascular stroma.
- Prognosis good, with recurrence rare if completely removed.

Neck lumps

Thyroglossal cyst

- Derived from persistent remnants of the thyroglossal duct.
- Presents as a 1- to 4-cm diameter lump in the anterior neck.
- Histologically lined by a pseudostratified columnar epithelium with a fibrous wall, often with a focus of thyroid tissue.

Branchial cyst

- Most are derived from second branchial arch remnants.
- Presents as a 2- to 5-cm diameter lump in the upper lateral neck.
- Most commonly seen in young adults aged 20–40.
- Histologically, the cysts are lined by stratified squamous or pseudostratified columnar epithelium, with a fibrous wall containing lymphoid tissue with prominent germinal centres.

▶ A cystic lymph node metastasis of squamous cell carcinoma is an important differential diagnosis to exclude.

Carotid body paraganglioma

- Rare tumour derived from the paraganglia of carotid bodies.
- Presents as a slow-growing, painless neck lump, arising at the bifurcation of the common carotid artery.
- Most commonly presents in fifth to sixth decades of life. F>M.
- Histologically composed of an organoid (Zellballen) pattern of chief cells with surrounding sustentacular cells in a delicate vascular network.
- Immunohistochemistry shows positivity for the neuroendocrine markers chromogranin, synaptophysin, and CD56. S100 stain highlights sustentacular cells around the nests.
- Germline mutations in the succinate dehydrogenase (SDH) gene found in ~30% of sporadic head and neck paragangliomas.
- Overall, normal life expectancy for non-malignant, sporadic paragangliomas which are completely resected.
- 5-year survival for locally metastasizing paraganglioma is 88% and patients with distant metastases or SDHB-mutation paragangliomas have the lowest 5-year survival rates of 11% and 36%, respectively.

Gastrointestinal pathology

Gastrointestinal malformations

Oesophageal atresia

- Occurs in 1 in 3500 live births.
- Results from faulty division of the foregut into the tracheal and oesophageal channels during the first month of embryonic life.
- In the majority of cases, there is a communication between the distal oesophagus and the trachea known as a tracheo-oesophageal fistula.
- Neonates present with coughing and choking during feeding due to aspiration.
- At least half of affected babies have other congenital abnormalities, and cardiac defects account for the majority of deaths in infants with oesophageal atresia.

Duodenal atresia

- Less common than oesophageal atresia.
- Associated with Down's syndrome in 30% of cases.
- Caused by failure of epithelial apoptosis and incomplete canalization of the duodenal lumen by 8 weeks of gestation.
- The obstruction is usually distal to the ampulla of Vater.
- Prenatal ultrasound shows dilation of the proximal duodenum and stomach with polyhydramnios.

Exomphalos

- An anterior abdominal wall defect at the umbilicus that causes abdominal contents to protrude through the umbilicus.
- The protrusion is covered by a delicate transparent sac composed of the amniotic membrane and peritoneum.
- Arises due to failure of the midgut to return to the abdomen from the umbilical coelom during embryogenesis.

Gastroschisis

- An anterior abdominal wall defect which lies to the side of the umbilicus through which loops of bowel protrude.
- Unlike exomphalos, there is no protective covering sac.

Malrotation

- Malpositioning of the intestine and mesentery due to failure of rotation of the developing gut as it returns from the umbilical coelom to the abdomen during development.
- A malrotated bowel is likely to have a narrow mesenteric base, predisposing to volvulus around the superior mesenteric artery.
- Compromised arterial blood supply leads to ischaemic necrosis of the entire midgut, extending from the duodenum to the transverse colon.
- Necrosis causes bleeding into the bowel and a high risk of perforation.
- Without prompt surgical intervention, the condition can be fatal.

Meckel's diverticulum

- A remnant of the vitellointestinal duct, the structure that connects the primitive gut to the yolk sac.

- Typically said to be '2 in (5 cm) long, 2 ft (60 cm) from the ileo-caecal valve in 2% of the population'.
- The mucosa of the diverticulum may contain areas of gastric or pancreatic tissue (heterotopia).
- Most children with a Meckel's diverticulum are asymptomatic.
- The most common symptom is painless rectal bleeding due to ulceration in a diverticulum containing acid-secreting gastric mucosa.
- Small bowel obstruction may also occur, related to intussusception or incarceration.

Imperforate anus

- Umbrella term for any atretic condition of the rectum or anus.
- Lesions range in severity from a stenosed anal canal to anorectal agenesis.
- Surgically, they are considered as either high or low anomalies, depending on the level of termination of the bowel with respect to the pelvic floor.
- Low defects are easier to correct and postoperative function is good.
- Higher defects are more difficult to correct as they are more likely to be associated with fistulae between the rectum and the genitourinary tract, as well as a deficient pelvic floor.

Hirschsprung's disease

- Not strictly a malformation, but a congenital gastrointestinal (GI) condition in which there is absence of ganglion cells from a variable length of the intestinal wall.
- Results from failure of neuroblasts to migrate from the oesophagus to the anal canal during weeks 5–12 of gestation.
- Absence of ganglion cells causes spasm in the aganglionic segment.
- Presents with intestinal obstruction and failure to pass meconium 24 h after birth.
- Rectal suction biopsy is the gold standard for the diagnosis of Hirschsprung's disease. The key feature is the absence of ganglion cells in the submucosa and abnormally thick nerve fibres in the mucosal layer. The diagnosis is made at the time of surgery by frozen section with histochemical staining for acetylcholinesterase.

Oesophagitis

Definition
- Inflammation of the oesophagus.

Presentation
- Burning retrosternal pain (heartburn).
- Dysphagia and hiccups may also occur.

Reflux oesophagitis
- Caused by gastric acid refluxing into the lower oesophagus.
- Very common. Most prevalent in adult white males but can occur in men and women of all races and in children.
- Predisposing conditions include obesity, alcohol, medications, hypothyroidism, pregnancy, hiatus hernia, and diabetes.
- Mucosal biopsy shows regenerative changes of the squamous epithelium demonstrated by basal cell hyperplasia and extension of vascular papillae into the upper part of the epithelium. Spongiosis (intercellular oedema) is a characteristic feature. Inflammation is typically mild with scattered neutrophils and eosinophils.
- ~10% of patients develop columnar metaplasia of the lower oesophagus which is visible endoscopically; this is known as **Barrett's oesophagus** or **columnar-lined oesophagus** (Fig. 7.1). There may also be intestinal metaplasia with goblet cells. This is associated with a higher risk of developing oesophageal adenocarcinoma. It should be noted that in the USA goblet cells are essential to make the diagnosis.

▶ Barrett's oesophagus is associated with a 50 times increased risk of oesophageal adenocarcinoma. Patients with Barrett's oesophagus should be considered for entry into a surveillance programme of regular endoscopy and biopsy to check for columnar epithelial dysplasia. Dysplasia is divided into high grade and low grade. This is a subjective assessment and current national guidelines state that it should always be made by two pathologists.

Drug-induced ('pill') oesophagitis
- Caused by direct toxicity of drugs to the oesophageal mucosa.
- Occurs mostly in the elderly.
- Common culprit drugs are bisphosphonates and iron tablets.
- Mucosal biopsy shows acute inflammation with erosion or ulceration of the surface epithelium. Encrusted golden brown iron pigment may be seen in cases caused by iron tablets.
- Usually resolves after discontinuation of the offending drug.

Eosinophilic oesophagitis
- Uncommon condition which occurs mostly in atopic individuals with a history of allergy, asthma, and drug sensitivities.
- Mucosal biopsy shows heavy infiltration of the mucosa by eosinophils (more than 15/high-powered field) which often form clusters ('micro-abscesses'). Note that smaller numbers of eosinophils are common in reflux oesophagitis. For this reason, it is helpful to take biopsies from all levels of the oesophagus.
- May coexist with reflux oesophagitis.

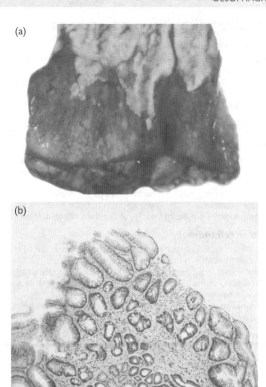

Fig 7.1 Barrett's oesophagus. (a) This segment from the lower oesophagus shows the white keratinized squamous epithelium at the top. The red area at the bottom represents an area of Barrett's oesophagus. (b) An oesophageal biopsy taken from an area of endoscopic Barrett's oesophagus, confirming the presence of glandular epithelium (see Plate 9).

Reproduced with permission from *Clinical Pathology* (Oxford Core Texts), Carton, James, Daly, Richard, and Ramani, Pramila, Oxford University Press (2006), p.139, Figure 8.1.

- Good outlook if diagnosed and treated early. If untreated, it can lead to severe oesophageal strictures.

Infectious oesophagitis

- More commonly seen in debilitated or immunocompromised patients, as the oesophagus is normally highly resistant to infection.
- Common infectious agents include herpes simplex virus (HSV), cytomegalovirus (CMV), and *Candida*.

Oesophageal polyps and nodules

Squamous papilloma

- Uncommon lesion, usually seen as a tiny white polyp in the distal oesophagus at endoscopy.
- Cases have been reported in association with human papillomavirus (HPV) infection.
- Dysplasia is uncommon.
- Histology shows a bland squamous epithelium forming papillary projections.

Leiomyoma

- Uncommon benign smooth muscle tumour arising from the muscular layers of the oesophagus. More common than GI stromal tumours at this site.
- Usually produces a polypoid mass covered by mucosa that may show surface ulceration.
- Histology shows interlacing fascicles of bland smooth muscle cells.

Granular cell tumour

- Uncommon neural tumour which can occur anywhere in the GI tract, but most frequently in the tongue and oesophagus.
- Forms a small firm, raised mucosal nodule in the lower oesophagus.
- Histologically characterized by aggregates of large polygonal cells with conspicuous granular cytoplasm.
- Almost all are benign, though very rare malignant cases have been reported.

Fibrovascular polyp

- Rare oesophageal lesion which typically presents with dysphagia.
- Can reach an alarmingly large size (up to 25 cm long!), such that it can regurgitate into the pharynx or mouth.
- Endoscopically visible as a pedunculated lesion on a long stalk.
- Histology shows a polypoid lesion covered by squamous epithelium with an underlying stromal core composed of loose fibrous tissue, fat, and a prominent vasculature.

Oesophageal carcinoma

Definition
- A malignant epithelial tumour arising in the oesophagus.
- Two major subtypes are distinguished: **squamous cell carcinoma** and **adenocarcinoma**.

Epidemiology
- Both types occur at a median age of 65 y.
- Oesophageal adenocarcinoma has attracted much attention in developed countries due to its dramatic and ongoing rise in incidence over recent decades.
- Squamous carcinomas are much more common in Asia and Africa.

Aetiology
- Heavy tobacco and alcohol use for squamous cell carcinoma.
- Chronic gastro-oesophageal reflux disease leading to Barrett's oesophagus is the most common precursor to adenocarcinoma.

Carcinogenesis
- Both types frequently harbour *p53* mutations.

Presentation
- Dysphagia, retrosternal or epigastric pain, and weight loss.
- By the time most patients present, the tumour is already advanced.

Macroscopy
- Tumour mass in the oesophagus which may grow into the lumen in an exophytic manner or infiltrate into the wall in a plaque-like fashion.
- Squamous cell carcinomas tend to occur in the middle oesophagus, whereas adenocarcinomas tend to occur in the lower oesophagus.
- At the time of resection, neo-adjuvant treatment may produce striking shrinkage of the tumour.

Histopathology
- Squamous cell carcinomas show infiltrating malignant epithelial cells, with evidence of squamous differentiation (i.e. intercellular bridges and/or keratinization).
- Adenocarcinomas show infiltrating malignant epithelial cells, with evidence of glandular differentiation (i.e. tubule formation and/or mucin production). The adjacent oesophageal mucosa may show high-grade dysplasia within an area of Barrett's oesophagus.

Prognosis
- Generally poor due to late presentation.
- 5-year survival rates ~10–20%.

Gastritis

Acute haemorrhagic gastritis

- Caused by an abrupt insult to the gastric mucosa.
- Often the result of drugs or a severe alcohol binge, but any acute medical illness which reduces gastric blood flow may also cause acute gastritis.
- Endoscopy shows numerous punctate erosions which ooze blood.
- Severe forms can cause significant upper GI haemorrhage.
- Histology shows neutrophilic infiltration of the gastric mucosa with haemorrhage and mucosal necrosis.
- Acute gastritis usually resolves rapidly and uneventfully.

Autoimmune gastritis

- Caused by autoimmune attack directed at parietal cells in fundic glands.
- Histology shows infiltration of the body mucosa by lymphocytes and plasma cells. The infiltrate is directed at fundic glands, with atrophy associated with loss of chief and parietal cells. Pyloric and intestinal-type metaplasia is common.
- Increased risk of gastric neuroendocrine tumours (which arise on a background of neuro-endocrine hyperplasia and are often multiple) and carcinoma.
- Some patients also develop antibodies to intrinsic factor, leading to depletion of vitamin B_{12} and megaloblastic anaemia.

Bacterial (*Helicobacter*) gastritis

- A very common cause of gastritis which is usually antral-predominant.
- Most are caused by *Helicobacter pylori*, a curved flagellate Gram-negative rod.
- *Helicobacter heilmannii*, which is larger and more tightly coiled, accounts for <1% of cases.
- Histology shows a heavy lymphoid inflammatory infiltrate in the lamina propria, often with lymphoid follicle formation, with neutrophilic infiltration of the superficial mucosa. Infection may be associated with intestinal metaplasia and dysplasia.
- The organisms can be identified on routine stains but are better visualized on special stains that highlight the bacteria.
- In most cases, the gastritis is healed by eradicating the organism.
- In a small proportion of untreated cases, the gastritis can be complicated by peptic ulceration, gastric carcinoma.

Chemical/reactive gastropathy

- Caused by any low-grade injury to the gastric mucosa.
- Seen mostly in the antrum in relation to bile reflux or non-steroidal anti-inflammatory drugs (NSAIDs).
- Endoscopically, there is erythema of the gastric mucosa.
- Histology shows vascular congestion, foveolar hyperplasia, and smooth muscle proliferation. Inflammation is minimal or absent. It is for this reason the term gastropathy is preferred to gastritis.
- It usually resolves without complication if the offending cause is removed.

Iron pill gastritis

- Caused by the corrosive effects of ingested iron tablets.
- Histology shows it causes acute inflammation with erosion or ulceration of the gastric mucosa. Yellow-brown iron pigment may be seen.

Gastric polyps

Hyperplastic polyp
- Common polyp which occurs mostly in the antrum or body.
- Non-neoplastic reactive lesion thought to represent an exaggerated regenerative response to mucosal injury.
- Often associated with an underlying gastric pathology such as *Helicobacter* or autoimmune gastritis.
- Histology shows a polyp containing a dilated, elongated, tortuous foveolar epithelium in an oedematous, inflamed lamina propria.

Fundic gland polyp
- Common polyp which occurs only in the body or fundus.
- Most frequently seen in patients taking proton pump inhibitors. Can occur sporadically or in association with familial adenomatous polyposis (FAP).
- FAP-associated polyps are more likely to be multiple and occur at a younger age.
- Sporadic polyps are not normally associated with any underlying mucosal pathology.
- Histology shows a polyp containing cystically dilated fundic glands lined by flattened parietal and chief cells.

Gastric adenoma
- Uncommon neoplastic polyp that can occur throughout the stomach.
- Microscopically composed of dysplastic glands with stratified hyperchromatic nuclei.
- Two main types are described—an intestinal and a foveolar type.
- Intestinal types are far more likely to show high-grade dysplasia or harbour gastric carcinoma than the foveolar type.

Gastric xanthoma
- Uncommon polyp that occurs anywhere in the stomach.
- Appears as a pale-yellow nodule due to its lipid content.
- Histology shows numerous lipid-laden macrophages in the lamina propria.

Inflammatory fibroid polyp
- Rare lesion which occurs mostly in the antrum.
- Histology shows a submucosal lesion composed of bland spindle cells arranged around prominent vessels, all set in a loose myxoid stroma containing conspicuous eosinophils.

Gastric carcinoma

Definition

- A malignant epithelial tumour arising in the stomach.

Epidemiology

- Marked geographical variability in incidence due to differences in diet.
- Changes in nutrition in countries with a traditionally high incidence is leading to a steadily declining global incidence.

Aetiology

- Diet is the most consistent factor. High salt intake is a strong risk factor, whilst fresh fruit and vegetables are protective due to their antioxidant effects.
- *H. pylori* and autoimmune gastritis are the other major risk factors, as they both promote a sequence of chronic gastritis, gastric atrophy, intestinal metaplasia, epithelial dysplasia, and carcinoma. This is referred to as the metaplasia–dysplasia of cancer development and is in contrast with the polyp–carcinoma pathway seen in the large bowel.

Carcinogenesis

- Free radicals, oxidants, and reactive oxygen species produced by *H. pylori* infection and dietary carcinogens cause DNA damage.
- Common gene targets include *p53* and *KRAS*.
- Diffuse-type carcinomas often show E-cadherin loss.

Presentation

- Early gastric cancer may be asymptomatic or cause non-specific symptoms such as dyspepsia.
- Advanced cases cause persistent abdominal pain with weight loss.
- Tumours may also bleed, causing haematemesis, or obstruct the gastric outlet leading to vomiting.

Macroscopy

- A tumour mass in the stomach wall which may be exophytic or diffusely infiltrative ('linitis plastica').

Histopathology

- Almost all are adenocarcinomas. The Lauren classification divides them into intestinal and diffuse.
- Intestinal-type adenocarcinoma shows infiltrating malignant epithelial cells forming recognizable glandular structures.
- Diffuse-type adenocarcinoma shows infiltrating malignant epithelial cells growing as poorly cohesive cells, with little or no gland formation. Individual malignant cells may contain intracytoplasmic vacuoles filled with mucin. Cells distended with mucin, such that the nucleus is displaced to one side, are also known as 'signet ring' cells. Tumours with abundant signet ring cells tend to be widely infiltrative.
- *Her-2* testing is now routinely carried out to predict response to Herceptin® (trastuzumab) therapy. Mismatch repair (MMR) immunohistochemical staining is also commonly requested.

Prognosis

- Dependent on the stage, but generally presents late with a poor prognosis.
- Tumour budding and the presence of extranodal lymph node deposits have recently been recognized as additional predictors of survival.

Gastrointestinal stromal tumours

Definition
- Mesenchymal tumours of variable malignant potential which arise within the wall of the GI tract and recapitulate the phenotype of the interstitial cell of Cajal, the pacemaker cell of the Auerbach plexus.

Epidemiology
- Incidence of about ~15 per million population per year.
- Most arise in adults at a median age of 50–60 y.

Aetiology
- Aetiology of sporadic cases unknown.
- A small proportion arise in association with neurofibromatosis type 1 and Carney's triad, and in families with germline *KIT* mutations.

Genetics
- The vast majority show activating mutations of the oncogene *KIT*.
- The remainder show activating mutations in the related gene *PDGFRA*.

Presentation
- Palpable upper abdominal mass, pain, or bleeding.
- Malignant tumours may cause symptoms related to metastasis.

Sites of involvement
- Can occur anywhere in the GI tract, from the oesophagus to the rectum.
- Most arise in the stomach (60–70%) or small intestine (20–30%).
- A small number appear to arise primarily within the omentum.

Macroscopy
- Well-defined tumour mass centred on the submucosal, muscular, or serosal layer of the bowel.
- Range in size from 1 to >20 cm.

Histopathology
- Composed of spindle cells, often with paranuclear vacuoles. Plumper epithelioid cells may also be present and some tumours may be entirely epithelioid in nature.
- Small intestinal tumours may also have so-called skeinoid fibres.
- Almost all express the markers CD117 (c-kit) and DOG-1. Tumours treated with imatinib often show diminished staining.
- Molecular detection of *CD117* or *PDGFRA* mutations may be necessary in a minority of cases and is indicted in cases which are CD117 negative.

Prognosis
- Based on location, size, and mitotic activity, they are stratified into very low risk, low risk, intermediate risk, and high-risk categories for progressive disease. Generally, those arising in the stomach carry a better prognosis than those arising in the rest of the gastrointestinal tract.

Peptic duodenitis

Definition

- Inflammation or ulceration of the duodenal mucosa due to excess gastric acid.

Epidemiology

- Common, affecting up to 10% of the population.
- Mostly seen in male patients aged >40 y.

Aetiology

- Chronic *H. pylori* infection is thought to be the key aetiological factor.
- Smoking and NSAIDs are also major risk factors.
- Recurrent multiple duodenal ulcers, particularly if present beyond the first part of the duodenum, should raise suspicion of possible Zollinger–Ellison syndrome (➲ Pancreatic endocrine tumours, p. 184).

Pathogenesis

- Increased gastric acid production causes injury to the duodenal mucosa, varying from mild erosions only through to severe ulceration.

Presentation

- Burning epigastric pain relieved by eating.
- Severe cases cause persistent epigastric pain, nausea, and vomiting.

Macroscopy

- Peptic duodenitis shows mucosal erythema ± superficial erosions.
- Peptic ulcers appear as well-circumscribed, punched-out mucosal defects with granulation tissue at the base.

Histopathology

- Peptic duodenitis shows acute inflammation, oedema, and haemorrhage in the lamina propria. The surface epithelium typically shows areas of gastric metaplasia. *H. pylori* organisms may be identified overlying the metaplastic gastric epithelium.
- Peptic ulcers show complete loss of the whole mucosal layer, with replacement by granulation tissue and underlying scar tissue.

Prognosis

- Eradication of *H. pylori* and acid suppressive therapy improves symptoms and leads to healing.
- Scarring of ulcers can lead to stricture formation and obstruction.
- Breach of a large vessel by a peptic ulcer is a common cause of acute upper GI haemorrhage.
- Free perforation causes acute generalized peritonitis, necessitating urgent surgical intervention.

Coeliac disease

Definition
- An autoimmune disorder caused by an abnormal immune response to dietary gluten.

Epidemiology
- Common, affecting ~1% of the population.

Aetiology
- Dietary gluten and related proteins.

Pathogenesis
- The culprit proteins are poorly digested by intestinal proteases.
- Intact peptides enter the lamina propria and are deamidated by tissue transglutaminase, rendering them negatively charged.
- Negatively charged peptides bind more efficiently to human leucocyte antigen (HLA) receptors on antigen-presenting cells which are recognized by intestinal T-cells.
- Activated T-cells stimulate an immune reaction in the intestinal wall.

Presentation
- Symptoms relating to the GI tract may be present such as weight loss, abdominal pain, and diarrhoea.
- However, many patients are asymptomatic and only diagnosed during investigation of an iron deficiency anaemia.

Serology
- Presence of serum IgA endomysial or transglutaminase antibodies is highly specific and sensitive for coeliac disease. Care must be taken in interpreting these results in patients who are IgA-deficient.

Macroscopy
- Blunting and flattening of villi may be visible under a dissecting microscope (and may be identified at endoscopy).

Histopathology
- Fully developed cases show increased intraepithelial lymphocytes (>20/100 epithelial cells), mainly at the tips of the villi, many lymphocytes and plasma cells in the lamina propria, villous atrophy, and crypt hyperplasia (Fig. 7.2).
- Milder cases may only show increased intraepithelial lymphocytes without villous atrophy. This is termed lymphocytic duodenitis.

▶ Note that none of these changes are specific to coeliac disease; identical changes can be seen in a number of other conditions, e.g. drugs, tropical sprue. Biopsy findings must be interpreted in light of the clinical and serological picture.

Prognosis
- Strict adherence to a gluten-free diet leads to resolution of symptoms and normalization of histology, although architectural changes may take

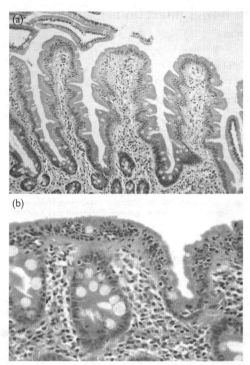

Fig 7.2 (a) Normal duodenal mucosa. The villi have a normal height and shape, and there is no increase in intraepithelial lymphocytes. (b) Duodenal biopsy from a patient with gluten-sensitive enteropathy. The villi have completely disappeared and the surface epithelium contains many intraepithelial lymphocytes (see Plate 10).

Reproduced with permission from *Clinical Pathology* (Oxford Core Texts), Carton, James, Daly, Richard, and Ramani, Pramila, Oxford University Press (2006), p.154, Figure 8.8.

some time to normalize. Cases which do not respond to a gluten-free diet need to be carefully assessed for the development of a lymphoma.
• Increased risk of type 1 diabetes, autoimmune thyroid disease, dermatitis herpetiformis, oropharyngeal and oesophageal carcinomas, small bowel adenocarcinoma, and a rare, but highly aggressive, form of T-cell lymphoma known as enteropathy-associated T-cell lymphoma (EATL) (→ Mature T-cell non-Hodgkin's lymphomas, p. 464).

Small bowel infarction

Definition
- Ischaemic necrosis of a segment of the small intestine.

Epidemiology
- Usually seen in patients aged >50 y.

Aetiology
- Thrombosis overlying an unstable atherosclerotic plaque in the superior mesenteric artery.
- Thromboemboli from the left ventricle or left atrium.
- Hypovolaemia.

Pathogenesis
- Sudden reduction in blood flow through the superior mesenteric artery leads to ischaemic necrosis of a segment of the small bowel.
- Massive haemorrhage into the infarcted bowel causes hypovolaemia.
- Bacteria rapidly permeate the devitalized intestinal wall, leading to sepsis.

Presentation
- Acute onset of severe abdominal pain with bloody diarrhoea and hypovolaemia.

Macroscopy
- The infarcted small bowel appears dusky purple (Fig. 7.3).
- On opening the segment of bowel, large amounts of blood are present in the lumen and the mucosal surface is friable and necrotic.

Histopathology
- Full-thickness necrosis of the bowel wall. Milder changes include crypt atrophy (withering).

Prognosis
- Early laparotomy is essential to resect the infarcted segment of bowel.
- Survival is generally poor due to the rapid development of hypovolaemia and sepsis, causing multiorgan failure.

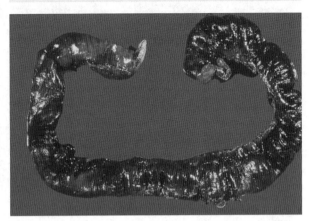

Fig 7.3 Small bowel infarction. Typical appearance of an infarcted segment of the small bowel. The dark colour is due to the intense congestion and haemorrhage within the intestine as a result of blockage to venous outflow (see Plate 11).

Reproduced with permission from *Clinical Pathology* (Oxford Core Texts), Carton, James, Daly, Richard, and Ramani, Pramila, Oxford University Press (2006)), p.159, Figure 8.11.

Intestinal infections

Campylobacter, Salmonella, Shigella, Escherichia coli
- Common bacterial causes of GI infection.
- Mucosal biopsies usually show an acute colitis, with neutrophils present in the lamina propria and within crypts.
- Enterotoxigenic *E. coli* (ETEC) is a common cause of diarrhoea in travellers. ETEC possesses fimbriae which allow the bacteria to adhere to small bowel epithelial cells and produce toxins, causing massive fluid loss.
- Enterohaemorrhagic *E. coli* produces a cytotoxin, leading to haemorrhagic necrosis of the colonic mucosa and bloody diarrhoea. Susceptible individuals, particularly children, are at risk of developing thrombotic microangiopathy, leading to haemolysis and ARF (haemolytic uraemic syndrome, HUS).

Clostridium difficile
- An important cause of colitis, often associated with broad-spectrum antibiotic use in hospitalized patients.
- The clinical picture is highly varied, ranging from mild diarrhoea to fulminant colitis with a risk of perforation and death.
- Macroscopically, the colitis leads to the formation of cream-coloured pseudomembranes on the mucosal surface of the colon (Fig. 7.4).
- Microscopically, crypts distended with neutrophils and mucin are covered by pseudomembranes composed of fibrin and neutrophils.

Mycobacterium avium
- Significant opportunistic pathogen in the immunosuppressed especially HIV positive patients with low CD4 counts).
- Disseminated infection throughout the small and large bowel causes chronic diarrhoea.
- Mucosal biopsy shows extensive infiltration of the lamina propria by macrophages filled with acid-fast bacilli.

Rotavirus
- Most common cause of severe diarrhoea in infants and young children.
- Faecal–oral transmission.
- Immunity develops during childhood, such that adult infection is rare.

Norovirus
- Common cause of epidemic outbreaks of gastroenteritis.
- Highly infectious with transmission through contaminated food or water, person-to-person contact, and contamination of surfaces.
- Often seen in close communities such as institutions, hospitals, and cruise ships.

Cytomegalovirus
- Usually associated with immunocompromise.
- CMV infection is an important cause of a sudden clinical deterioration in immunosuppressed patients with inflammatory bowel disease.

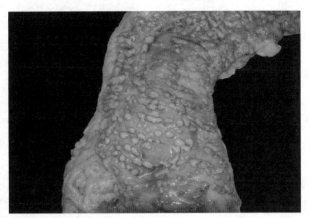

Fig 7.4 *Clostridium difficile* colitis. This is a freshly opened colon from a patient with profuse diarrhoea, following broad-spectrum antibiotic treatment. Note the large number of cream-coloured plaques studded across the mucosal surface, representing collections of neutrophils, fibrin, and cell debris (see Plate 12).

Reproduced with permission from *Clinical Pathology* (Oxford Core Texts), Carton, James, Daly, Richard, and Ramani, Pramila, Oxford University Press (2006), p. 163, Figure 8.14.

- Microscopically, the changes vary from mild inflammation to deep ulceration. CMV inclusions are found in endothelial and stromal cells.
- Immunohistochemical staining is very helpful in confirming the diagnosis.

Giardia lamblia
- Protozoan transmitted by drinking water contaminated with cysts of the organism.
- The mature pathogen attaches to the brush border of the epithelial cells of the upper small bowel and may be diagnosed on duodenal biopsy.
- The inflammatory reaction causes a mild diarrhoeal illness which lasts ~1 week and then resolves.
- Immunocompromised individuals may develop chronic infection.

Entamoeba histolytica
- Common protozoal infection, affecting ~10% of people worldwide.
- Symptoms range from mild diarrhoea and abdominal pain to severe fulminant colitis.
- The infection can disseminate to other sites such as the liver, and rarely large inflammatory masses can form (amoebomas).
- Mild cases show neutrophilic infiltration only, but more severe cases are associated with deep ulceration of the bowel.
- The organisms are round structures with a bean-shaped nucleus and foamy cytoplasm containing ingested red blood cells (RBCs).

Enterobius vermicularis
- Nematode pinworm transmitted by hand-to-mouth transfer of eggs.
- Larvae mature into adult organisms, residing mainly in the caecum.
- At night, female organisms migrate to the anus to deposit eggs which cause marked perianal itching.

Necator americanus **and** *Ancylostoma duodenale*
- Nematode hookworms which attach themselves to the jejunal mucosa.
- A pump mechanism is used to ingest blood and interstitial fluid from the host. High worm loads can lead to significant cumulative blood loss.
- Hookworm infestation is the most common cause of iron deficiency anaemia worldwide.

Intestinal obstruction

Definition
- Mechanical blockage to a segment of the bowel.

Epidemiology
- Common.

Aetiology
- Small bowel obstruction: adhesions, hernias, intussusception, volvulus.
- Large bowel obstruction: tumours, sigmoid volvulus, diverticular strictures.

Pathogenesis
- Mechanical blockage to the bowel prevents normal peristaltic movements.

Presentation
- Small bowel obstruction: acute colicky abdominal pain, abdominal distension, early onset of vomiting, later onset of absolute constipation (neither flatus nor faeces passed).
- Large bowel obstruction: acute colicky abdominal pain, abdominal distension, early onset of absolute constipation, later onset of vomiting.

Macroscopy
- The bowel proximal to the obstruction is usually dilated.
- The underlying cause of the obstruction is usually apparent (e.g. adhesions, tumour, intussusception).

Histopathology
- Ischaemic changes may be present in prolonged cases.
- Features of the underlying cause may also be seen.

Prognosis
- Depends on the underlying cause.
- Benign causes of obstruction generally have a good prognosis, following either spontaneous resolution or surgical intervention.
- Large bowel obstruction due to colorectal carcinoma generally implies advanced disease and poorer prognosis.

Acute appendicitis

Definition
- An acute inflammatory process of the appendix related to obstruction.

Epidemiology
- Peak incidence between ages 5 and 15, but can occur at any age.

Aetiology
- Believed to be the result of obstruction of the appendiceal lumen by a faecolith, undigested food, or enlarged lymphoid tissue.

Pathogenesis
- Obstruction to the appendiceal lumen leads to superimposed infection in the mucosa which then spreads through the whole wall of the appendix.

Presentation
- Right iliac fossa pain accompanied by fever and malaise.
- Many cases do not show typical features, possibly related to the precise positioning of the appendix within the individual.

Macroscopy
- The appendix may appear normal in early cases where the inflammation is confined to the mucosal layer.
- In more advanced cases, the appendix is dilated and a fibrinopurulent exudate may be seen on the serosal surface.

Histopathology
- Acute transmural inflammation is seen involving the mucosa, submucosa, and muscularis propria.
- Extensive necrosis of the muscularis propria can lead to perforation.
- In cases where there is peritonitis, but no underlying crypt inflammation, extra-appendicular causes of inflammation should be excluded.
- Other types of appendicitis include granulomatous and parasites (e.g. schistosomiasis).

Prognosis
- Prognosis is excellent, provided an appendectomy is performed promptly.
- Delayed treatment risks perforation of the inflamed appendix, with potential complications such as intra-abdominal abscess formation or generalized peritonitis.

Crohn's disease

Definition

- An idiopathic inflammatory bowel disease, characterized by multifocal areas of inflammation which may involve any part of the GI tract.

Epidemiology

- Uncommon.
- Major incidence between 20 and 30 y.

Aetiology and pathogenesis

- Thought to be caused by an abnormal mucosal immune response to luminal bacteria in genetically susceptible individuals.
- *NOD2* (nucleotide oligomerization binding domain 2) mutations are relatively common, although only 10% of individuals with risk-associated variants develop the disease.
- Smoking increases the risk.
- A true infectious aetiology remains unproven, although mycobacteria have been long suspected to play a role.

Presentation

- Crampy right iliac fossa pain and diarrhoea, which is usually not bloody.
- Fever, malaise, and weight loss are common.

Macroscopy

- Disease usually involves the terminal ileum and colon.
- Affected bowel is thickened with encroachment of mesenteric fat around the anti-mesenteric border of the bowel ('fat wrapping').
- Adhesions and fistulae may be seen between adjacent loops of bowel.
- The mucosal surface shows linear ulceration and 'cobblestoning'.

Histopathology

- Mucosal biopsies: variability of inflammation within a single biopsy and between several biopsies is the key feature. This is typically manifested by discrete areas of inflammation adjacent to histologically normal crypts. Surface erosions and ulceration may be present. Poorly formed granulomas may be seen, but these are generally uncommon.
- There may be evidence of chronicity with architectural changes, Paneth cell metaplasia, and loss of the inflammatory cell gradient. If not, the differential diagnosis of focal acute inflammation includes an infectious colitis.
- Resection specimens: deep fissuring ulcers separated by relatively normal mucosa. Lymphoid aggregates are present in the submucosa and muscular layers. Poorly formed granulomas may be seen. These need to be distinguished from a giant cell reaction associated with a ruptured crypt. Transmural inflammation is the key diagnostic feature, although it may be seen in the toxic megacolon associated with ulcerative colitis (UC).

Prognosis

- Relapsing and remitting course.
- Most patients require surgery at some point to relieve symptoms from obstruction or fistula formation.
- Increased risk of small and large bowel adenocarcinomas.
- Extra-GI manifestations include enteropathic arthropathy (◆ Spondyloarthropathies, p. 527), anterior uveitis, gallstones, primary sclerosing cholangitis, erythema nodosum (◆ Erythema nodosum, p. 489), and (◆ Pyoderma gangrenosum, p. 490).

Ulcerative colitis

Definition
- An idiopathic inflammatory bowel disease, characterized by inflammation restricted to the large bowel mucosa, which always involves the rectum and extends proximally in a continuous fashion for a variable distance.

Epidemiology
- Uncommon.
- Major incidence between 15 and 25 y.

Aetiology and pathogenesis
- Thought to be due to an abnormal mucosal immune response to luminal bacteria.
- The genetic link is weaker than for Crohn's disease (CD).
- Smoking appears to decrease the risk of UC.
- One unusual, but consistently confirmed, observation is the protective effect of appendectomy on the subsequent development of UC.

Presentation
- Recurrent episodes of bloody diarrhoea, often with urgency and tenesmus.

Macroscopy
- Erythematous mucosa with a friable, eroded surface and haemorrhage.
- Inflamed mucosa may form polypoid projections (inflammatory polyps).
- Disease always involves the rectum and extends continuously to involve a variable amount of colon (Fig. 7.5).

Histopathology
- Biopsies show almost always show evidence of chronic mucosal damage: crypt architectural distortion, Paneth cell metaplasia, and loss of the inflammatory cell gradient in the lamina propria. There is also mucosal inflammation with cryptitis and crypt abscess formation. Inflammation. The changes are usually more marked distally although the rectal changes may be mild if there has been topical treatment.
- Resection specimens show diffuse inflammation limited to the mucosal layer. Inflammatory polyps may be present.
- Extension of inflammation into the submucosa or muscle layers may occur in very severe acute UC, but the inflammation still remains heaviest in the mucosal layer.

Prognosis
- Generally good with treatment.
- Increased risk of colorectal carcinoma, so surveillance colonoscopy is usually recommended several years after diagnosis.
- Extra-GI manifestations include enteropathic arthropathy (➋ Spondyloarthropathies, p. 527), primary sclerosing cholangitis (➋ Primary sclerosing cholangitis, p. 160), erythema nodosum (➋ Erythema nodosum, p. 489), pyoderma gangrenosum (➋ Pyoderma gangrenosum, p. 490), uveitis, and AA amyloidosis.

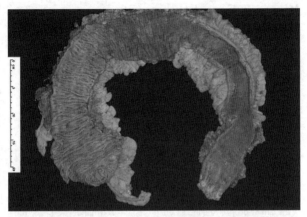

Fig 7.5 Ulcerative colitis. This is a colectomy specimen from a patient with ulcerative colitis. The right colon is on the left of the picture (note the appendix), and the left colon and rectum are on the right side of the picture. The inflamed mucosa, which looks red, begins at the rectum and continuously affects the left colon until the transverse colon where there is a sharp transition into normal mucosa (see Plate 13).

Reproduced with permission from *Clinical Pathology* (Oxford Core Texts), Carton, James, Daly, Richard, and Ramani, Pramila, Oxford University Press (2006), p. 163, Figure 8.15.

Microscopic colitis

Definition

- A chronic form of colitis, characterized by chronic watery diarrhoea, normal or near normal colonoscopy, and microscopic evidence of colonic inflammation.

Subtypes

- Two types are recognized: **lymphocytic and collagenous colitis, although they may coexist**. There is an association with NSAIDs and coeliac disease.

Lymphocytic colitis

- Incidence of 3 per 100 000 population.
- Equal sex incidence.
- Mean age of onset is 50 y.
- Strong association with coeliac disease.
- Mucosal biopsy specimens show increased numbers of plasma cells in the lamina propria and increased intraepithelial lymphocytes (>20/100 epithelial cells).
- Most patients respond to medical therapy.

Collagenous colitis

- Incidence of 1–2 per 100 000 population.
- Significant predilection for women ($\female$:$\male$ = 8:1).
- Mean age of onset is 60 y.
- Mucosal biopsy specimens show thickening of the subepithelial collagen plate and increased numbers of plasma cells in the lamina propria, and increased intraepithelial lymphocytes.
- Most patients respond to medical therapy.

Colorectal polyps

Hyperplastic polyps

- Very common polyps, occurring most frequently in the distal colon.
- Usually small lesions, <1 cm in size, found on the crest of a mucosal fold.
- Microscopically, they are composed of crypts which are dilated and serrated in the superficial portion and narrow at the base.
- Benign lesions with no risk of progression into carcinoma, unless they show dysplasia which is very uncommon. The hyperplastic polyposis syndrome, in which there are very large numbers of hyperplastic polyps, is also associated with an increased risk.

Sessile serrated lesions (or polyps)

- Relatively recently characterized polyps which tend to be >1 cm and more likely to be found in the right colon.
- Genetically, they tend to harbour mutations in mismatch repair genes.
- Microscopically, they show markedly dilated serrated crypts which are widened at their base: 'boot-shaped crypts'.
- There may be coexisting dysplasia.
▶ Associated with an increased risk of subsequent colorectal carcinoma.

Adenomatous polyps

- Very common polyps which may occur anywhere in the large bowel.
- Most occur sporadically, but they are also associated with **familial adenomatous polyposis** (FAP). FAP is an inherited condition in which the colon becomes carpeted with thousands of adenomas at a young age, with the inevitable development of colorectal carcinoma without prophylactic colectomy. There may be polyps in the duodenum as well. Gardener's syndrome, which is a variant of FAP, may be associated with extraintestinal manifestations such as desmoid tumours.
- Neoplastic polyps which harbour frequent mutations of *APC*, *KRAS*, and *p53*.
- Microscopically, the polyps contain dysplastic glands lined by epithelial cells with stratified hyperchromatic nuclei growing in complex tubules or finger-like villous projections. Depending on the relative proportion of tubules and villi, they are classified as tubular, tubulo-villous, and villous adenomas.
- The dysplasia is graded into low or high grade, according to the degree of cytological and architectural abnormality.
- ~10% of adenomas develop carcinoma.
- The likelihood of malignant transformation is higher with larger polyps, high-grade dysplasia, and a villous architecture. When carcinomas arise in pedunculated polyps, they are staged using the **Haggitt system** to assess the risk of the presence of lymph node metastasis.

Inflammatory polyps

- Thin, filiform lesions which occur following any mucosal injury, but are often seen in patients with inflammatory bowel disease.
- Microscopically, they are covered by mucosa on all sides, with only a tiny amount of submucosal tissue.

Mucosal prolapse ('solitary rectal ulcer syndrome')
- Prolapsed pieces of mucosa which appear as polypoid projections.
- Can occur at any point in the large bowel, but characteristically seen on the anterior rectal wall or in association with diverticular disease.
- Can ulcerate and mimic colorectal carcinoma.
- Microscopically, they show distorted angulated crypts set in the lamina propria containing bundles of smooth muscle running up from the muscularis mucosae.

Benign fibro-epithelial polyps
- Almost always incidental polyps picked up in adults undergoing screening colonoscopy.
- Microscopically, they show a bland spindle cell proliferation in the lamina propria. The spindle cells show no specific line of differentiation immunohistochemically.

Leiomyomas
- Benign smooth muscle tumours arising from the muscularis mucosae.
- Usually small polyps, located mostly in the distal large bowel.
- Microscopically, they show bundles of bland smooth muscle cells.

Juvenile (hamartomatous) polyps
- Most common colonic polyp found in children.
- Thought to be hamartomatous in nature.
- Microscopically, they show irregular, markedly dilated, disorganized colonic glands set in an oedematous stroma.
- Presence of multiple juvenile polyps may be a marker for **juvenile polyposis**, an autosomal dominant condition caused by germline mutations in either *SMAD4* or *BMPR1A*.

Colorectal carcinoma

Definition

- A malignant epithelial tumour arising in the colon or rectum.

▶ Note that only tumours that have penetrated through the muscularis mucosae into the submucosa are considered malignant at this site. This contrasts with carcinomas at other sites where a breach of the basement membrane directly underlying the epithelium is sufficient for the categorization of an epithelial tumour as malignant.

Epidemiology

- Third most common cancer in the UK, with a lifetime risk of 1 in 16 men and 1 in 20 women.
- Second most common cause of cancer-related deaths.

Aetiology

- A diet high in animal fat and low in fibre, together with a sedentary lifestyle, increases the risk.
- Other associations include idiopathic inflammatory bowel disease, FAP, and hereditary non-polyposis colorectal cancer (HNPCC).

Carcinogenesis

- Most develop through a sequence of aberrant crypt focus (dysplasia in a single crypt) → adenomatous polyp → invasive carcinoma.
- Common genetic aberrations include the loss of *APC, TP53,* and *SMAD4.*
- Some tumours are characterized by the inactivation of mismatch repair genes, recognized by the epiphenomenon of microsatellite instability.

Presentation

- Change in bowel habit, tenesmus, abdominal pain, iron deficiency anaemia.
- Asymptomatic tumours may be discovered via screening or surveillance programmes.

Macroscopy

- Most tumours grow as polypoid masses projecting into the bowel lumen, often with areas of surface ulceration (Fig. 7.6). Some tumours, particularly in the distal colon, form circumferential stenosing lesions.
- The cut surface shows a firm, white tumour mass in the bowel wall.
- Large pools of gelatinous material are seen in mucinous carcinomas.

Histopathology

- The vast majority are adenocarcinomas, i.e. infiltrating malignant epithelial tumours showing evidence of glandular differentiation.
- Well-differentiated tumours show plentiful tubular formation, whereas poorly differentiated tumours show minimal gland formation.
- Most tumours are well/moderately differentiated and often contain abundant necroinflammatory debris within the glandular spaces (so-called 'dirty' necrosis).

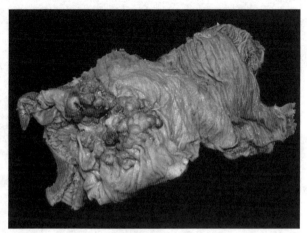

Fig 7.6 Adenocarcinoma of the caecum. This is a right hemicolectomy specimen, in which a small piece of the terminal ileum, the caecum, the appendix, and the ascending colon have been removed. A large tumour is seen in the caecum, which was confirmed on microscopy to be an adenocarcinoma. This tumour was picked up at colonoscopy performed because the patient was found to have an unexplained iron deficiency anaemia (see Plate 14).

Reproduced with permission from *Clinical Pathology* (Oxford Core Texts), Carton, James, Daly, Richard, and Ramani, Pramila, Oxford University Press (2006), p.168, figure 8.20.

- ~10% of colonic and 30% of rectal tumours show extensive mucin production, such that the malignant cells are seen floating in large pools of extracellular mucin; these are termed **mucinous adenocarcinomas**.
- Patients with tumours which have a pushing margin and/or associated with a marked increase in tumoural lymphocytes have a better prognosis.
- Tumour regression, with fibrosis, is assessed using the Mandard Grade.

Molecular markers

- Current guidelines suggest that all patients with colorectal cancer should be screened for HNPCC by immunohistochemistry for loss of expression of the mismatch repair proteins MLH1, MSH2, MSH6, and PMS2. This is usually carried out on the biopsy on which the diagnosis is made.
- *K-ras* and *BRAF* mutational status is routinely requested in patients with metastatic disease and increasingly in patients with localized disease.

Prognosis

- 5-year survival rate ~50%.
- Important prognostic factors include the stage (particularly the lymph node status), presence of venous invasion, differentiation of the

tumour, and completeness of surgical excision. Tumour budding and the presence of extranodal lymph node deposits are additional, prognostic factors.

NHS bowel cancer screening programme

- Two types of screening are offered by the NHS:
- **Faecal occult blood** (FOB) testing is offered every 2 y to men and women aged 60–74. This is a home test kit sent through the post that looks for evidence of blood in the stool.
- **Bowel scope screening** has been, more recently, introduced in England as a one-off test to men and women at age 55. This involves direct sigmoidoscopy to look for polyps.

Diverticular disease

Definition
- The presence of outpouchings of the colonic mucosa that have herniated through the circular muscular layer of the large bowel and are therefore only pseudodiverticula.
- The vast majority of cases are seen in the sigmoid colon.

Epidemiology
- Very common. Mostly a disease of patients aged >60 y.

Aetiology
- A diet low in fibre and high in meat is the strongest risk factor.

Pathogenesis
- Firm stools require higher intraluminal pressures to propel.
- High intraluminal pressure forces pouches of the colonic mucosa through an anatomical weak point in the muscular layer where blood vessels pass through to supply the mucosal layers.

Presentation
- Intermittent abdominal pain, altered bowel habit, iron deficiency anaemia. ▶ Note these symptoms may closely mimic colorectal carcinoma.
- Acute inflammation in a diverticulum (acute diverticulitis) presents with severe left iliac fossa pain.
- Occasionally, erosion of a large submucosal vessel can cause severe rectal bleeding.

Macroscopy
- Diverticula are seen herniating out between the taenia coli of the sigmoid colon.
- The circular muscle layer is often markedly thickened and numerous redundant mucosal folds are present, projecting into the lumen.
- In acute diverticulitis, an inflammatory mass may be visible surrounding a diverticulum.
- Diverticular strictures cause fibrous narrowing of the bowel lumen which can closely mimic a stenosing carcinoma.

Histopathology
- Diverticula are seen herniating through a thickened circular muscle layer. Only a thin coating of longitudinal muscle separates the diverticulum from the pericolic fat.
- In cases of acute diverticulitis, there is superimposed acute inflammation associated with a diverticulum; severe cases may show pericolic abscess formation.

Prognosis
- Acute diverticulitis can be complicated by pericolic abscess formation, fistula formation, and free perforation.
- Free perforation causes generalized peritonitis which can be fatal in frail elderly patients.

Anal pathology

Haemorrhoids

- Abnormally dilated and prolapsed anal cushions.
- Extremely common.
- Thought to be due to disruption of the normal suspensory mechanisms caused by chronic straining at stool.
- Cause bright red rectal bleeding and discomfort.
- Excised haemorrhoids examined microscopically contain large, dilated blood vessels, which may show evidence of thrombosis and recanalization, with an overlying hyperplastic squamous epithelium.

Anal tags

- Polypoid projections of the anal mucosa and submucosa.
- Unrelated to haemorrhoids, but frequently confused with them.
- Microscopically composed of a fibrovascular core covered by squamous epithelium. The fibrovascular core lacks the typical ectatic vessels of haemorrhoids.

Anal fissure

- A tear in the mucosa of the lower anal canal which is almost always located posteriorly in the midline.
- Cause is unclear, but chronic infection may lead to loss of the normal elasticity of the mucosa, such that passage of hard faeces may precipitate the tear.
- Usually presents with severe pain.
- The presence of granulomas (rather than a foreign body reaction to foreign material) should raise the possibility of CD.

Anorectal abscess

- A collection of pus within deep perianal tissue.
- A complication of infection within a deep anal gland.
- Presents with perianal erythema, swelling, and pain.

Anorectal fistula

- An abnormal epithelial-lined tract connecting the anal canal to the perianal skin.
- Usually the result of infection in an anal gland tracking to the skin surface.
- Multiple perianal fistulae can also be a manifestation of CD.

Anal cancer

- Uncommon cancer which is invariably associated with HPV infection (including types 16 and 33) infection.
- Vast majority are squamous cell carcinomas which arise from areas of squamous dysplasia known as either anal intraepithelial neoplasia (AIN), which is graded 1–3 or anal squamous intraepithelial lesion (SIL), which is divided into low and high grade. They are often associated with similar pathology in the vagina and cervix.
- These tumours metastasize to inguinal lymph nodes.

Chapter 8

Hepatobiliary pathology

Acute viral hepatitis

Definition

- Infection of the liver by hepatitis A, B, C, or E, lasting less than 6 months.

Epidemiology

- Hepatitis A virus (HAV) is especially common in Africa and India. Hepatitis B virus (HBV) is especially common in Africa and Asia.
- Hepatitis C virus (HCV), Hepatitis D virus (HDV) and Hepatitis E virus (HEV) are common worldwide.
- All ages may be affected.

Virology

- HAV is a positive-sense, single-stranded ribonucleic acid (RNA) picornavirus transmitted orally by faecal contamination of food or water.
- HBV is a partially double-stranded DNA hepadnavirus transmitted through contaminated needles, sexual contact, or vertically from an infected mother to her baby.
- HCV is a positive-sense, single-stranded RNA hepacivirus transmitted from contaminated needles, mostly through intravenous drug abuse.
- HEV is positive-sense, single-stranded RNA hepevirus transmitted orally by faecal contamination of food or water.

Immunopathogenesis

- The viruses localize to the liver. After a variable incubation period, a specific T-lymphocyte response to the virus is mounted.
- The necro-inflammatory activity in the liver causes an episode of acute hepatitis.

Presentation

- Many cases are clinically silent or cause a non-specific, flu-like illness.
- Clinically apparent cases cause nausea, vomiting, malaise, and jaundice.

Serology

- Presence of serum anti-hepatitis IgM antibodies confirms a recent infection.

Macroscopy

- The liver may be swollen and discoloured with bile.

Histopathology

- Liver lobules are infiltrated by mononuclear inflammatory cells.
- Hepatocyte injury is manifested morphologically by swelling ('swelling') or shrinkage and pyknosis (apoptotic/acidophil bodies).
- Severe cases show confluent areas of hepatocyte necrosis and parenchymal collapse: 'spotty necrosis'.

▶ Note these histological changes are not specific to viral hepatitis and may be seen in acute liver injury from other causes.

Prognosis
- Acute HAV never progresses to chronic infection.
- Acute HBV progresses to chronic infection in ~10% of cases.
- Acute HCV progresses to chronic infection in ~90% of cases.

Chronic viral hepatitis

Definition
- Infection of the liver by hepatitis B, C, or D lasting longer than 6 months.

Epidemiology
- Chronic HCV is common worldwide, with ~3% of the world's population infected.
- Chronic HBV shows more geographical variation, being rarer in western countries, but very common in areas of Africa and Asia where infection rates are as high as 15%.

Immunopathogenesis
- Chronic viral hepatitis is the result of an immune response that fails to clear the virus following infection.
- 10% of people fail to clear HBV infection.
- 90% of people fail to clear HCV infection.
- HDV is an incomplete DNA virus which can only cause infection in patients who already have HBV. If the two infections occur together, this is co-infection; if the HDV follows HBV, this is superinfection. The latter produces more serious diseases.

Presentation
- Often asymptomatic and diagnosed incidentally on abnormal liver function tests (LFTs).
- Many patients do not present until advanced cirrhosis with ascites.

Serology
- Chronic HBV: presence of serum HBsAg (hepatitis B surface antigen) and anti-HBcAg (hepatitis B core antigen) antibodies.
- Chronic HCV: presence of serum anti-HCV antibodies and HCV RNA by PCR.
- HDV: presence of serum IgM anti-HDV antibodies or the detection of the virus in liver biopsies.

Macroscopy
- The liver may feel slightly firm due to fibrosis.

Histopathology
- Portal inflammation is dominant and composed mostly of lymphocytes.
- Interface hepatitis ('piecemeal necrosis') refers to the extension of the portal inflammatory infiltrate into the hepatocytes at the limiting plate, associated with hepatocyte degeneration.
- Lobular inflammation is usually focal and mild in chronic viral hepatitis (compare with acute viral hepatitis where it is the dominant site). In cases of HBV with superinfection with HDV, lobular changes may be prominent.
- Fibrosis is a marker of how advanced the disease is. Extensive bridging fibrosis through the liver terminates in cirrhosis.

- A liver biopsy report should include a description of the degree of inflammation (stage) and how advanced the fibrosis is (grade). These can be summarized using a semi-quantitative scoring system (e.g. Ishak or METAVIR).

▶ Note that all of these changes may be seen in chronic liver injury from a number of causes. Clues to a viral aetiology may be present, however, 'ground glass' hepatocytes in hepatitis B and portal lymphoid aggregates, in-flammatory bile duct damage, and fatty change in hepatitis C. As described earlier, HDV is characterized by lobular damage. It should be noted that because of the availability of markedly improved treatment, patients with HCV are, now, infrequently biopsied.

Prognosis

- Prognosis largely depends on the extent of fibrosis present on liver biopsy.
- Viral genotype is also important in hepatitis C.
- High risk of hepatocellular carcinoma (HCC), especially in patients with cirrhosis. This may occur, especially in endemic areas, in patients without cirrhosis.

Alcoholic liver disease

Definition
- Liver disease due to excessive alcohol consumption.
- Three patterns of disease are recognized: **steatosis**, **alcoholic steatohepatitis** (ASH), and **cirrhosis**.

Epidemiology
- Extremely common.

Pathogenesis
- Alcohol metabolism in the liver generates high levels of nicotinamide adenine dinucleotide dehydrogenase (NADH) which stimulates fatty acid synthesis and production of triglycerides, leading to steatosis.
- In some individuals, oxidative stress from metabolism of alcohol leads to hepatocyte injury and necro-inflammatory activity (ASH).
- Ongoing necro-inflammatory activity causes liver fibrosis which may progress to cirrhosis.

Presentation
- Steatosis and mild ASH are usually asymptomatic but are a common cause of mildly abnormal LFTs.
- Severe alcoholic hepatitis following binge drinking causes malaise and fever, with marked elevation of LFTs. Jaundice may occur if there is marked loss of liver function.
- Alcoholic cirrhosis presents with complications of cirrhosis (e.g. ascites or ruptured oesophageal varices).

Macroscopy
- Steatosis causes an enlarged soft greasy liver.
- ASH may cause a firm texture due to fibrosis in the liver.
- Cirrhosis causes diffuse nodularity of the liver.

Histopathology
- All the changes are most severe in zone 3 near the central vein.
- Steatosis shows large droplets of fat in hepatocytes which displace the nucleus to one side (macrovesicular / large droplet steatosis).
- ASH shows ballooned hepatocytes which may contain Mallory–Denk bodies (clumps of dense pink material derived from the cytoskeleton) and an inflammatory infiltrate rich in neutrophils.
- Fibrosis in ASH is typically pericellular but eventually forms fibrous bridges. Cirrhosis shows diffuse replacement of the liver by nodules of regenerating hepatocytes surrounded by fibrous bands.
- Fatty change, ballooning, and cirrhosis may-co-exist.

Prognosis
- Simple steatosis is fully reversible if alcohol consumption ceases.
- Alcoholic hepatitis may resolve with cessation of alcohol consumption or may progress to fibrosis and cirrhosis. It is more likely to be progressive in women.
- Alcoholic cirrhosis has a poor prognosis, with 5-year survival rates of only 50%.

Non-alcoholic fatty liver disease

Terminology
- The hepatic manifestation of the metabolic syndrome (central obesity, abnormal glucose tolerance, hyperlipidaemia).
- Non-alcoholic fatty liver disease (NAFLD) covers a range of conditions, including simple **steatosis** (fatty liver), **non-alcoholic steatohepatitis** (NASH), and **cirrhosis**.
- The term metabolic associated fatty liver (MAFLD) and steatohepatitis (MASH) disease has, recently, been suggested as being preferred terms as they are defined by a positive feature and also because they co-exist with alcoholic live disease.

Epidemiology
- Very common and increasing in incidence due to rising obesity rates.
- Now the most common cause of abnormal LFTs.
- Many cases of cirrhosis once thought to be cryptogenic are now thought to represent end-stage NAFLD.

Aetiology
- Obesity and diabetes are the most common associations.
- Also associated with some drugs and parenteral nutrition.

Pathogenesis
- Insulin resistance seems to be the key factor and is linked to obesity.
- Insulin resistance causes the accumulation of fat and hepatocyte injury.
- Inflammation in response to hepatocyte injury leads to fibrosis, and eventually cirrhosis in some individuals.

Presentation
- Most cases are asymptomatic and discovered because of abnormal LFTs.
- Occasional cases present with complications related to cirrhosis.

Macroscopy
- The liver is enlarged, soft, and greasy.
- Cirrhotic livers are diffusely nodular.

Histopathology
- Steatosis shows accumulation of fat within hepatocytes without significant inflammatory activity.
- NASH shows large droplet steatosis, together with the presence of ballooned hepatocytes (which may contain Mallory–Denk bodies) and mixed acute and chronic inflammatory infiltrate. Variable fibrosis may be present, depending on the stage of the disease. Generally, although the features are the same, the changes are milder than in alcoholic hepatitis.

▶ Ruling out alcoholic liver disease can sometimes be difficult, as many patients significantly under-report their alcohol intake.

Prognosis
- Steatosis has a very low risk of progression to chronic liver disease.

- NASH progresses to cirrhosis in ~10–15% of cases over 8y.
- The most important determinant of prognosis is the degree of fibrosis.
- Patients with cirrhosis due to NAFLD generally have a better survival rate than patients with cirrhosis due to alcoholic liver disease.
- Liver cell cancer is being increasingly recognized in patients without cirrhosis.

Autoimmune hepatitis

Definition
- A liver disease due to an autoimmune response targeted against the liver.

Epidemiology
- Uncommon.
- Typically affects middle-aged females.

Aetiology
- Unknown for certain, but thought to be triggered by infection or drugs.

Pathogenesis
- Current thinking suggests that liver damage from an infection or a drug causes genetically susceptible people to become sensitized to their liver and mount an immune response against it.

Presentation
- Most cases are asymptomatic in the early stages but may be diagnosed incidentally due to abnormalities of LFTs.
- Some patients present late with symptoms and signs of chronic liver disease or terminal cirrhosis.
- ~25% of cases present suddenly with an episode of acute hepatitis with jaundice.
- Rarely, massive acute liver damage occurs and the patient presents with acute hepatic failure.

Serology
- Serum IgG is usually raised.
- A variety of autoantibodies may be present (e.g. anti-nuclear antibodies, liver–kidney microsomal (LKM) antibodies, and smooth muscle antibodies). LKM antibody associated disease is commoner in children.

Macroscopy
- Few macroscopic changes, except in patients with cirrhosis or in cases of severe acute hepatitis with massive hepatocyte necrosis.

Histopathology
- Chronic hepatitis pattern of injury with portal inflammation, interface hepatitis, lobular inflammation, and variable fibrosis.
- In contrast with chronic viral hepatitis, interface hepatitis and lobular inflammation tend to be more prominent. Plasma cells are often a conspicuous component of the inflammatory cell infiltrate.

Prognosis
- Most cases respond well to immunosuppressive therapy.
- Long-term prognosis is dependent on the extent of fibrosis in the liver at the time of diagnosis.
- Biopsy is necessary to assess the response to treatment as disease may progress with normal serum biochemistry.

Primary biliary cholangitis

Definition
- A chronic liver disease characterized by the destruction of small intrahepatic bile ducts and the presence of anti-mitochondrial antibodies.

Terminology
- Previously called primary biliary cirrhosis.
- The name has changed because less than half of patients with this condition have cirrhosis.
- There are cases which have serological features of an autoimmune hepatitis, but pathological features of primary biliary cholangitis (PBC) and these cases are best termed autoimmune cholangitis unless the biopsy shows a severity of inflammation beyond that seen in PBC in which case it is an 'overlap syndrome'.

Epidemiology
- Uncommon.
- Occurs most frequently in middle-aged women and is associated with other autoimmune conditions.

Aetiology
- Unknown, but may be triggered by infection with organisms that show molecular mimicry to antigens on the biliary epithelium.

Pathogenesis
- Thought to be an autoimmune disease in which the immune system mounts an abnormal response to the biliary epithelium.

Presentation
- Asymptomatic in its early stages, although may be picked up by elevated alkaline phosphatase levels. It should be noted that a rise in bilirubin is a late feature.
- Patients presenting with symptoms usually do so with fatigue or pruritus due to the accumulation of bile salts.

Serology
- >95% of cases are associated with the presence of anti-mitochondrial antibodies directed at a component of the pyruvate dehydrogenase enzyme complex located in the inner mitochondrial matrix.

Macroscopy
- Early disease shows few macroscopic changes in the liver.
- In advanced disease, the liver is cirrhotic and bile-stained.

Histopathology
- Earliest feature is the infiltration and destruction of interlobular bile ducts by lymphocytes and macrophages ('florid duct lesion'). The macrophages may coalesce into clusters and form granulomas.
- Copper accumulates in the liver as it cannot be excreted via the biliary tree.

- As the disease progresses, there is inflammation and destruction of hepatocytes at the edges of the portal tracts (interface hepatitis) which begins a sequence of periportal fibrosis → portal–portal bridging → cirrhosis.

Prognosis

- Gradual progression towards cirrhosis over 15–20 y.
- Ursodeoxycholic acid therapy decreases the rate of progression.

Primary sclerosing cholangitis

Definition
- A chronic liver disease characterized by inflammation and scarring in the biliary tree.
- Usually, the entire biliary tree is affected, but occasionally only small interlobular bile ducts are affected (small duct PSC).

Epidemiology
- Uncommon.
- Seen predominantly in young men with ulcerative colitis. There is a less strong association with Crohn's Disease.
- ~70% of patients with PSC also have ulcerative colitis.

Aetiology
- Unknown, although there is a genetic link with certain human leukocyte antigen (HLA) types.

Pathogenesis
- Chronic biliary inflammation is followed by fibrotic scarring which narrows the affected bile ducts. Obstruction within the biliary system leads to progressive fibrosis within the liver which terminates in cirrhosis. Biliary stasis also promotes infection and stone formation.

Presentation
- Asymptomatic in its early stages and is often picked up when elevated alkaline phosphatase levels are found in a patient with UC.

Radiology
- Demonstration of strictures and dilations within the biliary tree on imaging is highly suggestive of PSC.

Macroscopy
- Early PSC usually causes no macroscopic changes. Advanced disease causes a cirrhotic liver with bile staining. Fibrotic biliary strictures may be apparent in the major bile ducts.

Histopathology
- Explanted liver specimens show fibrosis and inflammation in large bile ducts with inspissated bile and stones. There is a biliary pattern of cirrhosis with large, irregular, jigsaw-like nodules of hepatocytes.
- Liver biopsy specimens show variable features, depending on the biopsy site. If the biopsy is taken from an area unaffected by the primary disease, but distal to a large duct stricture, the liver shows features of duct obstruction (i.e. portal oedema with proliferation of bile ductules). If the biopsy comes from an area affected by PSC, then medium-sized bile ducts show periductal oedema and concentric fibrosis, whilst small bile ducts are often completely absent. Copper accumulates in periportal hepatocytes.

Prognosis

• Progressive liver disease eventually terminating in cirrhosis.

▶▶ Patients are at high risk of bile duct carcinoma, which develops in ~20% of patients (◑ Extrahepatic bile duct carcinoma, p. 172) and has a very poor prognosis.

Wilson's disease

Definition
- An inherited disorder of copper metabolism, leading to the accumulation of toxic levels of copper in the liver and brain.

Epidemiology
- Uncommon.
- Most cases present in childhood or young adulthood; however, the diagnosis should be considered as a possible cause of liver disease presenting at any age.
- Males and females are equally affected.

Genetics
- Autosomal recessive disorder due to mutations in the gene *ATP7B* which codes for a copper-transporting ATPase.
- ~100 different mutations have been described and the majority of patients are compound heterozygotes (i.e. they have two differently mutated alleles). This makes genetic screening difficult.

Pathogenesis
- Possession of two mutated *ATP7B* alleles causes disruption of normal copper transport and accumulation of toxic levels of copper in hepatocytes and basal ganglia.

Presentation
- Most patients present in childhood or early adulthood with chronic liver disease or cirrhosis.
- A small proportion of patients present in hepatic failure.
- About half of patients also develop neuropsychiatric symptoms due to copper accumulation in the brain, though this usually occurs after the liver disease presents.

Macroscopy
- By the time of presentation, most patients have advanced disease and the liver is firm due to extensive fibrosis or cirrhotic.

Histopathology
- Liver biopsies show a chronic hepatitis pattern with portal inflammation, scattered lobular inflammation, and variable amounts of fibrosis, depending on the stage of the disease.
- The diagnosis is strongly suggested by the presence of high levels of stainable copper or copper-associated protein in hepatocytes, though this can only be demonstrated in 50% of cases. The diagnosis is best made by measuring tissue copper levels which are higher than those seen in PBC or PSC.

Prognosis
- Progressive disease which terminates in cirrhosis, if untreated.
- Lifelong treatment with metal-chelating agents prevents this progression if the diagnosis is made early enough.
- Risk of HCC is low.

Hereditary haemochromatosis

Definition
- An inherited disorder characterized by increased intestinal absorption of iron, leading to iron overload in multiple organs, particularly the liver, and sometimes leading to organ damage.

Epidemiology
- Genetic prevalence of the mutated gene is 0.4% in white races, making it the most common genetic disease in people of Celtic origin, though the clinical penetrance is much lower.
- Males and females are affected equally, though women usually present later in life due to menstrual and pregnancy iron loss.

Genetics
- Autosomal recessive disorder caused by mutations of the *HFE* gene on chromosome 6p.
- *HFE* encodes an iron regulatory hormone called **hepcidin**.
- Most common mutation is a missense mutation at codon 282, causing a cysteine residue to be switched for a tyrosine (C282Y).

Pathogenesis
- Hepcidin controls plasma iron concentrations by inhibiting iron export by ferroportin from duodenal enterocytes and macrophages.
- Deficiency of hepcidin results in raised plasma iron concentrations and accumulation in multiple organs, including the liver, pancreas, heart, joints, and pituitary.

Presentation
- Early symptoms are non-specific (e.g. fatigue and arthropathy)
- Later, there may be skin pigmentation, cirrhosis, hypogonadism, cardiac failure, and diabetes mellitus.
- If transferrin saturation and serum ferritin are raised, then testing for the C282Y mutation should be performed.

Macroscopy
- Advanced cases cause diffuse nodularity due to cirrhosis.

Histopathology
- The earliest histological change is the accumulation of iron within periportal hepatocytes, highlighted by Perl's stain.
- As the disease progresses, iron accumulates within hepatocytes throughout the liver lobules, associated with expansion of portal tracts by fibrosis. The gradings system is based on how extensively iron is found in hepatocytes.
- Eventually, bridging fibrosis occurs which terminates in cirrhosis.

Prognosis
- Overall mortality is not higher in patients with timely diagnosis and adequate iron depletion therapy.
- ~5% of men and 1% of women develop cirrhosis. This has a worse prognosis, even with treatment, and carries a significant risk of HCC (➔ Hepatocellular carcinoma, p. 168).

Cirrhosis

Definition
- Irreversible replacement of the normal liver architecture by bands of fibrous tissue separating nodules of regenerating hepatocytes.

Epidemiology
- Common and increasing in incidence due to alcohol and obesity.

Aetiology
- Alcohol, chronic viral hepatitis, and NAFLD are the most common causes.
- Less commonly, PBC, PSC, autoimmune hepatitis (AIH), Wilson's disease, and haemochromatosis.
- In some cases, the cause remains unclear (cryptogenic cirrhosis) although many of these are thought to be secondary to NAFLD.

Pathogenesis
- Persistent liver injury causes Kupffer cells lining the vascular sinusoids to release cytokines which activate hepatic stellate cells.
- Activated stellate cells proliferate and secrete large quantities of dense collagen, leading to irreversible liver fibrosis and hepatocyte loss.
- Cirrhosis causes a number of functional defects: reduced synthesis of coagulation factors; low glycogen reserves; reduced clearance of organisms by Kupffer cells; portal hypertension with hypersplenism and oesophageal varices; and splanchnic vasodilation → decreased renal blood flow → secondary hyperaldosteronism → ascites.

Presentation
- Non-specific symptoms of tiredness and malaise.
- Signs of chronic liver disease are usually present on clinical examination and LFTs are usually abnormal.
- Patients often present with a complication related to the presence of cirrhosis (e.g. upper GI haemorrhage).

Macroscopy
- The liver may be normal in size, enlarged, or shrunken.
- The cut surface has a firm texture and shows diffuse nodularity (Fig. 8.1).

Histopathology
- The entire liver is replaced by nodules of regenerating hepatocytes surrounded by fibrous bands.
- The size of the nodules is related to the cause: micronodular cirrhosis in alcoholic liver disease and macronodular cirrhosis secondary to viral hepatitis.
- The fibrous bands contain a variable inflammatory infiltrate and reactive bile ductular proliferation.
- In some cases, the features may point to a particular aetiology.

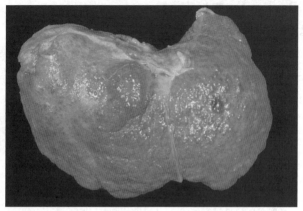

Fig 8.1 The cirrhotic liver. This liver was removed at post-mortem from a patient known to abuse alcohol. The whole of the liver is studded with nodules. Microscopically, the liver showed nodules of regenerating hepatocytes separated by dense bands of fibrosis, confirming established cirrhosis (see Plate 15).

Reproduced with permission from *Clinical Pathology* (Oxford Core Texts), Carton, James, Daly, Richard, and Ramani, Pramila, Oxford University Press (2006), p. 168, Figure 9.9.

Prognosis

- Generally poor, with a high risk of significant complications such as infections (including bacterial peritonitis), upper GI bleeding, renal failure, and HCC.

▶ Development of complications may tip the patient into terminal hepatic failure, characterized by deep jaundice, severe coagulopathy, hepatic encephalopathy, and high risk of mortality.

Benign liver lesions

Haemangioma

- Most common tumour of the liver.
- Macroscopically, well-circumscribed red tumours with a spongy texture due to the numerous vessels within them.
- Microscopically, composed of numerous dilated blood vessels lined by bland endothelial cells.
- Benign lesions which are usually asymptomatic and require no treatment. Larger lesions closer to the surface are associated with a higher risk of bleeding and, therefore, are more likely to come to surgery.

Hepatic adenoma

- Rare tumour seen almost exclusively in young women of reproductive age.
- Associated with oral contraceptive use.
- Macroscopically, solitary lesions, often >10 cm in size, with a softer consistency and a lighter colour than the adjacent liver.
- Microscopically, hepatocytes arranged in plates 1–3 cells thick. Large vessels are often present within the lesion, but portal tracts are absent. On the basis of their histological appearances and underlying genetic changes they are divided into inflammatory, HNF1A (Hepatic Nuclear Factor 1A) -mutated and β-catenin activated.
- Surgical resection is often performed to prevent the potentially fatal complication of rupture and haemoperitoneum.
- There is a low, but definite risk of progression to liver cell cancer especially in tumours with a the B-catenin mutation.

Focal nodular hyperplasia

- Benign, non-neoplastic lesion usually seen in young women of reproductive age.
- Thought to represent a localized area of liver hyperplasia in response to changes in blood flow associated with a pre-existing arterial malformation.
- Macroscopically, a well-defined nodular area with a lighter colour than the adjacent liver. Most lesions have a characteristic central scar.
- Microscopically, nodules of hepatocytes separated by fibrous stroma containing bile ductules. Large, thick-walled vessels are very often present and a helpful diagnostic clue.
- Benign and not associated with a risk of haemorrhage.

Biliary microhamartoma (von Meyenberg's complex)

- Thought to be a ductal plate malformation.
- Macroscopically, it is a small (<5 mm), irregular, grey lesion of the liver which may be multifocal.
- Microscopically, it is composed of small, irregular ductules embedded in a dense fibrous stroma. Inspissated bile may be present within the ductules.
- May be associated with other forms of fibro-polycystic liver disease: congenital hepatic fibrosis, polycystic liver diseases, Carol's

disease (dilatation of intrahepatic bile ducts), and choledochal cyst (dilatation of extrahepatic bile ducts).
• These conditions are associated with an increased risk of cholangiocarcinoma.

Bile duct adenoma

• May not be a true neoplasm, but rather a reactive proliferation of ductular structures (peribiliary hamartoma).
• They often present as small white lesions on the surface of the liver, which are noted at the time of abdominal surgery. A frozen section is often required to exclude a metastasis.
• Macroscopically, small (but usually larger than biliary microhamartomas), firm, white lesions which are often subcapsular.
• Microscopically, small uniform ductules which are more closely packed than a biliary hamartoma. Bile is not present in the ductules.

Hepatocellular carcinoma (liver cell cancer)

Definition
- A malignant epithelial neoplasm of the liver derived from hepatocytes.

Epidemiology
- Common worldwide, but with a wide geographical variation.
- Incidence figures largely parallel rates of infection with HBV, making HCC particularly common in parts of Africa and Asia.

Aetiology
- HCC usually arises on a background of liver cirrhosis.
- Chronic hepatitis B and haemochromatosis are particularly carcinogenic substrates.
- Dietary ingestion of aflatoxins produced by *Aspergillus* fungi which are also known to be potent liver carcinogens.

Carcinogenesis
- Loss of function of tumour suppressor genes, such as *TP53*, is common.
- Activating mutations of oncogenes appear to be rare.
- Hepatitis B X gene product disrupts p53 function and inhibits nucleotide excision repair.

Presentation
- Presents late with non-specific weight loss and abdominal pain.
- Known cirrhotics may be diagnosed following investigation of a rising serum alpha-fetoprotein (AFP) or on ultrasound surveillance.

Macroscopy
- Expansile tumour mass in the liver, often with satellite deposits (Fig. 8.2).
- Tumour may have a green tinge due to the production of bile.
- Distinguishing tumour deposits from dysplastic nodules in cirrhotic livers can be difficult.

Histopathology
- Classical HCC is composed of epithelial cells resembling hepatocytes, which typically grow in trabeculae that resemble thickened liver cell plates. Bile production may be seen by the tumour. A very typical feature is the loss of reticulin fibres.
- HepPar 1 and CD10 staining (to demonstrate canaliculi) can be useful to confirm a tumour as being an HCC.
- Glypican 3 staining is useful especially in poorly differentiated tumours.
- It is increasingly apparent that many tumours have features of both HCCs and cholangiocarcinomas.
- A number of histological variants of HCC are now recognized: clear cell, steatohepatitic, scirrhous, macrotrabecular, chromophobe, and fibro-lamellar.
- Fibrolamellar HCC is a rare, but distinctive, variant which typically arises in young patients without background cirrhosis. Histologically,

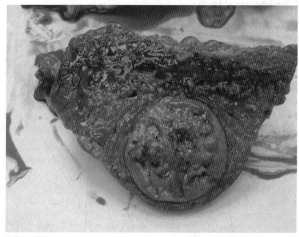

Fig. 8.2 Liver cell cancer arising in a cirrhotic liver (see Plate 16).

the tumour is composed of nests of very large neoplastic cells with abundant granular pink cytoplasm separated by dense fibrous bands.

Prognosis

- Generally very poor, with 5-year survival rates <5%. HCCs of stem cell origin are CK19-positive and carry a worse prognosis.
- Fibrolamellar HCC has a slightly better prognosis, with 5-year survival rates ~60%.

Cholecystitis

Definition
- Inflammation of the gall bladder.

Epidemiology
- Very common.

Aetiology
- Most cases are caused by gallstones (calculous cholecystitis).
- Acalculous cholecystitis also occurs, particularly in the elderly.

Pathogenesis
- Thought to be due to chemical injury to the mucosa caused by bile.
- Biliary stasis may be caused by obstruction of the gall bladder outlet by a gallstone or poor gall bladder motility.

Presentation
- Biliary colic, characterized by severe upper abdominal pain which resolves spontaneously after several hours.
- Acute cholecystitis is a more severe illness with prolonged upper abdominal pain, fever, and tachycardia.

Macroscopy
- The gall bladder wall is thickened and the mucosa may be friable.
- Gallstones are usually present.

Histopathology
- Acute cholecystitis shows oedema, acute inflammatory cells, and granulation tissue.
- Chronic cholecystitis shows muscular hypertrophy and fibrosis, mild chronic inflammation, and the presence of mucosal diverticula herniating through the muscular layer (Rokitansky–Aschoff sinuses).
- Xanthogranulomatous cholecystitis is a variant of chronic cholecystitis, in which sheets of macrophages and fibroblasts are present, probably in reaction to a ruptured Rokitansky–Aschoff sinus.
- Hyaline cholecystitis ('porcelain gall bladder') carries a significantly higher risk for developing gall bladder cancer.

Prognosis
- Most patients with calculous cholecystitis are cured by cholecystectomy.

Cholangiocarcinoma

Definition

- A malignant epithelial neoplasm arising in the biliary tree. They can be divided into intrahepatic and extrahepatic cholangiocarcinomas. The pre-invasive stage is termed biliary-intraepitheial neoplasia and, as elsewhere in the gastro-intestinal tract, is divided into high grade and low-grade dysplasia

Epidemiology

- Rare in most populations. In areas where environmental risk factors (e.g. worms) are especially common (e.g. Thailand) it is much commoner.

Aetiology

- Liver flukes (*Clonorchis sinensis* and *Opisthorchis viverrini*).
- Hepatolithiasis.
- PSC (➡ Primary sclerosing cholangitis, p. 160).
- Exposure to Thorotrast (a contrast medium used from 1930 to 1955).
- Biliary malformations (e.g. choledochal cyst).
- Cirrhosis.

Carcinogenesis

- Mutations of *RAS* and *TP53* are the most common genetic abnormalities.

Intrahepatic cholangiocarcinoma

Presentation

- Most present late, as they can grow to a large size within the liver before causing symptoms of malaise, weight loss, and abdominal pain.
- Tumours infiltrating the hilar region of the liver may present with obstructive jaundice.

Macroscopy

- The liver contains large confluent nodules of a grey-white tumour, often with satellite deposits.
- The background liver is usually non-cirrhotic.

Histopathology

- Adenocarcinomas in which the infiltrating malignant epithelial cells form glandular and papillary structures.
- A typical feature is the presence of abundant fibroblastic stroma.
- There is a strong propensity for perineural invasion.
- It is increasingly apparent that many tumours have features of both HCCs and cholangiocarcinomas.

Prognosis

- Generally poor, with 5-year survival rates of 40–50%, depending on the stage.

Extrahepatic bile duct carcinoma

Presentation
- Obstructive jaundice.
- Superimposed cholangitis may cause fevers and rigors.

Macroscopy
- The involved bile duct contains a tumour which may be polypoid, stenosing, or diffusely infiltrative.

Histopathology
- Most are well- or moderately differentiated adenocarcinomas, in which the infiltrating malignant epithelial cells form glandular structures resembling biliary ducts.

Prognosis
- The 5-year survival in patients with resectable tumours and clear surgical margins is in the order of 20–40%.
- Tumours arising on a background of PSC have a particularly poor outlook, with 5-year survival rates of <10%.

Pancreatic pathology

Pancreatic malformations

Ectopic pancreas

- Common developmental anomaly in which pancreatic tissue is located outside the usual position of the pancreas.
- The duodenum is the most common site, but it can be seen in the jejunum and ileum and within a Meckel's diverticulum (● Meckel's diverticulum, p. 108).
- Most cases are incidental findings, but some patients present with symptoms relating to bleeding or obstruction.

Pancreas divisum

- Common developmental anomaly in which the dorsal and ventral pancreatic buds fail to fuse.
- The duct of Santorini becomes the dominant ductal system of the pancreas. As this duct drains into the duodenum via the smaller minor papilla, there is a tendency to stasis of pancreatic secretions and susceptibility to pancreatitis.
- Usually asymptomatic and discovered incidentally on imaging, though some patients may present with pancreatitis in adulthood.

Annular pancreas

- Rare developmental anomaly in which the dorsal and ventral pancreatic buds fuse around the duodenum.
- The ring of the pancreas can cause obstruction to the duodenum.
- Most patients present around 1y of age with vomiting and abdominal distension after meals.

Acute pancreatitis

Definition
- Acute inflammation of the pancreas and peripancreatic tissues.

Epidemiology
- Uncommon.

Aetiology
- Gallstones (the commonest cause) and alcohol account for the majority of cases.
- Other causes include abdominal trauma, endoscopic retrograde cholangiopancreatography (ERCP), drugs (e.g. thiazides), hypercalcaemia, hyperlipidaemia, pancreas divisum, and viral infection (including mumps).
- Many cases are idiopathic.

Pathogenesis
- Injury to the pancreas leads to release and activation of digestive enzymes, causing necrosis of pancreatic and peripancreatic tissue.
- Exudation of plasma into the retroperitoneal space leads to hypovolaemia and cardiovascular instability.
- Paralytic ileus may also occur as a reaction to extensive inflammation occurring in the vicinity of the bowel.

Presentation
- Sudden onset of severe upper abdominal pain radiating to the back, associated with nausea, vomiting, and fever.
- Hypotension is often present which, in severe cases, causes shock.

Biochemistry
- A significantly raised serum amylase is virtually diagnostic of acute pancreatitis in the correct clinical setting.
- Hypocalcaemia is common (except in cases due to hypercalcaemia).

Macroscopy
- The pancreas is swollen and soft.
- White flecks of fat necrosis are present in peripancreatic tissues.
- In severe cases, there is haemorrhage into the necrotic pancreas.

Histopathology
- Milder cases show acute inflammation, oedema, and focal necrosis within the pancreas.
- Surrounding peripancreatic tissue shows fat necrosis.
- Severe cases show widespread necrosis and haemorrhage into the gland.

Prognosis
- Many cases are mild and resolve with supportive treatment.
- Severe cases can be life-threatening and require organ support.

- Superadded infection of the necrotic pancreatic tissue is an ominous complication, often leading to disseminated intravascular coagulation (DIC) and multiple organ failure.
- Pancreatic pseudocyst (a collection of fluid within the region of the pancreas not lined by epithelium) is a common late complication.

Chronic pancreatitis

Definition
- A chronic inflammatory process of the pancreas, leading to irreversible loss of pancreatic function.

▶ Chronic pancreatitis can closely mimic pancreatic carcinoma clinically, radiologically, and pathologically.

Epidemiology
- Uncommon.

Aetiology
- Almost all cases are associated with alcohol abuse.
- A small proportion is thought to be autoimmune in origin (which includes IgG4-related disease).

Pathogenesis
- Chronic inflammation in the pancreas leads to the replacement of functional pancreatic tissue by fibrous scar tissue.

Presentation
- Persistent upper abdominal pain and weight loss.
- Steatorrhoea and diabetes mellitus occur late once most of the gland is destroyed.

Macroscopy
- The pancreas is replaced by firm fibrous tissue, within which are dilated ducts and areas of calcification.

▶ The scarred mass is so firm, it can closely mimic carcinoma macroscopically.

Histopathology
- The pancreas shows a chronic inflammatory cell infiltrate with scarring and loss of exocrine tissue. The endocrine tissue is typically spared until late in the disease. Large ducts are dilated and contain inspissated secretions. Calcification is also common. ▶ Small residual atrophic ducts set in a fibrous background can closely mimic an infiltrating pancreatic carcinoma.
- A recently recognized variant of chronic pancreatitis has been described, **IgG4-related disease**, in which there is a prominent periductal and perivenular chronic inflammatory cell infiltrate rich in IgG4 positive plasma cells. Patients often have raised serum IgG4 levels. It may involve any part of the hepato-biliary system but the pancreas is the commonest site.

Prognosis
- Alcoholic chronic pancreatitis tends to be associated with a fairly poor outcome. Treatment is supportive only and most patients will have other alcohol-related pathology.
- The outlook is better for patients with autoimmune pancreatitis, as this responds to steroid therapy.

Pancreatic ductal carcinoma

Definition
- A malignant epithelial tumour arising in the pancreas, composed of infiltrating duct-like structures.

Epidemiology
- Most common type of pancreatic neoplasm.
- Usually seen in people >60 y and slightly more commonly in men.
- Incidence in developed countries ranges from 1 to 10 per 100 000.

Aetiology
- Smoking is the main recognized risk factor.

Carcinogenesis
- Activating mutations of *KRAS*.
- Loss of function of *TP53*, *P16*, and *DPC4*.
- Pancreatic ductal carcinomas may arise from **pancreatic intraepithelial neoplasia** (PanIN). PanIN is now graded as low or high grade, with reference to increasing cytological and architectural atypia.
- Tumours may also arise from intrapancreatic mucinous neoplasms.

Presentation
- Persistent upper abdominal pain and profound weight loss.
- Many present as metastatic adenocarcinomas to the liver.
- Tumours in the head may cause obstructive jaundice and, therefore, may present earlier.
- Sudden onset of diabetes mellitus is also a suspicious finding.

Macroscopy
- A poorly defined, firm tumour mass is present within the pancreas.
- Most arise within the head, but they can occur anywhere in the pancreas.

Histopathology
- Most pancreatic carcinomas are ductal carcinomas (90%) are well to moderately differentiated adenocarcinomas. Other variants, such as acinar carcinomas, are much rarer.
- A typical feature is the presence of abundant fibroblastic stroma around the infiltrating glands.
- Perineural invasion is also common and probably accounts for the high rates of peripancreatic tumour extension.

Prognosis
- Extremely poor, with 5-year survival rates of <5%.

Pancreatic cystic tumours

Intraductal papillary mucinous neoplasm
- A grossly visible, benign, mucin-producing tumour that grows within the pancreatic ductal system.
- Most arise within the head of the pancreas in men.
- Macroscopically, there are mucin-filled cysts within the pancreas that communicate with the duct system.
- Histologically, the cysts are lined by mucin-secreting columnar epithelial cells which form papillary projections into the cyst. The epithelial cells may show a range of atypia from low to high grade. Invasive carcinoma can arise within this lesion.

Mucinous cystic neoplasms
- A range of lesions, most of which are benign.
- Almost all occur in women and present with symptoms of an abdominal mass.
- Macroscopically, they are well-circumscribed cystic tumours with large locules containing mucoid material. The cysts do not communicate with the pancreatic ductal system.
- Histologically, the cysts are lined by mucus-secreting columnar epithelial cells, beneath which there is a densely cellular, ovarian-like stroma as do their counterparts when they occur in other sites. The epithelial component may show a range of atypia from low to high grade. Invasive carcinomas can arise within these lesions.
- They need to be distinguished from intraductal papillary neoplasms (IPMNs) which involve the pancreatic ducts and lack the ovarian-type stroma. IPMNs may progress to invasive adenocarcinoma.

Serous cystic neoplasms
- A range of lesions, the majority of which are benign.
- Almost all occur in women and present with symptoms of an abdominal mass.
- The most common type is the **serous microcystic adenoma**, which gives rise to a well-circumscribed pancreatic mass containing numerous small cysts with a central scar. Histologically, the small cysts are lined by cuboidal cells with a round nucleus and clear cytoplasm due to the accumulation of glycogen.

Solid pseudopapillary neoplasm
- A neoplasm of the pancreas which often shows cystic change.
- Occurs in young women with symptoms of an abdominal mass.
- The tumours may occur anywhere in the pancreas as a solid mass with cystic areas and haemorrhage.
- Histologically, the tumour is composed of uniform round cells which form sheets and cords. The cells tend to be poorly cohesive and fall apart, creating pseudopapillary and cystic areas.
- The tumours generally have very low-grade biological behaviour, with most patients remaining tumour-free many years after resection.

Acinar cell carcinoma

Definition
- A malignant epithelial neoplasm of the pancreas, demonstrating evidence of enzyme production by the neoplastic cells.

Epidemiology
- Rare tumour, accounting for ~1% of all pancreatic tumours.
- Most occur in older adults.

Aetiology
- Unknown.

Carcinogenesis
- Abnormalities have been described in the APC/β-catenin pathway.
- Genetic mutations typically found in ductal adenocarcinomas are absent.

Presentation
- Non-specific symptoms of abdominal pain, weight loss, nausea, and diarrhoea.
- ~10% of patients have a syndrome of multifocal fat necrosis and polyarthralgia due to lipase secretion.

Macroscopy
- Large, well-demarcated, soft-tan tumour arising within the pancreas.
- Extension outside the pancreas may be present.

Histopathology
- Cellular tumours composed of neoplastic epithelial cells growing in sheets, trabeculae, and acini.
- Some cells have abundant eosinophilic, finely granular cytoplasm.
- The cells show positive immunoreactivity for lipase, trypsin, and chymotrypsin.

Prognosis
- Aggressive malignant tumours.
- Median survival 18 months from diagnosis, with 5-year survival rates of <10%.

Pancreatic neuroendocrine tumours

Definition
- A group of epithelial tumours of the pancreas showing endocrine differentiation. Tumours may be functioning or non-functioning, depending on whether a syndrome of inappropriate hormone secretion is present.

Epidemiology
- Rare tumours, accounting for ~2% of all pancreatic tumours.
- Peak incidence between 30 and 60 y.

Aetiology
- Unknown in sporadic cases.
- ~15% associated with multiple endocrine neoplasia (MEN)-1.

Genetics
- Accumulation of further alterations is associated with malignant behaviour.

Presentation
- Functioning tumours present with features related to excess hormone production, for example, hypoglycaemia (insulin-producing tumours—the commonest hormone to be secreted), recurrent duodenal ulceration (gastrin-producing tumours), a skin condition known as necrolytic migratory erythema (glucagon-producing tumours).
- Non-functioning tumours are either picked up incidentally on imaging or present when they grow large enough to produce symptoms of local disease or metastasis.

Macroscopy
- Most are well-demarcated tumours within the pancreas. They are relatively more common in the tail of the pancreas.

Cytopathology
- Fine-needle aspiration (FNA) smears are cellular and composed of a monotonous population of cells present singly, in loose clusters, or as pseudorosettes.
- The nuclei usually have a distinct granular chromatin pattern ('salt-and-pepper').

Histopathology
- Most tumours are composed of cells with granular cytoplasm, forming solid nests, trabeculae, glands, or rosettes.
- Immunostaining confirms the endocrine nature of the cells with reactivity for the markers CD56, chromogranin, and synaptophysin.
- Tumours are classified according to their Ki-67 labelling index which is a marker of their proliferative activity: grade 1 = 2% or less, grade 2 = >2% but <10%, grade 3 = 10% or more.
- Functional tumours can also be stained for the hormones they secrete.

Prognosis

- Often difficult to predict with certainty.
- All tumours should be considered potentially malignant, and long-term follow-up is essential as metastases may develop many years after removal of the primary lesion. The Ki-67 labelling index is not entirely reliable.

Renal pathology

Acute kidney injury (AKI)

Definition

- A sudden decrease in glomerular filtration rate (GFR) manifested by an increase in serum creatinine or oliguria over a period of 48 hours to 7 days.
- The severity (stage) of AKI determined by the severity of increase in serum creatinine or oliguria.
- AKI is one manifestation of the more generic 'acute kidney disease' (AKD), which also includes disorders presenting with haematuria, pyuria, and urinary tract obstruction, in which the rate of decline in GFR is not as rapid as in AKI.

Epidemiology

- Common.
- Often occurs as a complication of a pre-existing illness causing circulatory disturbance.

Aetiology

- **Pre-renal**: hypoperfusion (e.g. hypovolaemia, sepsis).
- **Renal** ('intrinsic'): this can be due to diseases in any of the renal compartments: glomerular compartment (e.g. glomerulonephritis, thrombotic microangiopathy; tubulointerstitial compartment: e.g. acute tubular injury, acute interstitial nephritis; vascular compartment: e.g. cholesterol emboli).
- **Post-renal**: urinary tract obstruction (e.g. stones, cancer, etc.).
- The cause of AKI should be determined promptly, with special attention to reversible causes. Several causes may coexist. By far, the most common causes are hypoperfusion (e.g. sepsis, hypovolaemia) and acute tubular injury (e.g. injury to the tubular epithelial cells caused by drugs and toxins such as contrast, aminoglycosides, etc.).
- A renal biopsy may be required to ascertain the cause of AKI (e.g. if the diagnosis is unclear; if there is associated proteinuria and/or haematuria or features of a systemic disease such as systemic lupus erythematosus (i.e. suspicion of glomerular disease); if there is persistent injury despite reversal of cause; or if the serum creatinine does not return to baseline with 7–14 d of injury onset).

Presentation

- Most cases are heralded by the onset of oliguria (passing of small volumes of urine), though some cases may produce few symptoms or signs.
- Very severe cases cause marked pulmonary oedema, encephalopathy, and pericarditis.

Biochemistry

- Elevated serum urea and creatinine.
- Hyperkalaemia and metabolic acidosis are also commonly present.

❶ Severe hyperkalaemia is pro-arrhythmic and can lead to a cardiac arrest, so it must be treated promptly.

Prognosis

- Pre-renal and post-renal AKI may be reversible if treated promptly (e.g. by restoring circulating volume or relieving obstruction).
- Treatment is supportive whilst the cause is treated, and dialysis may be needed whilst renal function recovers.
- Prognosis of the intrinsic causes of AKI depends on the underlying disease.

Chronic kidney disease (CKD)

Definition

- Abnormalities of kidney structure or function, present for >3 months, with implications for health. Most cases of CKD are irreversible, but some cases may be partially or even entirely reversible.
- Abnormalities of kidney function/structure include decreased GFR (<60 ml/min per 1.73 m^2), increased albuminuria, urinary sediment abnormalities, electrolyte, and other abnormalities due to tubular disorders, abnormalities detected by histology, and structural abnormalities detected by imaging.
- CKD is classified based on the cause, GFR category, and albuminuria category.

Epidemiology

- Common, with a significant impact on health worldwide.

Aetiology

- Diabetic nephropathy and hypertensive nephropathy are the most common causes, particularly in developed countries.
- As for AKI, diseases affecting any of the three renal compartments (glomeruli, tubulointerstitium, arteries) can cause CKD.
  Examples: adult polycystic kidney disease (APKD), dysplastic kidneys, reflux nephropathy, obstructive nephropathy, infections, drugs, systemic diseases that affect the kidney (e.g. systemic lupus erythematosus (SLE), amyloidosis, monoclonal gammopathy, gout), and intrinsic renal diseases (e.g. glomerulonephritis or focal segmental glomerulosclerosis (FSGS)).
- A kidney biopsy may be required to establish the cause of CKD and inform the treatment plan, for example in cases that present with a rapid elevation in serum creatinine on a background of early stage CKD, or new-onset haematuria or proteinuria.

Pathogenesis

- Injury may primarily affect glomeruli, vessels, or the tubulo-interstitium, eventually leading to loss of nephrons.
- Loss of nephrons is visible in a biopsy as globally sclerosed glomeruli and atrophy or loss of the associated tubule, with expansion of the interstitium by fibrous tissue.
- Nephron loss is associated with an attendant reduction in GFR.
- Nephron loss leads to haemodynamic stress in remaining nephrons, leading to further nephron loss.

Presentation

- Early disease is asymptomatic and can only be picked up if GFR is measured, in particular in at-risk patients (e.g. diabetics, hypertension).
- With progression, patients feel tired and develop bony pain.
- Some patients present with high-risk CKD requiring immediate renal replacement therapy ('end-stage renal failure'), with fluid overload and metabolic derangement.

Biochemistry

- ↑ urea and creatinine due to impaired excretion of waste products.
- ↓ calcium due to lack of active calcitriol.
- ↑ phosphate due to impaired excretion of phosphate.
- Secondary hyperparathyroidism due to hypocalcaemia.
- ↓ haemoglobin (Hb) due to reduced erythropoietin secretion.

▶ Note that loss of acid-base and sodium/potassium balance occurs late in CKD.

Prognosis

- CKD is classified based on the cause, GFR category, and albuminuria category. Albuminuria and GFR are used to group cases into four risk categories, according to their associations with risks for various outcomes (all-cause and cardiovascular mortality, kidney failure requiring replacement therapy, AKI, and CKD progression).

Complications

- High incidence of cardiovascular disease due to a combination of hypertension, vascular calcification, and hyperlipidaemia.
- Derangement of calcium and phosphate metabolism leads to renal bone disease, which is a complex mixture of hyperparathyroid bone disease, osteomalacia, and osteoporosis (Fig. 10.1).

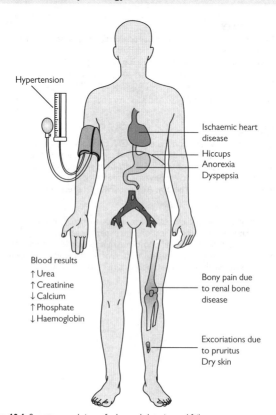

Fig. 10.1 Symptoms and signs of advanced chronic renal failure.

Reproduced with permission from *Clinical Pathology* (Oxford Core Texts), Carton, James, Daly, Richard, and Ramani, Pramila, Oxford University Press (2006), p. 208, Figure 10.4.

Nephrotic syndrome

Definition
- Combination of nephrotic-range proteinuria (>3.5 g/1.73 m² body surface area/24 h), hypoalbuminaemia (<30 g/L), hyperlipidaemia, and oedema.

Aetiology
- Primary renal diseases, most commonly: minimal change disease (MCD), FSGS, and membranous glomerulonephritis (GN).
- Systemic diseases (e.g. diabetes and amyloidosis; ➔ Primary amyloidosis, p. 468).
- A biopsy is usually required to determine the cause; in children with nephrotic syndrome, where MCD is the likely cause and the clinical course is typical, empiric treatment is often given without the need for a biopsy.

Pathogenesis
- Dysfunction of the glomerular filtration barrier, which normally prevents loss of protein in the urine.
- Podocyte injury plays a major role in loss of the glomerular filtration barrier function.

Presentation
- Abrupt onset of heavy proteinuria and oedema with hypoalbuminaemia.
- Hyperlipidaemia.
- Increased risk of thrombosis related to loss of proteins regulating coagulation.

Biochemistry
- Creatinine can be normal or elevated.
- Heavy proteinuria (>3.5 g/1.73 m² body surface area/24 h).
- Hypoalbuminaemia (<30 g/L).
- Hyperlipidaemia.

Prognosis
- Depends on the cause.
- Procoagulant state due to loss of anticoagulant proteins in the urine may lead to vein thrombosis and life-threatening pulmonary embolism.

Haematuria and non-nephrotic-range proteinuria

Definition

- Kidney disease can present with variable combinations of proteinuria (above the upper limit of normal, usually defined by a urinary protein to creatinine ratio of >50 mg/mmol), and/or macro- or micro-haematuria, with or without acute or chronic renal dysfunction.

Aetiology

- Primary renal diseases, most commonly glomerulonephritides, tubulointerstitial diseases, either acquired or inherited.
- Systemic diseases can also present with isolated urinary abnormalities (e.g. early stages of diabetic nephropathy present with non-nephrotic proteinuria; some forms of amyloidosis present with only low-level proteinuria and renal dysfunction).
- A biopsy may or may not be needed to determine the cause, depending on clinical and biochemical findings.
- A biopsy is usually indicated in patients with haematuria with presence of acanthocytes or red blood cell casts with an elevated serum creatinine level or proteinuria; in patients with proteinuria >1 g/d on multiple visits with no clear comorbidity (e.g. diabetes or hypertension), especially if accompanied by an increase in serum creatinine; and in patients with proteinuria>3 g/d in the absence of diabetes or a rapid increase in proteinuria even in patients with diabetes.
- A biopsy is usually not necessary in the case of diabetic patients showing a typical clinical course of progressive proteinuria and CKD, or in patients with isolated haematuria with neither dysfunction nor proteinuria, who usually have a benign clinical course (other non-kidney diseases of the genitourinary tract will need to be excluded).

Pathogenesis

- Glomerular disease: dysfunction of the glomerular filtration barrier with leakage of protein and/or red blood cells into the urine. Dysmorphic red blood cells and heavy proteinuria are suggestive of glomerular disease.
- Tubular epithelial cell injury can lead to low-level proteinuria and low-level haematuria.

Presentation

- Can be asymptomatic and picked up at a routine medical examination (e.g. urinary dipstick test).
- Can be picked up through the appearance of macroscopic haematuria or frothy urine.

Biochemistry
- Creatinine can be normal or elevated.
- Proteinuria may be present.
- Macro- or microhaematuria may be present.

Prognosis
- Depends on the cause; see individual causes.

Acute tubular injury

Definition
- Acute injury to renal tubules leading to AKI.
- The equivalent terminology 'acute tubular necrosis' is less accurate, as only the most severe of cases of acute tubular injury have necrosis as a histological feature.

Epidemiology
- One of the most common causes of AKI.

Aetiology
- Ischaemia due to prolonged hypoperfusion (e.g. hypotension, sepsis).
- Nephrotoxins such as specific nephrotoxic drugs (e.g. calcineurin inhibitors), radiological contrast, haemoglobin, myoglobin, oxalate crystals (e.g. hereditary hyperoxaluria or ethylene glycol poisoning), etc.

Pathogenesis
- Tubular epithelial cells are metabolically active and very sensitive to damage from ischaemia or toxins.

Presentation
- AKI.

Histopathology
- The injured tubules are dilated, with flattening of tubular epithelial cells and loss of the brush border (Fig. 10.2).

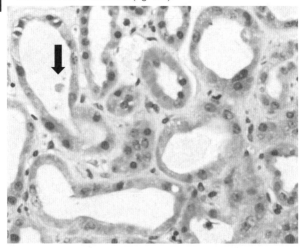

Fig. 10.2 Acute tubular injury. Haematoxylin and eosin stain. The epithelial cells are flattened and the tubular lumen is widened. Arrow indicates a sloughed tubular epithelial cell in the lumen of a tubule (see Plate 17).

- Sloughed epithelial cells may be seen in the lumen of distal tubules, sometimes combining to form 'granular casts'.
- The interstitial compartment is expanded by oedema, with few or no inflammatory cells.
- Clues to the underlying cause may be present (e.g. birefringent intraluminal oxalate crystals in ethylene glycol poisoning or typical myoglobin casts in rhabdomyolysis).

Prognosis

- Depends on underlying cause and reversibility of the cause.
- When seen in the context of ischaemic injury, often associated with a severe circulatory disturbance and a significant mortality rate.

Acute tubulointerstitial nephritis

Definition
- Immune injury to the tubules and interstitium leading to AKI.

Aetiology
- The main causes are drugs, autoimmune diseases (e.g. SLE, Sjogren's), and infections.
- Drug-related tubulointerstitial nephritis (TIN) causes tubular injury through immune hypersensitivity to the drug, rather than through direct nephrotoxic effect of the drug.
- Any drugs can cause acute TIN, but the most common culprits are:
  - NSAIDs;
  - antibiotics;
  - diuretics;
  - allopurinol;
  - proton pump inhibitors.

Pathogenesis
- A hypersensitivity-type immune reaction to a drug or to an infection, or an autoimmune reaction to local antigens causes a predominantly monocytic tubulointerstitial inflammatory infiltrate. Inflammatory cells cause injury to the tubules and interfere with their normal function.

Presentation
- The typical presentation is AKI.
- In drug-related TIN, presentation often occurs within days of starting the drug, though occasionally it only occurs after several months of exposure. Patients often have fever, rash, eosinophilia, eosinophiluria, and raised serum IgE levels.
- Patients with NSAID-induced disease may also show heavy proteinuria related to the concomitant development of MCD.

Histopathology
- The interstitium is expanded by oedema and a predominantly monocytic inflammatory cell infiltrate.
- Lymphocytes are seen infiltrating into the tubules ('tubulitis') (Fig. 10.3).
- In drug-related TIN, there are often eosinophils.
- Granulomatous TIN is a subtype of TIN in which histiocytic granulomas are present in the interstitium, sometimes with giant cells, with or without central necrosis. The most common causes are drug-related TIN, sarcoidosis, and mycobacterial infections.

Prognosis
- Successful treatment of the underlying autoimmune disease or infection, or cessation of the offending drug, may result in complete recovery. A short course of steroids is given to clear the local inflammatory infiltrate and therefore halt further injury to the tubules.

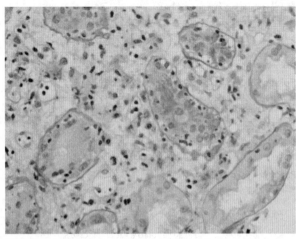

Fig. 10.3 Active tubulointerstitial nephritis. Periodic acid–Schiff stain. Lymphocytes and cells of monocytic lineage appear as small dark nuclei amongst the tubular epithelial cells, which have larger nuclei with more dispersed chromatin. Tubulitis is defined by inflammatory cells within the spaces delimited by the tubular basement membranes, seen on this PAS stain as bright pink lines around individual tubular profiles (see Plate 18).

Reflux nephropathy

Definition
- Renal scarring associated with vesicoureteric reflux (VUR), a congenital disorder in which urine regurgitates from the bladder into the upper urinary tract.

Epidemiology
- An important cause of CKD, responsible for up to 30% of cases in children and 10% of cases in adults.

Aetiology
- VUR.
- ▶ Note not all VUR cases are complicated by reflux nephropathy.

Pathogenesis
- Thought to be the result of reflux of infected urine into the kidney.
- Intra-renal reflux tends to occur at the poles of the kidneys where compound papillae are found.
- Compound papillae are more susceptible to reflux, as the papillary ducts open at less oblique angles onto a flat or concave surface.
- Repeated inflammatory response to the infection causes tubulointerstitial injury and nephron loss, with replacement of nephrons by scarring.
- As more and more nephrons are lost, CKD progresses.

Presentation
- Patients typically present with hypertension and/or proteinuria and/or CKD.

Macroscopy
- The poles of the kidneys show macroscopic areas of renal cortical scarring.

Histopathology
- The scarred areas show features of chronic tubulointerstitial nephritis, with or without features of chronic pyelonephritis.
- In chronic tubulointerstitial nephritis, there is tubular atrophy and interstitial fibrosis, associated with a predominantly mononuclear inflammatory cell infiltrate. Some tubules show regular atrophy with thickened basement membranes and a reduced diameter, whereas others may be dilated and filled with proteinaceous material ('thyroidization'). There is extensive global sclerosis of glomeruli; non-sclerosed glomeruli may show hypertrophy and secondary focal and segmental glomerulosclerosis.
- The microscopic features of chronic tubulointerstitial nephritis are not specific to reflux nephropathy and may be seen in other causes of CKD.
- In chronic pyelonephritis, neutrophils may be present in tubules and/or in the interstitium in the case of ongoing infection. The collecting system shows marked chronic inflammation often with lymphoid aggregates and follicles.

Complications
- Recurrent urinary tract infection (UTI).
- Renal stones.
- CKD.

Obstructive nephropathy

Definition
- Renal damage caused by obstruction in the urinary tract.

Epidemiology
- Predominantly seen in children (due to congenital anomalies of the urinary tract) and elderly men (due to prostatic hyperplasia).

Aetiology
- Obstruction may occur anywhere in the urinary tract (➔ Urinary tract obstruction, p. 254).
- Common causes include urinary calculi, pelviureteric junction obstruction, prostatic hyperplasia, urothelial tumours, and compression of the ureters by abdominal/pelvic masses.

Pathogenesis
- Renal damage is thought to be predominantly a pressure-related phenomenon, though superimposed infection may also be contributory.

Presentation
- Depends on the extent of disease and laterality.
- Patients may be asymptomatic or present with hypertension and renal failure.

Macroscopy
- In CKD due to obstructive uropathy, the kidney shows diffuse cortical thinning and pelvicalyceal dilation with blunting of papillae.

Histopathology
- The scarred areas show features of chronic tubulointerstitial nephritis, with or without features of chronic pyelonephritis. For a description of these features, see Reflux Nephropathy.

▶ Note that the microscopic features of reflux nephropathy and obstructive nephropathy are similar. Distinction is usually possible, based on the clinical picture and macroscopic features.

Prognosis
- Patients with significant bilateral disease are at risk of developing progressive renal impairment.

Hypertensive nephropathy

Definition
- CKD in patients with hypertension.

Epidemiology
- A common cause of CKD.

Aetiology
- Hypertension.

Pathogenesis
- Two pathophysiological theories have been suggested, which may not be mutually exclusive.
- The first suggests that narrowing of arteries and arterioles causes glomerular ischaemia and global glomerular scarring.
- The second suggests that glomerular hypertension leads to glomerular haemodynamic stress, leading to focal and segmental glomerulosclerosis.

Presentation
- Renal dysfunction and proteinuria in a long-standing hypertensive patient, in the absence of other causes of renal disease.
- Other signs of hypertension may be present (e.g. left ventricular hypertrophy).

Macroscopy
- Both kidneys are shrunken with finely granular cortical surfaces.

Histopathology
- Hyaline deposits are seen in the walls of afferent arterioles.
- Interlobular and larger arteries show medial hypertrophy and fibrous intimal thickening (Fig. 10.4).
- Glomeruli may show wrinkling and shrinkage (due to ischaemia), followed by scarring of the whole tuft (global sclerosis; see first pathogenetic mechanism) and/or enlargement of glomerular tufts with focal and segmental glomerular sclerosis (see second pathogenetic mechanism).
- This constellation of pathological features is often referred to as hypertensive nephrosclerosis, a term meaning scarring of the kidney due to hypertension.

▶ Note that hypertension develops as a consequence of renal failure of any cause. Therefore before attributing CKD to hypertensive nephrosclerosis in patients with hypertension, other causes of renal disease should be considered, excluded and treated.

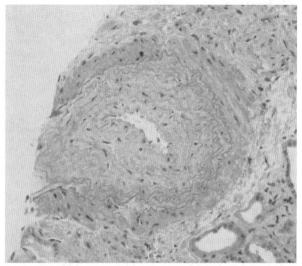

Fig. 10.4 Fibrous arterial intimal thickening. Hematoxylin and eosin stain. A thick layer of fibrous tissue is present under the endothelium and above the duplicated layers of elastic lamina, which appear as thin wavy dark pink lines. In a normal artery, the endothelium is much more closely apposed to the elastic lamina, with only a thin intervening layer of matrix (see Plate 19).

Prognosis
- Patients with persistent poorly controlled hypertension progress to renal failure, which may result in the need for renal replacement therapy.
- The decline in renal function can be slowed by aggressive control of blood pressure.

Diabetic nephropathy

Definition
- CKD caused by diabetes mellitus.

Epidemiology
- Common cause of CKD.

Aetiology
- Type 1 or type 2 diabetes mellitus.
- Only 30–40% of diabetics develop nephropathy. This is largely dependant on glycaemic control; however other factors are involved, as the severity of renal involvement is variable from patient to patient.

Pathogenesis
- Complex and multifactorial.
- High glucose levels are thought to be directly injurious, at least partly through abnormal glycosylation of extracellular proteins, oxidative stress, and enhanced production of TGF-β, which promotes fibrosis.

Presentation
- Onset of proteinuria in a patient with diabetes mellitus.
- Typically, this starts as microalbuminuria but progresses to overt proteinuria, which may be heavy enough to cause the nephrotic syndrome.
- Hypertension is often present.

Histopathology
- Glomerular changes develop progressively and are classified by severity, from early to late lesions:
  - Class I: thickening of the glomerular basement membranes on electron microscopy only (light microscopy normal or near normal);
  - Class II: increase in mesangial matrix, without nodules (IIa, mild; IIb, severe);
  - Class III: nodular glomerulosclerosis/Kimmelstiel–Wilson lesion (Fig. 10.5);
  - Class IV: advanced diabetic glomerulosclerosis (many globally sclerosed glomeruli).
- Hyalinization of arterioles, typically affecting both afferent and efferent arterioles.
- Tubulointerstitial fibrosis proportional to the degree of glomerular damage.

▶ Note that a renal biopsy is not necessary to confirm a diagnosis of diabetic nephropathy, provided the clinical picture is typical. Biopsy is usually reserved for atypical cases where an alternative or additional diagnosis is suspected (e.g. new-onset of nephrotic-range proteinuria without antecedent proteinuria).

Immunofluorescence
- Linear enhancement of glomerular and tubular basement membranes with IgG may be seen.

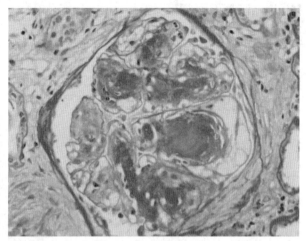

Fig. 10.5 Nodular diabetic glomerulosclerosis (periodic acid–Schiff stain). The mesangial matrix is expanded by nodules of matrix referred to as Kimmelstiel–Wilson nodules (see Plate 20).

Electron microscopy

- Diffuse glomerular basement membrane thickening and increase of mesangial matrix.
- No electron-dense deposits are present.

Prognosis

- Patients with poor glycaemic control, hypertension, and proteinuria show gradual deterioration in renal function, which may result in the need for renal replacement therapy.
- Control of blood pressure and glycaemic control can slow disease progression.

Minimal change disease

Definition
- A glomerulopathy characterized clinically by the nephrotic syndrome and histologically by podocyte injury, with glomeruli that appear normal on light microscopy ('minimal change' in glomeruli).

Epidemiology
- Main cause of nephrotic syndrome in children.
- Frequent cause of nephrotic syndrome in adults.

Aetiology
- As a primary disease: aetiology uncertain; current evidence points towards an immune dysfunction causing podocyte injury.
- As a secondary disease, MCD can occur in association with drug administration (e.g. NSAIDs), bee stings/other allergens, venom exposure, and lymphoma.

Pathogenesis
- Podocyte injury.
- Loss of normal podocyte function leads to a defective glomerular filtration barrier with excessive permeability to proteins.

Presentation
- Nephrotic syndrome.

Light microscopy
- By definition, the glomeruli appear normal on light microscopy.

Immunofluorescence
- Negative for immunoglobulins (IgG, IgA, and IgM) and complement components (C3 and C1q), as well as for light chains (kappa and lambda).

Electron microscopy
- Extensive effacement of podocyte foot processes, often with microvillous change on the podocyte cell surface (Fig. 10.6).
- No electron-dense deposits are present.

Prognosis
- Complete recovery usually occurs in MCD treated with steroids, particularly in children.
- Adults with steroid-resistant disease should be carefully monitored, as they may turn out to have FSGS which was not apparent on biopsy due to sampling issues in a disease that is focal in nature.

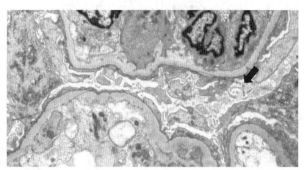

Fig. 10.6 Electron micrograph showing diffuse effacement of podocyte foot processes along the outside of the glomerular basement membrane, and microvillous change on the podocyte cell surface (arrow).

Focal segmental glomerulosclerosis

Definition

- Characterized histologically by sclerosis involving some but not all glomeruli (focal) and affecting only a portion of the glomerular tuft (segmental).
- As a primary glomerular disease, focal and segmental glomerulosclerosis (FSGS) is, like MCD, characterized clinically by the nephrotic syndrome and histologically by podocyte injury. However, in FSGS there is focal and segmental glomerular scarring on light microscopy.
- FSGS can also occur as a pattern of scarring secondary to glomerular injury of any type and cause; therefore, segmental glomerular scarring can be seen in many clinical contexts and does not always indicate primary FSGS.

▶ Careful exclusion of other underlying diseases through histological examination and clinical correlation is essential before making a diagnosis of primary FSGS.

Epidemiology

- Primary FSGS is a common cause of nephrotic syndrome in adults.
- Patients of African origin or ancestry are at increased risk of FSGS; this is related to more frequent risk alleles of *APO-L1* in these populations.

Aetiology

- Idiopathic primary FSGS: unknown; rapid recurrence of the disease after kidney transplantation suggests a circulating factor.
- Rare cases are due to genetic mutations, particularly in podocyte proteins involved in the slit diaphragm, cytoskeleton, and signalling pathways. Genetic causes are more frequently seen in children then adults (e.g. congenital nephrotic syndrome of Finnish type due to mutations of *NPHS1*, or diffuse mesangial sclerosis/Dennis Drash syndrome/Frasier syndrome related to mutations of *WT-1*).
- Podocyte injury and FSGS can also develop in association with viral infections (e.g. HIV), drugs (e.g. pamidronate) and tumours (in particular lymphoid).
- Haemodynamic stress to the glomerulus can also cause podocyte injury leading to secondary FSGS, either through increased workload on a normal-size nephron population (e.g. obesity, anabolic steroids, sickle-cell anaemia), or through reduced nephron mass of any cause with related increased work in remaining nephrons.
- APO-L1 risk allele associated FSGS: in patients with African ancestry, risk alleles confer an increased risk of FSGS of any aetiology.

Pathogenesis

- Podocyte injury and loss cause heavy proteinuria and segmental glomerular scarring.

Presentation

- Primary FSGS, genetic FSGS, FSGS related to viral infections, drugs and tumours: nephrotic syndrome.
- Secondary FSGS: heavy proteinuria without the nephrotic syndrome; variable degree of renal failure depending on cause.

Light microscopy

- Involved glomeruli show replacement of a segment of the glomerular tuft by sclerosis (Fig. 10.7).
- The sclerotic segment often shows adhesion to Bowman's capsule.
- Glomerulosclerosis is usually accompanied by tubulointerstitial fibrosis around the involved glomerulus.
- There are five morphological patterns of FSGS: not otherwise specified (NOS), tip variant, cellular variant, collapsing variant, and perihilar variant. The collapsing variant is most often seen in association with drugs (e.g. pamidronate) and viruses (e.g. HIV). The perihilar variant is usually seen in secondary FSGS related to haemodynamic stress (e.g. obesity).

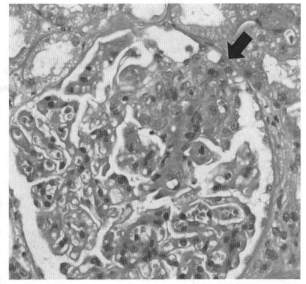

Fig. 10.7 Focal and segmental glomerulosclerosis, not otherwise specified (NOS). Haematoxylin and eosin. A portion of the tuft between 1 and 2 o'clock is replaced by fibrous stroma, with closure of the capillary lumens. This part of the glomerulus also adheres to Bowman's capsule (arrow) (see Plate 21).

Table 10.1 Classification of FSGS by cause with histological findings

Type	Putative aetiology	Pathology findings
Primary FSGS	Putative circulating factor, possibly an autoantibody or a cytokine	Usually NOS, tip, or cellular variants; widespread foot process effacement on EM
Secondary: Maladaptive FSGS	Reduced number of functioning nephrons and/or abnormal stress on an initially normal nephron population	Most often peri-hilar variant; foot process effacement is segmental on EM
Secondary: Infection (viral) and inflammation-associated FSGS	Possibly due to interferon and other cytokines Associated with HIV, and possibly others: CMV, parvovirus B19, EBV, HCV Also adult Still's disease, haemophagocytic syndrome and NK cell leukaemia	Often collapsing variant
Secondary: Drug induced FSGS	some antivirals, mTOR inhibitors, calcineurin inhibitors, anthracyclines, bisphosphonates, heroin, lithium, interferon, anabolic steroids	Often collapsing variant
High penetrance genetic (renal limited or syndromic; mendelian or mitochondrial)	Many different genetic mutations described	Variable
APO-L1 related	High-risk allele(s) of APO-L1; FSGS can be triggered by one of the other aetiologies above in patients with risk alleles	Variable

Immunofluorescence

- Non-specific entrapment of IgM and C3 may be seen in areas of sclerosis.

Electron microscopy

- Primary FSGS: extensive podocyte foot process effacement, often with microvillous change, as for MCD. There are no electron-dense deposits.
- Secondary FSGS: segmental podocyte foot process effacement; there may also be evidence of an underlying disease causing the scarring, such as immune complex glomerulonephritis (in which case, electron-dense deposits may be seen).

Prognosis

- Depends on whether primary or secondary FSGS, and on the histological variant: tip variant has a better outcome, and collapsing variant has a worse outcome.
- Commonly leads to progressive renal insufficiency.
- Primary FSGS has a high rate of recurrence in kidney transplants and without appropriate pre-emptive treatment often leads to rapid loss of the graft function.

Membranous glomerulonephritis

Definition

- Glomerulopathy caused by subepithelial (between the podocyte and glomerular basement membrane) immune complex deposition.

Epidemiology

- Most common primary renal cause of nephrotic syndrome in adults, except in patients of African origin or ancestry, where APOL1-related FSGS is more common.

Aetiology

- Membranous glomerulonephritis (GN) has historically been divided into 'primary' (an autoimmune disease characterized by autoantibodies against podocyte antigens) and 'secondary' (developed in association with malignancies, autoimmunity, drugs, and infections). Many target antibodies have now been described: PLA2R, THSD7A, SEMA3B, NELL-1, PCDH7, EXT1/EXT2, and NCAM-1. Future classifications may rely more on the target antigen involved.
- In primary/idiopathic membranous GN, the most commonly incriminated antigen is PLA2R (phospholipase A2 type M receptor, a protein expressed in podocytes). Antibodies against PLA2R are found in about 75% of cases of membranous glomerulopathy. The second most frequent antigen is THSD7A (~5% of cases).
- Secondary membranous GN can develop in association with malignancies (in particular, epithelial malignancies), drugs (e.g. captopril, gold, penicillamine), infections (e.g. hepatitis B, syphilis, and malaria), and SLE. In these cases, the immune complexes can form in situ in reaction to 'planted' antigens, or are present in the circulation and deposit in the glomeruli. EXT1 and EXT2 antigens, and to a lesser extent NCAM, are more commonly seen in membranous in the context of SLE.

Pathogenesis

- Immune complexes within the subepithelial space injure podocytes and disrupt the normal filtration barrier, causing heavy proteinuria.

Presentation

- Nephrotic syndrome.

Light microscopy

- Glomeruli show thickened, rigid capillary walls.
- Silver staining shows 'holes' in the glomerular basement membrane which represent the immune deposits, and 'spikes' which represent the glomerular basement membrane reaction to the deposits (Fig. 10.8(a)).
- More advanced cases may also show glomerular segmental sclerosis and tubulointerstitial fibrosis.

Immunofluorescence

- Granular deposits of IgG and C3 along the capillary walls (Fig. 10.8(b)).
- If deposits of IgA, IgM, and C1q are also present, then membranous nephropathy secondary to SLE should be considered.

Electron microscopy

- Subepithelial electron-dense immune complex deposits are present with a variable reaction of the adjacent basement membrane, which may surround them (Fig. 10.8(c)).
- Podocytes show diffuse foot process effacement.

Prognosis

- About one-third of patients develop renal failure requiring renal replacement therapy.

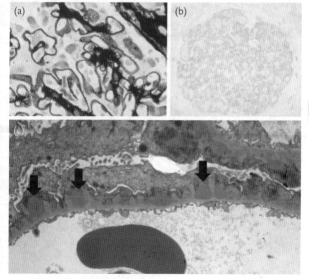

Fig. 10.8 Membranous glomerulonephritis. (a) Silver stain showing 'spikes' and 'holes' (irregularities) along the glomerular capillary walls. (b) Immunoperoxidase staining for IgG showing granular capillary wall staining in brown. (c) Electron microscopy showing subepithelial 'electron-dense deposits' (arrows) corresponding to the immune complex deposition (see Plate 22).

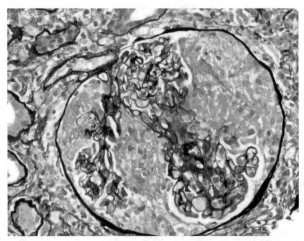

Fig. 10.9 Crescentic GN: Segmental glomerular necrosis with cellular crescent (Jones silver stain). Bowman's space is filled with/obliterated by cells and fibrin strands (see Plate 23).

Glomerulonephritis

Definition

- Glomerulonephritis (GN) is characterized by increased glomerular cellularity, caused by proliferation of indigenous glomerular cells and/or leucocyte infiltration.

Aetiology

- On the basis of aetiology, there are five classes of GN:
  - immune complex GN (e.g. IgA nephropathy (IgAN), post-infectious GN, lupus nephritis, cryoglobinaemic GN, etc.);
  - pauci-immune GN; usually related to ANCA (anti-neutrophil cytoplasm antibodies) vasculitis;
  - anti-glomerular basement membrane antibody (anti-GBM) GN;
  - monoclonal immunoglobulin-related GN;
  - C3 glomerulopathy.
- These are primarily autoimmune diseases, some with a genetic predisposition/aetiology. Monoclonal immunoglobulin GN is due to monoclonal immunoglobulins produced by clonal B-cell populations.

Pathogenesis

- Damage to the glomerulus with leakage of protein and blood into the urine. There may be rupture of the glomerular basement membrane, with a cellular reaction in the Bowman's space (crescent formation). The cause of the damage to the glomerulus depends on the cause:
- immune complex GN and monoclonal immunoglobulin GN: deposition of polyclonal or monoclonal immune complexes, respectively, within the glomerulus; these deposits lead to local complement activation, cellular proliferation, inflammation and injury;
- pauci-immune GN: 80–90% of patients have serologic evidence of ANCA with multi-system vasculitis. There is necrosis of the glomerular tuft; the pathogenetic link between ANCA and glomerular inflammation is not fully characterized;
  - anti-GBM GN: circulating antibodies against the GBM cause glomerular damage;
  - C3 glomerulopathy: abnormalities in regulation of the alternative pathway of complement activation lead to deposition of complement component C3 in the glomerulus, with glomerular inflammation and injury.

Presentation

- Haematuria (microscopic or macroscopic), proteinuria, and a variable degree of renal dysfunction.

Light microscopy

- Cases with immune complex or C3 deposition most often show glomerular hypercellularity. This can be limited to the mesangium (mesangial hypercellularity), and/or can involve the capillary lumina (endocapillary hypercellularity), and/or the extracapillary Bowman's space (crescents).
- Pauci-immune and anti-GBM GN typically show necrosis of the glomerular tuft and crescents, most often without hypercellularity in the unaffected glomerular portions.

- Crescents (Fig. 10.9) may be seen in all types of GN but are particularly large and common in pauci-immune and anti-GBM GN.

Immunofluorescence

- Immune complex GN: granular deposits of immunoglobulins, often with complement, in glomeruli. The type and location of the immune deposits point to the underlying aetiology—IgAN shows dominant or co-dominant staining with IgA; lupus nephritis shows a 'full-house' pattern with IgG, IgM, IgA, C3, and C1q positivity. In the case of monoclonal immunoglobulin GN, there is restriction of light chains to one type (kappa or lambda).
- C3 GN: dominant C3 granular deposits in the glomeruli with minimal or no Ig deposits.
- ANCA: negative for immunoglobulins and complement.
- Anti-GBM GN: linear deposition of IgG and C3 along glomerular basement membranes.

Electron microscopy

- Immune complex and C3 GN: electron-dense immune deposits are present; variable distribution (mesangial, subendothelial, subepithelial). In some cases, the deposits have a substructure on EM (e.g. fibrils or microtubules, e.g. in fibrillary GN).
- ANCA and anti-GBM GN: no electron-dense deposits.

Prognosis

- Variable, depending on the underlying cause.
- Cases presenting with crescents and rapidly progressive AKI require urgent treatment. The cause of a crescentic GN can be ascertained using Table 10.2.

Table 10.2 Differential diagnosis of different glomerulonephritides causing crescents

Diagnosis	Light microscopy	Immuno-fluorescence	Electron microscopy	Serology
Anti-GBM	Synchronous crescents Glomerular necrosis present Normal glomeruli also present	Linear capillary wall IgG and C3	No electron-dense deposits (EDD)	Circulating anti-GBM antibody
ANCA vasculitis	Acute and chronic glomerular lesions both present Glomerular necrosis present Arteries may also show vasculitis Normal glomeruli are also present	Scanty/negative	No or few EDD	ANCA

(Continued)

Table 10.2 (Contd.)

Diagnosis	Light microscopy	Immuno-fluorescence	Electron microscopy	Serology
Immune complex GN	Most/all glomeruli are hypercellular Necrosis may be present or not	Positive (various, depending on cause, e.g. 'full house' in lupus nephritis)	EDD in various locations	Various (e.g. positive lupus serology, cryoglobulin, etc.)

IgA nephropathy

Definition

- Immune complex GN related to glomerular deposition of immune complexes containing IgA.

Epidemiology

- The most common GN worldwide.

Aetiology

- Primary: incompletely understood; an abnormal mucosal immune system and the production of abnormally glycosylated IgA molecules play a role.
- Secondary: IgA can be deposited in glomeruli in patients with liver disease, bowel disease, and dermatitis herpetiformis.
- Systemic form with small-vessel vasculitis (Henoch–Schönlein purpura).

Typical pathological features

- IgAN can cause a number of changes in the glomeruli, ranging from mild mesangial hypercellularity only to global glomerular hypercellularity. Secondary FSGS is often be present. Crescents may be seen in severe cases.
- Immunofluorescence / immunoperoxidase: by definition, there is dominant or co-dominant staining with IgA in the mesangial region of the glomeruli (Fig. 10.10).

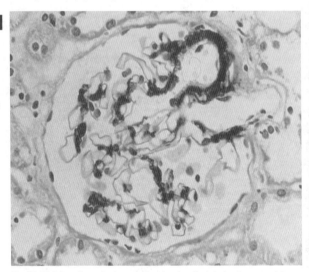

Fig. 10.10 IgA nephropathy. Immunohistochemistry for IgA showing mesangial positivity in a case of IgA nephropathy (see Plate 24).

- Electron microscopy: electron-dense immune deposits are present, mainly in the mesangium.

Prognosis

- About one-third of patients develop progressive renal disease.
- A number of clinical features can help predict the risk of progression (proteinuria, hypertension, renal function).
- The Oxford Classification of IgA Nephropathy (MESTC score) documents 5 features known to provide independent prognostic value in predicting the outcome: mesangial hypercellularity (M), endocapillary hypercellularity (E), segmental glomerulosclerosis (S), tubular atrophy/interstitial fibrosis (T), and crescents (C) (Table 10.3).

Table 10.3 Oxford classification of IgA nephropathy

M score	Mesangial hypercellularity absent (M0) or present (M1)
E score	Endocapillary hypercellularity absent (E0) or present (E1)
S score	Glomerular segmental scars absent (S0) or present (S1)
T score	Tubular atrophy interstitial fibrosis <25% (T0), 26-50% (T1) or >50% (T2)
C score	Crescents absent (C0), in <25% of glomeruli (C1) or in >25% of glomeruli (C2)

Lupus nephritis

Definition

- Immune complex GN related to SLE with glomerular deposition of immune complexes.

Epidemiology

- Up to 40% of patients with SLE will develop renal involvement. Renal involvement is usually indicated by the presence of haematuria, proteinuria or decreased renal function, and requires a renal biopsy for confirmation
- Can develop in patients with known SLE, or be the first manifestation of SLE.

Aetiology

- Circulating immune complexes deposit in the kidney, lead to complement activation and glomerular inflammation.
- The pattern of glomerular involvement depends on where the immune complexes deposit.

Typical pathological features

- Lupus nephritis can cause a number of changes in the glomeruli, ranging from mild mesangial hypercellularity to global glomerular hypercellularity. Secondary FSGS may be present. In severe cases, there are crescents and necrosis of the glomerular tuft. In some cases, the immune complex deposits are so large they can be seen on light microscopy along the capillary walls ('wire-loop') and/or within capillary lumens ('hyaline thrombi') (Fig. 10.11).

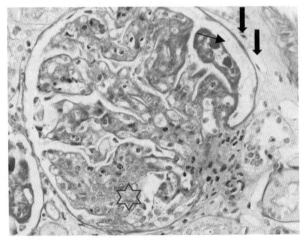

Fig. 10.11 Lupus nephritis showing endocapillary hypercellularity (star), hyaline thrombi within capillary loops (thick arrows) and 'wireloops' (thin arrow) along a capillary wall (see Plate 25).

- Patterns of involvement are classified using the Renal Pathology Society/International Society of Nephrology Lupus Nephritis classification (Table 10.4).
- Immunofluorescence: most often there is a 'full house' deposition of IgG, IgA, IgM, C3, and C1q, although other patterns can be observed. The presence of C1q indicates activation of the classical pathway of complement activation and its presence in a GN must always raise suspicion for lupus nephritis.
- Electron microscopy: electron-dense immune deposits are present. Their distribution depends on the pattern of involvement. Presence of at least a small number of deposits in all three sites (mesangial, subendothelial, and subepithelial) is typical and when noted must always raise suspicion for lupus nephritis.
- SLE can also lead to renal pathologies other than GN: lupus podocytopathy resembles MCD; SLE is a cause of active TIN and can be associated with immune complex deposits within the tubular basement membrane; arteries can show involvement by immune complex deposits (lupus vasculopathy) or vasculitis (necrotizing arteritis).

Prognosis

- 10–20% of patients progress to end-stage renal failure within 5 years of diagnosis of lupus nephritis.
- With adequate treatment, remission is achieved in about 50–70% of patients, but relapses occur.
- The RPS/ISN Classification of Lupus Nephritis documents 6 types of glomerular involvement (see Table 10.4). Proliferative lupus nephritis (classes III and IV) have a worse outcome.
- As for other renal diseases, persistent proteinuria, increased creatinine, and hypertension are clinical features of poor prognosis.
- In addition to the class system, activity and chronicity indices are given to quantify changes in lupus nephritis. The activity index relates to extent of 'active', potentially treatable lesions (endocapillary hypercellularity, karyorrhexis, 'wire loops', and hyaline thrombi, cellular

Table 10.4 Renal Pathology Society/International Society of Nephrology Lupus Nephritis classification

Class I	Minimal mesangial lupus nephritis (normal glomeruli on light microscopy)
Class II	Mesangial proliferative lupus nephritis
Class III	Focal lupus nephritis (endocapillary proliferative affecting <50% of glomeruli)
Class IV	Diffuse lupus nephritis (endocapillary proliferative affecting ≥50% of glomeruli)
Class V	Membranous lupus nephritis
Class IV	Advanced sclerotic lupus nephritis (>90% glomeruli globally sclerosed without residual activity)

crescents, fibrinoid necrosis, interstitial inflammation), and the chronicity index indicates the extent of chronic, likely irreversible lesions (global and segmental scarring, fibrous crescents, and tubular atrophy/ interstitial fibrosis).

Infection-related glomerulonephritis

Definition
- Immune complex GN related to infection.

Aetiology
- Acute post-streptococcal GN: group A streptococcal upper respiratory tract infection (e.g. pharyngitis), followed a few weeks later by AKI.
- *Staphylococcus Aureus* infection-associated GN (SAGN) (including methicillin-resistant *Staphylococcus aureus*, MRSA): infections of the viscera, skin, bones, and teeth, shunts, and heart valves (endocarditis) are associated with GN with a variety of patterns. The infections are often synchronous with the GN but may be occult. MRSA-related occur most commonly in elderly patients in iatrogenic settings or in relation to IVDU.
- Other microorganisms (bacterial, viral, and parasitic) can also cause GN.

Typical pathological features
- Acute post-streptococcal GN: global glomerular hypercellularity with neutrophils; predominant C3 on immunofluorescence; typical subepithelial 'humps' (dome-shaped electron-dense deposits) on electron microscopy (Fig. 10.11).
- SAGN often shows IgA predominance on IF, often with a lot of C3 positivity as well.
- Some infection-related GN (e.g. in the setting of endocarditis) have less typical findings, with variable glomerular proliferation, occasional necrosis of the glomerular tuft, immunoglobulins and complement on immunofluorescence, and electron-dense deposits on electron microscopy without 'humps'. It is important to keep a high index of suspicion for infection in unexplained GN.

Prognosis
- Mostly self-limiting; disappears after treatment of infection.
- Rare cases are progressive.

C3 glomerulopathy

Definition

- C3 glomerulopathy comprises C3 GN and dense deposit disease (DDD); both are characterized by C3-predominant deposits within glomeruli, and sometimes tubules, with little or no immune complexes.

Aetiology

- These diseases are related to dysregulation of the alternative pathway of complement activation (inherited or acquired) and can be due to mutation or autoimmune dysregulation of various components of the alternative pathway (e.g. DDD is often due to a C3 nephritic factor which is an autoantibody against C3; C3 GN can be due to mutations in factor H, a protein that regulates activation of the alternative pathway).

Typical pathological features

- Variable glomerular hypercellularity.
- Immunofluorescence: C3 predominance, with or without immunoglobulins.
- Electron microscopy: electron-dense deposits in variable locations within the glomeruli; DDD is characterized by electron-dense transformation of the glomerular and tubular basement membranes (Fig. 10.12).

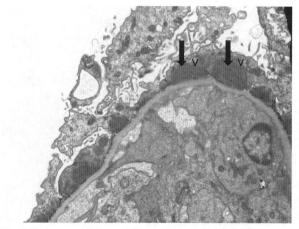

Fig. 10.12 Acute post-streptococcal GN on electron microscopy: electron-dense deposits in a subepithelial location with a 'hump'-like shape (arrows)

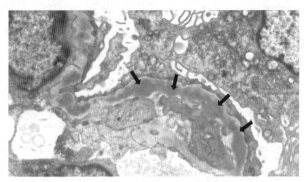

Fig. 10.13 Dense deposit disease on electron microscopy. Long areas of electron density are present within the glomerular basement membrane (arrows)

Prognosis
- Depends on the underlying pathogenetic mechanism; cases with autoantibodies may respond well to immunosuppression or removal of the antibody by plasmapheresis, whereas cases due to defective proteins may respond well to replacement of the defective proteins by fresh plasma.

ANCA vasculitis

Definition
- Systemic small-vessel vasculitis related to ANCA.

Epidemiology
- Rare disease affecting mainly elderly (peak incidence 60–70 years old).
- Four different syndromes:
  - Renal limited
  - Microscopic polyangiitis—necrotizing vasculitis also affecting other systems (e.g. skin, mucous membranes, lungs, brain, gastrointestinal tract, and muscle)
  - Granulomatosis with polyangiitis—necrotizing vasculitis along with necrotizing granulomas of the upper and lower respiratory tract
  - Eosinophilic granulomatosis with polyangiitis—necrotizing vasculitis along with history of asthma or allergic rhinitis and blood eosinophilia
- The kidney is frequently involved. Patients present with acute renal failure (often rapidly progressive) along with haematuria and a degree of proteinuria.

Aetiology
- ANCA are pathogenic and cause small-vessel inflammation including most notably pulmonary, dermal, and glomerular capillaries.
- Not entirely known; genetic and environmental factors play a role (smoking/pollution).

Typical pathological features
- Segmental necrotizing GN with fibrinoid necrosis of the glomerular tuft and crescents in most cases (Fig. 10.14).
- Mix of active and chronic lesions (secondary FSGS) most often present due to remitting relapsing course.
- Immunofluorescence: most often negative ('pauci-immune').
- Electron microscopy: no or few small electron-dense immune deposits are present ('pauci-immune').

Prognosis
- Rapid instigation of treatment is critical.
- Histological predictors of good long-term renal function are: higher number of normal glomeruli, and lower glomerulosclerosis and interstitial fibrosis/tubular atrophy.
- Histological predictors of response to treatment: presence of crescents, fibrinoid necrosis, and interstitial inflammation.

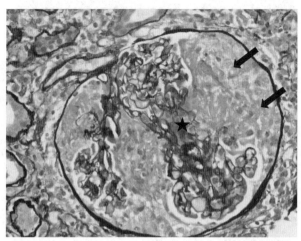

Fig. 10.14 ANCA vasculitis affecting a glomerulus. There is a large cellular crescent (arrows) and there is fibrinoid necrosis (star) of the glomerular tuft (see Plate 26).

Anti-glomerular basement membrane disease

Definition
- Severe GN caused by the development of autoantibodies to the glomerular basement membrane.

Epidemiology
- Rare disease. Two age peaks of incidence, the first around 30 years old and the second (larger) around 60–70 years old.

Aetiology
- Autoantibodies to the C-terminal domain of type IV collagen, a component of the glomerular basement membrane.

Pathogenesis
- Autoantibodies bind to the glomerular basement membrane and initiate inflammation and injury.
- Autoantibodies are thought to arise in genetically susceptible patients, after an environmental factor (e.g. infection) leads to exposure of cryptic epitopes in the lung or kidney.

Presentation
- AKI due to severe acute GN, usually presents as rapidly progressive renal failure.
- Some patients also present with pulmonary haemorrhage if the autoantibody cross-reacts with the alveolar basement membrane ('Goodpasture disease').

Light microscopy
- Glomeruli show a segmental, necrotizing GN with breaches in the glomerular basement membrane and formation of crescents in the Bowman's space.
- Unaffected segments of the glomeruli appear normal.

Immunofluorescence
- Strong linear staining of IgG and C3 is seen in the glomerular basement membrane (Fig. 10.15).

Electron microscopy
- No electron-dense deposits are present.

Prognosis
- Although prompt immunosuppressive therapies can halt ongoing disease activity with good recovery, severe cases or cases caught too late may be irreversible.
- Anti-GBM is often a 'one hit' disease, with no subsequent recurrence.

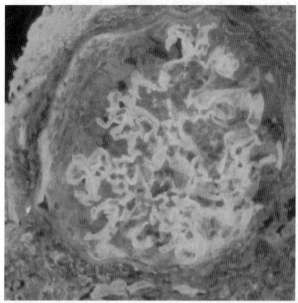

Fig. 10.15 Anti-GBM disease on immunofluorescence for IgG: there is bright linear positivity along the glomerular basement membrane (see Plate 27).

Monoclonal gammopathy-associated kidney disease

Definition

- The production of monoclonal immunoglobulins or free light chains by clonal proliferations of plasma cells or B-cells can cause a range of renal lesions, referred to collectively as monoclonal gammopathy-associated kidney disease.

Epidemiology

- Monoclonal gammopathy-associated kidney disease can be seen in association with myeloma, monoclonal gammopathy of unknown significance, and lymphomas and, rarely, in the absence of any of these.

Aetiology

- Abnormal light and/or heavy chains accumulate in the glomeruli, the tubules, the interstitium, and/or vessels.

Pathogenesis

- Free light chains can accumulate in the tubular lumen as casts (light chain cast nephropathy), the tubular epithelium (proximal light chain tubulopathy), or as amyloid fibrils (AL amyloidosis).
- Complete monoclonal immunoglobulins can deposit in glomeruli, leading to an immune complex GN, either with structured deposits in the form of microtubules or crystals (immunotactoid GN, cryoglobulinaemic GN) or with linear granular deposits (monoclonal immunoglobulin deposition disease) or with circumscribed granular electron-dense deposits (proliferative GN with monoclonal immunoglobulins).
- The different patterns that develop are mostly determined by the physicochemical properties of the monoclonal proteins produced. Rate of production of the monoclonal proteins is also important (e.g. light chain cast nephropathy is often related to high monoclonal light chain production).

Presentation

- Variable: for example, tubular dysfunction in proximal light chain tubulopathy, AKI in light chain cast nephropathy, nephrotic syndrome in AL amyloidosis, and nephritic syndrome in immune complex GN.

Light microscopy

- Light chain cast nephropathy: casts in tubules with 'cracks' and a cellular reaction at the periphery, staining weakly with periodic acid–Schiff (PAS) (Fig. 10.16).
- Proximal light chain tubulopathy: vacuolation of proximal tubular epithelial cells or crystals within epithelial cells.
- AL amyloidosis: amorphous deposits in glomeruli, interstitium, and vessels; Congo Red stain-positive.
- Immune complex GN: variable glomerular hypercellularity.

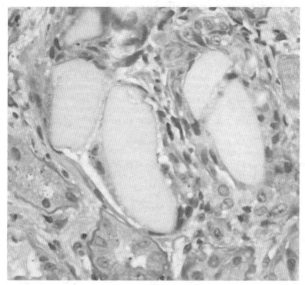

Fig. 10.16 Light chain cast nephropathy (PAS stain). The casts stain weakly with PAS in contrast to usual hyaline casts or granular casts. They often have angular edges, 'cracks' and a border of cells around the edge (see Plate 28).

Immunofluorescence
- Monoclonal immunoglobulin and/or light chains can be identified by light chain restriction (i.e. staining for only kappa or only lambda light chain).
- Distribution will depend on the type of lesion (i.e. tubular, glomerular, etc.).

Electron microscopy
- Microtubular, amorphous granular, and/or crystalline electron densities are seen, with a variable distribution.

Prognosis
- Successful treatment of the underlying clonal population is necessary for renal recovery.

Hereditary renal diseases

Definition
- A number of hereditary conditions may affect the kidney primarily or as part of a systemic disease.
- In addition, patients may be predisposed to developing kidney failure because of underlying genetic traits; most importantly, high-risk alleles of *APOL1* confer an increased risk of renal failure to some patients with African ancestry. Specific human leukocyte antigen (HLA) haplotypes are also associated with certain kidney diseases—for example, anti-GBM disease is strongly associated with an HLA-DR2 haplotype.

Epidemiology
- Uncommon.
- The prevalence of risk alleles in patients of African origin or descent is variable, between a few % and up to 40% of the population.

Examples
- Cystic kidney diseases such as autosomal dominant polycystic kidney disease.
- Alport's syndrome and thin basement membrane lesion: mutations in the alpha chains of type IV collagen.
- Hereditary FSGS/congenital nephrotic syndrome (see FSGS).
- Sickle-cell nephropathy.
- Storage disorders (e.g. Fabry disease).
- Autosomal dominant tubulointerstitial kidney disease (ADTKD): group of conditions with autosomal dominant inheritance and slowly progressive CKD. Several genes have been incriminated: *UMOD, REN, MUC1 HNF1B*.

Presentation
- Cystic kidney disease may present with renal impairment and/or symptoms related to an increased kidney size.
- Alport's syndrome and thin basement membrane lesion typically present with microhaematuria; some cases progress to FSGS and CKD.
- Hereditary FSGS/congenital nephrotic syndrome: nephrotic syndrome *in utero*, in infancy, or later in life.
- Fabry disease: kidney dysfunction is part of a systemic picture with involvement of the skin (angiokeratomas), nerves, heart, brain, and gastrointestinal (GI) tract.
- ADTKD: Patients have a bland urinary sediment with slowly progressive CKD. Biopsy shows non-specific findings of tubular atrophy/interstitial fibrosis. In UMOD-associated kidney disease, there is typically also hyperuricaemia and gout, sometimes with renal cysts.

Prognosis
- Depends on the cause; renal transplantation may cure the disease.

Alport's syndrome and thin basement membrane lesion

Definition
- Mutations of the alpha chains of type IV collagen, leading to structural defects in the glomerular basement membrane.

Aetiology
- Most cases of Alport's syndrome are X-linked dominant and due to mutations of the alpha 5 chain of type IV collagen.
- Mutations affecting the alpha 3 and alpha 4 chains of type IV collagen may lead to autosomal dominant or recessive forms of Alport's syndrome or to thin basement membrane lesion.

Presentation
- Typically presents with microhaematuria.
- Patients with Alport's syndrome often have deafness and ocular abnormalities.
- Alport's syndrome is typically a progressive disease, with CKD in middle age.
- Thin basement membrane lesion may be entirely benign ('benign familial haematuria') or may progress to renal failure, depending on the underlying mutation.

Histopathology
- Light microscopy: normal or progressive scarring in glomeruli (FSGS) and tubules.
- Immunofluorescence: no immunoglobulin or complement deposition; depending on the mutation, some cases how abnormal staining patterns using antibodies directed against the alpha chains of type IV collagen, either within the kidney or within a skin biopsy.
- Electron microscopy: Alport's syndrome shows a typical 'basket-weave' pattern to the glomerular basement membranes; thin basement membrane lesion shows marked and diffuse thinning of glomerular basement membranes (Fig. 10.17).

Prognosis
- Depends on the exact genetic mutation and family history of renal failure; renal transplantation may cure the disease.

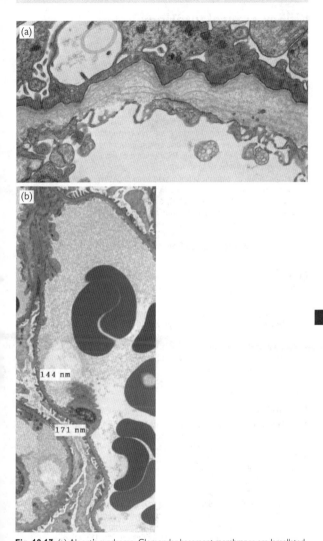

Fig. 10.17 (a) Alport's syndrome. Glomerular basement membranes are lamellated and thickened. (b) Thin basement membrane disease. Glomerular basement membranes are diffusely thinned (<200 nm).

Kidney transplantation

Introduction

- Kidney transplantation is the treatment of choice for most patients with end-stage kidney failure. It offers decreased morbidity and mortality, and improved quality of life, compared to other renal replacement therapies (various types of dialysis).
- Although improved tissue matching (predominantly of blood group type and of HLA antigens) and improved immunosuppressive drugs have led to longer kidney transplant survival, kidney transplants have a limited life span, due to a number of factors, the most important being alloimmune rejection, where the host immune system mounts an immune response against mismatched antigens in the donated organ.
- Other causes of loss of graft function are mostly related to complications of immunosuppression to prevent rejection: drug toxicity (e.g. calcineurin inhibitors have direct renal toxicity); infection (pyelonephritis; BK nephropathy); cardiovascular disease (transplant renal artery stenosis; ischaemia due to hypoperfusion).
- The cause of the initial failure of renal function can recur in the transplant (e.g. recurrent FSGS or GN).
- Disease can also be inherited from the donor (e.g. vascular disease, especially from older donors).

Presentation

- Transplant function is monitored regularly through serum creatinine and proteinuria.
- Transplant patients are also monitored for the development of antibodies against the donor antigens as these are associated with a poor outcome, especially if they lead to antibody-mediated rejection.
- When a transplant patient presents with increased creatinine, new or worsening proteinuria or a new antibody against the donor antigens, an indication biopsy is taken.
- In some centres, 'protocol' or 'surveillance' biopsies are also taken, to monitor for subclinical disease.

Histopathology

- An important consideration in a transplant biopsy is whether there is evidence of rejection or not. Two main types of rejection are recognized: T-cell-mediated rejection and antibody-mediated rejection.
- The histological findings in transplant biopsies are documented using an internationally agreed classification system: The Banff Classification for Allograft Pathology.
- T-cell-mediated rejection is due to a cognate T-cell response against mismatched donor antigens, leading to a tubulointerstitial infiltrate of T-cells and monocytes. The light microscopy appearances are very similar to those of active tubulointerstitial nephritis, with a predominantly monocytic interstitial infiltrate and tubulitis (Fig. 10.18). In some cases the inflammation also involves the arteries, in the form of intimal arteritis (Fig. 10.19).
- Antibody-mediated rejection is characterized by fixation of antibodies to donor antigens on the surface of the endothelium, leading to

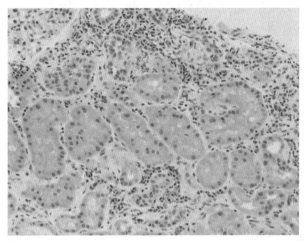

Fig. 10.18 T-cell-mediated rejection is characterized by a chronic inflammatory infiltrate (predominantly T lymphocytes and monocytes) in the interstitium, with tubulitis (see Plate 29).

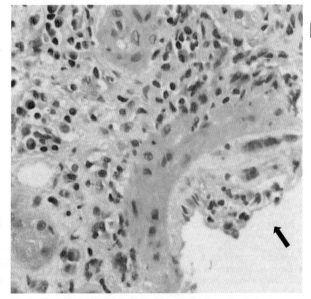

Fig. 10.19 In both T-cell-mediated rejection and antibody-mediated rejection, endarteritis can be seen. This is characterized by inflammatory cells beneath the endothelium, within the intima (arrow) (see Plate 30).

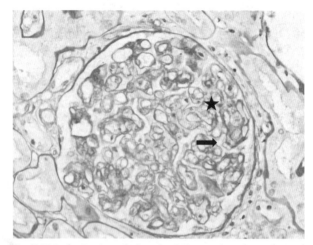

Fig. 10.20 In chronic active antibody-mediated rejection, a 'transplant glomerulopathy' develops in response to fixation of an antibody against donor HLA antigens on the endothelium: there is endocapillary hypercellularity (star) and double contours along capillary wall (two parallel lines instead of one, arrow) (see Plate 31).

inflammation in the capillaries of the glomeruli and peritubular capillaries, with or without activation of the complement system with deposition of complement fragment C4d on the endothelial cell surface. In some cases of antibody-mediated rejection, the large vessels are also involved, with intimal arteritis (Fig. 10.19). In the long term, the endothelial activation that ensues leads to deposition of new matrix, in the form of double contours of basement membrane along capillary walls (Fig. 10.20).

- Infection in the graft can take the form of a bacterial neutrophilic pyelonephritis; or can be related to viral infection. In BK nephropathy there is chronic tubulointerstitial inflammation resembling T-cell-mediated rejection, but viral inclusions are noted, either on light microscopy, and/or with the help of immunohistochemistry for SV40 large T antigen (expressed by several members of the polyoma virus family, including BK virus).

- If signs of calcineurin inhibitor (CNI) toxicity are noted, CNI levels can be reduced (if no rejection is noted). In the acute phase CNI toxicity is associated with acute tubular injury with fine vacuolation of the tubular epithelial cells. In the chronic phase, arterioles show hyaline transformation of the vessel wall (hyalinosis).

- Glomeruli should be assessed for recurrent disease, if necessary including immunohistochemical studies and electron microscopy.

Further reading

Colvin RB, Change A (2019). *Kidney Diseases*, third edition. Philadelphia: Elsevier.

Fogo AB, Kashgarian M (2012). *Diagnostic Atlas of Renal Pathology*, second edition. Philadelphia: Elsevier Saunders.

Jennette JC, Olson JL, Silva FG, D'Agati VD (2015). *Heptinstall's Pathology of the Kidney*, seventh edition. Philadelphia: Wolters Kluwer.

Levey K, et al. Nomenclature for Kidney Function and Disease: Report of a Kidney Disease: Improving Global Outcomes (KDIGO) Consensus Conference. *Kidney Int* 2020:97:1117–1129.

Luciano RL, Moeckel GW. Update on the Native Kidney Biopsy: Core Curriculum. *AJKD* 2019;73(3):404–415.

Sethi S, Haas M, Markowitz GS, *et al.* Mayo Clinic/Renal Pathology Society Consensus Report on Pathologic Classification, Diagnosis and Reporting of Glomerulonephritis. *J Am Soc Nephrol* 2016;**27**:1278–1287.

Urological pathology

Genitourinary malformations

Renal agenesis
- Absence of one or both kidneys.
- Bilateral renal agenesis is uniformly fatal *in utero* or shortly after birth.
- Unilateral renal agenesis is usually asymptomatic, though it is often associated with other anomalies of the genital tract.

Renal fusion
- May involve some or all portions of each kidney.
- The most common form of renal fusion is the **horseshoe kidney**, in which the lower poles of each kidney are fused into a single renal mass in the midline.
- Patients are prone to developing obstruction.

Rotational anomalies
- Occur due to failure of the renal pelvis to rotate from an anterior position to a medial position.
- May occur in an otherwise normal kidney or accompany renal fusion or ectopia.

Renal dysplasia
- Refers to a kidney with abnormal development.
- Unilateral disease causes renal enlargement and a flank mass in infancy.
- Bilateral disease is usually fatal.
- Grossly, the kidney may be enlarged and cystic or small and solid.
- Histologically, the kidney contains abnormally formed nephron structures, often with cystic change. The presence of fetal cartilage is a characteristic feature.

Pelviureteric junction obstruction
- A common cause of congenital obstructive uropathy.
- Due to an intrinsic malformation of the smooth muscle of the wall of the outflow tract at that site.
- More common in boys.
- Usually unilateral, more common on the left.
- May present in childhood with abdominal pain.

Ureteral duplication
- Common anomaly in which the kidney has two separate renal pelves, accompanied by partial to complete reduplication of the ureter.
- When there is complete reduplication, the upper ureter typically enters the bladder posteriorly at the normal site of the ureteric orifice on the trigone of the bladder. The lower ureter usually enters the bladder laterally with a short intramural course, predisposing it to VUR.

Vesicoureteric reflux
- Failure of the vesicoureteric valve causes abnormal reflux of urine into the ureter when the bladder contracts.

- Predisposes to urinary tract infection (UTI) in children. In severe cases, may be complicated by intra-renal reflux and renal scarring, a condition known as **reflux nephropathy** (→ Reflux nephropathy, p. 202).

Posterior urethral valves

- Abnormal mucosal folds in the posterior prostatic urethra that cause obstructive uropathy.
- Their presence is usually indicated when bilateral hydronephrosis is detected on antenatal ultrasound.

Cryptorchidism

- Occurs when the testis fails to descend into its normal position in the scrotum.
- Mobilization of the testis and fixation in the scrotum (orchidopexy) should be performed by the age of 2y to preserve fertility.
- Cryptorchidism is important due to its association with a higher risk of testicular germ cell tumours (→ Testicular germ cell tumours, p. 272).

Hypospadias

- The most common anomaly of the penis.
- Refers to the abnormal opening of the urethral meatus on the undersurface of the penis.
- Usually an isolated defect, though the incidence of cryptorchidism appears to be higher in boys with hypospadias.

Urinary tract infection

Pathogens

- *Escherichia coli* is the main organism.
- *Staphylococcus saprophyticus* and *Proteus mirabilis* are other causes.

Epidemiology

- Extremely common.
- ~60% of women will have a UTI at some point in their life.

Transmission

- Ascending spread of endogenous gut bacteria into the urethra.
- The shorter urethra of women and its closer proximity to the anus are thought to be the main reason why females are more susceptible.

Risk factors

- Female gender, sexual intercourse, pregnancy, diabetes, catheterization, urinary tract obstruction, or malformation.

Pathogenesis

- Pathogenic strains of *E. coli* have pili which allow them to bind to galactose-containing receptors on the surface of urothelial cells.
- Other important virulence factors include haemolysin which allows invasion of tissues and the K antigen which protects the organism from neutrophil phagocytosis.

Presentation

- Bladder infection (**cystitis**) causes frequency, urgency, dysuria, haematuria, and suprapubic pain.
- Ascending spread into the kidneys (**acute pyelonephritis**) causes a more severe illness with fever, rigors, vomiting, and loin pain.
- ▶ May present with acute confusion in the elderly.

Diagnosis

- Urinalysis showing leucocytes or nitrites is a useful quick screening test.
- The gold standard is microbiological culture of a correctly collected midstream urine specimen. A pure growth of $>10^5$ organisms/mL of urine is considered diagnostic.

Urinary tract obstruction

Definition

- Urinary tract obstruction (**obstructive uropathy**) is a blockage to the flow of urine at some point in the urinary tract (Fig. 11.1).

Epidemiology

- Seen mostly in older men (due to benign prostatic hyperplasia (BPH)) and children (due to congenital anomalies of the urinary tract).

Aetiology

- Urinary stones.
- Urothelial tumours.

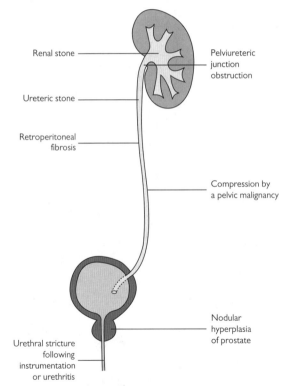

Fig. 11.1 Common causes of obstruction in the urinary tract.

Reproduced with permission from *Clinical Pathology* (Oxford Core Texts), Carton, James, Daly, Richard, and Ramani, Pramila, Oxford University Press (2006), p. 226, Figure 11.2.

- Extrinsic compression by abdominal/pelvic masses.
- Prostatic hyperplasia.
- Urinary tract malformations.
- Strictures.

Presentation

- Symptoms directly suggestive of obstruction (e.g. ureteric colic).
- Impaired renal function.
- Recurrent UTIs.

The precise clinical picture will depend on whether the obstruction is acute or chronic, whether it involves the upper or lower urinary tract, and whether it is unilateral or bilateral.

Macroscopy

- There is dilation of the urinary tract above the level of the obstruction, causing hydroureter, and hydronephrosis.
- Renal damage is associated with loss of renal tissue and scarring.

Complications

- Obstruction increases the risk of infection, stone formation, and renal damage (**obstructive nephropathy**) (Obstructive nephropathy, p. 204).

Urinary calculi

Definition
- Crystal aggregates which form in the renal collecting ducts but may become deposited anywhere in the urinary tract.

Epidemiology
- Common, with a lifetime incidence of up to 15%.
- Males are at higher risk than females (3:1).

Stone types
- Calcium oxalate (75%).
- Magnesium ammonium phosphate (15%).
- Uric acid stones (5%).

Pathogenesis
- Calcium stones are associated with hypercalciuria. Most patients have absorptive hypercalciuria, in which too much calcium is absorbed from the gut. Others have renal hypercalciuria, in which calcium absorption from the proximal tubule is impaired. Only a minority have hypercalciuria due to hypercalcaemia which is usually due to primary hyperparathyroidism.
- Triple stones are formed largely as a result of infections with organisms such as *Proteus* that produce the enzyme urease which splits urea to ammonia. The ammonia alkalinizes the urine and promotes precipitation of magnesium ammonium phosphate salts. Triple stones can become very large and may form branching masses filling the entire renal pelvis and calyces (**staghorn calculus**).
- Uric acid stones may form in patients with hyperuricaemia (e.g. patients with gout and conditions of rapid cell turnover, e.g. leukaemias). However, most patients do not have hyperuricaemia nor increased urinary excretion of uric acid. It is thought that these patients have a tendency to make slightly acidic urine which is prone to forming uric acid stones.

Presentation
- Large stones tend to remain confined to the kidney. They may be asymptomatic or picked up following investigation of haematuria or recurrent UTIs.
- Smaller stones may pass into the ureter and become impacted, causing ureteric colic. Common points of impaction are the pelviureteric junction, the pelvic brim, and the vesicoureteric junction.

Complications
▶ Complete obstruction of the urinary tract requires urgent intervention to remove the stone.
▶▶ Superadded infection in an obstructed urinary tract or any obstruction within the tract of a solitary kidney is a urological emergency requiring immediate intervention.

Cystic renal diseases

Adult (dominant) polycystic kidney disease

- Most common cystic renal disease, with a frequency of up to 1 in 500 and a leading cause of end-stage renal failure.
- 90% of cases are caused by an inherited mutation in the *PKD1* gene on chromosome 16.
- Defects in the function of the PKD1 protein lead to cystic change in renal tubules and loss of normal renal tissue.
- Most patients present aged 30–40, with hypertension, flank pain, and haematuria.
- Grossly, the kidneys are massively enlarged (weighing >2 kg) and completely replaced with cysts.
- Histologically, both kidneys contain numerous cysts lined by flattened cuboidal epithelium with little intervening normal renal parenchyma.
- Extra-renal manifestations include liver cysts and berry aneurysms.

▶ Subarachnoid haemorrhage from a ruptured berry aneurysm can cause sudden death.

Infantile (recessive) polycystic kidney disease

- A rare, inherited condition causing bilateral polycystic kidneys and congenital hepatic fibrosis.
- Caused by mutations in the gene *PKHD1* on chromosome 6p which encodes a component of the cilia on collecting duct epithelial cells.
- Grossly, the kidneys are enlarged and contain numerous cysts.
- Histologically, the cysts are lined by flattened cuboidal epithelium.
- Severe cases cause neonatal death from pulmonary hypoplasia.
- Children with less severe renal disease who survive suffer from congenital hepatic fibrosis and complications of portal hypertension.

Medullary cystic disease

- Congenital presence of numerous cysts at the corticomedullary junction which vary in size from <1 mm to 2 cm.
- The childhood disease (juvenile nephronophthisis) is autosomal recessive and associated with mutations in the genes *NPH1*, *2*, or *3*.
- The adult disease (uraemic medullary cystic disease) is autosomal dominant and associated with mutations in the genes *MCDK1* or *2*.

Medullary sponge kidney

- Associated with an irregular enlargement of the collecting ducts, leading to microcystic change of the renal medullae and papillae with calcification.
- The condition usually presents in adult life with recurrent infections.

Acquired renal cystic disease

- Development of multiple bilateral cortical and medullary cysts in patients with end-stage kidneys on dialysis.
- An important additional feature is the increased occurrence of renal tumours which are often papillary in type and may be multiple.

Benign renal tumours

Papillary adenoma

- Benign unencapsulated renal epithelial tumour with a papillary or tubulopapillary architecture and size ≤15 mm.
- Frequently found incidentally in nephrectomy specimens or at autopsy.
- Macroscopically, they are well-circumscribed, unencapsulated cortical nodules which measure ≤15 mm.
- Histologically, they are composed of bland epithelial cells growing in papillary or tubulopapillary patterns.

Oncocytoma

- Benign oncocytic renal epithelial tumour which is usually discovered incidentally in adults.
- Most cases are sporadic, but some are associated with genetic syndromes (e.g. Birt–Hogg–Dubé syndrome).
- Macroscopically, they are well-circumscribed tumours with a mahogany brown colour, often with central scarring.
- Histologically, they are characterized by cells with abundant granular eosinophilic cytoplasm, growing in nests within an oedematous stroma.
- Immunohistochemically they are positive for pancytokeratin, Pax8, and CD117. Staining with CK7 characteristically stains scattered single positive cells only.
- Oncocytomas are benign tumours with no capacity for metastatic spread. Large tumours are nevertheless often excised as they are more likely to be symptomatic.
- Infiltration of tumour cells into perinephric fat may be seen and this has no adverse consequence.

Angiomyolipoma

- Benign mesenchymal tumour of the kidney composed of variable amounts of fat, smooth muscle, and thick-walled blood vessels.
- Most occur sporadically in adults, but a small proportion is associated with tuberous sclerosis. These are more likely to be multiple and bilateral.
- Although most are picked up incidentally, occasionally they present with flank pain due to haemorrhage into the tumour.
- Macroscopically, they are lobulated renal masses which may appear rather yellow if their fat content is high.
- Histologically, they are composed of a mixture of adipose tissue, smooth muscle bundles, and thick-walled blood vessels in variable amounts.

Cystic nephroma

- Benign cystic renal tumour which shows a marked predilection for women.
- Macroscopically, they are encapsulated multicystic lesions without a solid component.

- Microscopically, the cysts are lined by a single layer of attenuated cuboidal epithelial cells.
- The septa may show cellular areas resembling ovarian stroma, and interestingly the nuclei of the cells within the septa often react with antibodies to oestrogen and progesterone receptors.

Leiomyoma

- Benign smooth muscle tumours which usually arise from the renal capsule.
- Most occur in adults as incidental small, well-circumscribed, capsular tumours.
- Histologically, they show bundles of bland smooth muscle cells.

Renomedullary interstitial cell tumour

- Common benign renal tumours often encountered incidentally in kidneys at autopsy.
- Macroscopically, they are small (1–5 mm) white nodules centred on a medullary pyramid.
- Histologically, they are composed of small stellate or polygonal cells set in a loose stroma. Entrapped tubules may be found at the edge of the lesion.

Renal cell carcinoma

Definition
- A malignant epithelial tumour arising in the kidney.

Epidemiology
- Accounts for ~2% of all cancers worldwide.
- More common in developed countries, with an average incidence of ~10 per 100 000 in men and 3 per 100 000 in women.

Aetiology
- Recognized risk factors include smoking, hypertension, obesity, environmental chemicals, and long-term dialysis.
- Some genetic syndromes are associated with renal cell carcinoma (RCC) (e.g. von Hippel–Lindau and tuberous sclerosis).

Presentation
- About half of all cases present with painless haematuria.
- Most of the remainder is picked up incidentally on imaging.
- A small proportion presents with metastatic disease.

Subtypes
- 70% clear cell RCC.
- 15% papillary RCC.
- 5% chromophobe RCC.
- A number of rare subtypes make up the remainder of cases.

Clear cell renal cell carcinoma
- Macroscopically, heterogenous tumours with golden yellow and haemorrhagic areas (Fig. 11.2).
- Histologically composed of epithelial cells with clear or eosinophilic cytoplasm, set within a delicate vascular network.
- Immunohistochemically positive for AE1/AE3, EMA, CD10, vimentin, Pax8, RCC, and CAIX.
- Immunohistochemically negative for CK7 and CD117.
- Genetically demonstrates losses at chromosome 3p.

Papillary renal cell carcinoma
- Macroscopically, well-circumscribed, friable tumours with a surrounding fibrous pseudocapsule.
- Histologically composed of epithelial cells arranged in a papillary or tubulopapillary growth pattern and a size >15 mm.
- Immunohistochemically positive for AE1/AE3, CK7, Pax8, and racemase.
- Genetically shows trisomy of chromosomes 7 and 17 and loss of chromosome Y in men.

Chromophobe renal cell carcinoma
- Macroscopically, well-circumscribed, solid light brown tumours.
- Histologically composed of sheets of large, round epithelial cells with distinct cell borders and finely reticulated cytoplasm. The vasculature within the tumour is thick-walled.
- Immunohistochemically positive for CK7, Pax8, E-cadherin, and CD117.

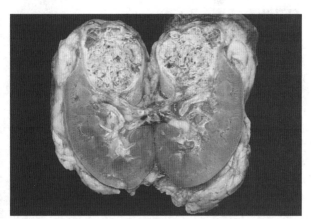

Fig 11.2 This patient presented with macroscopic haematuria and was found to have a solid renal mass on CT imaging. Anephrectomy was performed and sent to pathology. The kidney has been sliced open by the pathologist to reveal a large tumour in the upper pole of the kidney. Subsequent microscopic examination of samples of the tumour revealed this to be a clear cell renal cell carcinoma (see Plate 32).

Reproduced with permission from *Clinical Pathology* (Oxford Core Texts), Carton, James, Daly, Richard, and Ramani, Pramila, Oxford University Press (2006), p.233, Figure 11.6.

- Immunohistochemically negative for CAIX.
- Genetically shows extensive chromosomal losses.

Prognosis

- Overall 5-year survival rate is ~60%.
- Stage and grade are the most important prognostic factors.
- The recommended grading system for clear cell RCC and papillary RCC is the ISUP (International Society of Urologic Pathologists) nucleolar grade. Grade 1 has the best prognosis, and grade 4 the worst. Chromophobe RCC is not graded.
- The Leibovich risk model may also be used for clear cell RCC to predict the likelihood of progression. Tumour stage, size, grade, and necrosis are each scored to give a maximum possible total of 11: 0–2 = low risk, 3–5 = intermediate risk, 6 or more = high risk.

ISUP nucleolar grading system for clear cell and papillary RCC

Grade 1: nucleoli are inconspicuous or absent at high-power magnification.

Grade 2: nucleoli are clearly visible at high-power magnification but are not prominent.

Grade 3: nucleoli are prominent and are easily visualized at low-power magnification.

Grade 4: presence of tumour giant cells and/or marked pleomorphism.

Childhood renal tumours

Nephroblastoma (Wilms' tumour)

- A malignant childhood renal neoplasm.
- Second most common childhood malignancy, with an incidence of ~1 in 8000.
- Most children present aged 2–5 years old with an abdominal mass.
- Macroscopically, they are well-demarcated tumours with a grey or tan colour.
- Histologically, most nephroblastomas contain a mixture of undifferentiated small, round, blue cells (blastema), with areas of more differentiated epithelial and stromal components (so-called 'triphasic' tumours).
- Most nephroblastomas are of low stage with a favourable histology and have an excellent prognosis with treatment.
- ~5% of cases show unfavourable histology, characterized by nuclear anaplasia or the presence of multipolar mitotic figures; these cases are associated with an adverse outcome.

Clear cell sarcoma

- A rare childhood renal sarcoma with a marked propensity to metastasize to bone.
- Most children present between 1 and 2 years of age.
- Macroscopically, they are typically large tumours centred on the renal medulla.
- Histologically, the classical pattern is of nests or cords of cells separated by fibrovascular septae.

Rhabdoid tumour

- A rare, highly malignant renal tumour of young children.
- Most present around 1 year of age with haematuria or symptoms of disseminated disease.
- Macroscopically, tumours are large and infiltrative with necrosis.
- Histologically, the malignant cells have vesicular chromatin, prominent cherry red nucleoli, and hyaline pink intracytoplasmic inclusions. Extensive vascular invasion is usually evident.
- Prognosis is extremely poor, with mortality rates in excess of 80% within 2y of diagnosis.

Congenital mesoblastic nephroma

- A low-grade fibroblastic renal sarcoma arising in young children.
- May be diagnosed on antenatal ultrasound or present within the first year of life with an abdominal mass.
- Macroscopically, the tumour is centred on the renal sinus and has either a firm, whorled appearance or a softer cystic cut surface.
- Histologically, two types are recognized: a 'classic' type composed of fascicles of bland spindled cells and a 'cellular' type composed of sheets of densely packed rounder cells.
- Prognosis is generally excellent when the tumour is completely excised by nephrectomy.

Urothelial carcinoma

Definition
- A group of urothelial neoplasms arising in the urothelial tract.

Epidemiology
- Common with over 250 000 new cases worldwide.
- Can occur anywhere in the urothelial tract, but the vast majority arises in the bladder, then the renal pelvis, then the ureters (50:3:1, respectively).

Aetiology
- Cigarette smoking.
- Occupational exposure to aromatic amines.

Presentation
- Most present with haematuria.

Subtypes
- Non-invasive urothelial carcinoma (low-grade and high-grade).
- Invasive urothelial carcinoma.
- Urothelial carcinoma *in situ* (CIS).

Genetics
- Low-grade, non-invasive urothelial carcinomas show relatively few genetic alterations, the most common being losses of chromosome 9.
- High-grade, non-invasive urothelial carcinomas, invasive urothelial carcinomas, and urothelial CIS are genetically unstable lesions with many chromosomal aberrations, including *TP53* and *RB* mutations.

Non-invasive papillary urothelial carcinoma
- Macroscopically appear as exophytic frond-like masses.
- Histologically composed of atypical urothelium growing in papillary fronds. Low-grade tumours show mild disorganization and low-grade nuclear atypia. High-grade tumours show marked disorganization and high-grade nuclear atypia.

Invasive urothelial carcinoma
- Macroscopically appear as solid masses which infiltrate into underlying tissues.
- Histologically composed of an atypical urothelium growing as tumour nests infiltrating into the bladder wall.
- Tumours showing divergent differentiation (usually squamous or glandular) show more aggressive biology.
- Immunohistochemically show a CK7+ p63+ GATA3+ phenotype.

Urothelial carcinoma *in situ*
- Macroscopically may be invisible or manifest as an erythematous area of mucosa.
- Histologically, a flat lesion in which the urothelium displays unequivocally high-grade nuclear atypia.

Urine cytology

- Poorly sensitive at picking up low-grade urothelial carcinomas.
- Good at detecting high-grade lesions where shed severely atypical urothelial cells can be visualized due to their large pleomorphic nuclei with dark coarsely granular chromatin.

Prognosis

- All show a tendency to multifocality and recurrence.
- Non-invasive, low-grade papillary urothelial carcinomas carry a very low risk of progression to invasion and death (<5%).
- Non-invasive, high-grade papillary urothelial carcinomas and urothelial CIS carry a much higher risk of progression.
- The prognosis of infiltrating urothelial carcinoma is mostly dependent on disease stage.

Benign prostatic hyperplasia

Definition
- Enlargement of the prostate gland due to an increase in cell number.

Epidemiology
- Very common.
- Symptomatic disease affects ~3% of men aged 45–49, rising to nearly 25% of men by age 80.
- Histological evidence is present in 90% of men by age 80.

Aetiology
- Unclear.

Pathogenesis
- Androgens are critical in the development of BPH, more specifically increased levels of dihydrotestosterone locally in the prostate.
- Current evidence suggests that increased oestrogen levels in blood (which rise with age) induce androgen receptors in prostate tissue and stimulate hyperplasia.

Presentation
- Frequency, urgency, nocturia, hesitancy, poor flow, and terminal dribbling (collectively known as lower urinary tract symptoms or 'LUTS').
- Some patients present with UTI, acute urinary retention, or renal failure.

Macroscopy
- The prostate shows nodular enlargement which usually involves the transition zone.
- There is a poor correlation between the size of the prostate and the severity of symptoms.

Histopathology
- There is nodular proliferation of epithelial and stromal elements of the prostate.
- The proportion of epithelial and stromal elements varies considerably between cases, with some being predominantly epithelial and some being predominantly stromal.

Complications
- Urinary retention.
- Recurrent UTIs.
- Bladder stones.
- Obstructive nephropathy.

Prostate carcinoma

Definition
- A malignant epithelial tumour arising in the prostate.

Epidemiology
- The most common malignant tumour in men, accounting for about 25% of all male cancers.
- About 1 in 8 men will develop prostate cancer in their lifetime.
- Prevalence rising due to longer life expectancy and increased detection rates.
- A less prominent cause of cancer-related deaths, as many cases behave in a relatively indolent fashion.

Aetiology
- Racial background and genetic factors are important, with a 5- to 10-fold increased risk in men with two or more affected first-degree relatives.
- Dietary association with animal products, particularly red meat.

Carcinogenesis
- Arises from a precursor lesion known as **prostatic intraepithelial neoplasia** (PIN), characterized by neoplastic transformation of the epithelium lining of the prostatic ducts and acini.
- Harbour mutations in a number of genes, including *GST-pi, PTEN, AMACR, p27,* and *E-cadherin* (note these are not classical tumour suppressor genes or oncogenes).

Presentation
- The vast majority of prostate cancers are diagnosed early following investigation of a raised serum prostate-specific antigen (PSA) level.
- More advanced localized disease may be present with a suspicious-feeling prostate on digital rectal examination or lower urinary tract symptoms.
- Rarely, patients present with symptoms of metastatic disease.

Diagnosis
- Patients with raised PSA are usually referred for MRI of the prostate to identify suspicious areas that may be targeted for biopsy.
- Prostate biopsy may be performed via a transperineal or transrectal route. The transperineal route carries a much lower risk of introducing infection into the prostate gland.

Histopathology
- The most common type of prostate cancer is acinar adenocarcinoma, in which the malignant epithelial cells form glandular structures.
- One of the key diagnostic features of prostate cancer is the abnormal architecture of the malignant glands which are crowded and show infiltration between benign glands and ducts.
- Malignant epithelial cells have enlarged nuclei with prominent nucleoli and denser amphophilic cytoplasm.

- Malignant glands often have intraluminal crystalloids (dense crystal-like structures), amorphous pink secretions, or blue-tinged mucin.

Gleason scoring

- Prostate cancers are graded using the Gleason scoring system.
- Gleason **scores** are expressed in the format $x + y = z$ and are based on the two most common Gleason **patterns** present in the tumour.
- Gleason patterns range from 1 to 5 and are based on the architectural growth of the tumour.
- In practice, patterns 1 and 2 are never diagnosed, and so all prostate cancers have a Gleason score of between 6 and 10.
- Gleason pattern 3 is composed of well-formed discrete glandular units (Fig. 11.3).
- Gleason pattern 4 is composed of poorly formed, fused, or cribriform glands (Fig. 11.4).
- Gleason pattern 5 is composed of solid sheets, cords, or single cells showing no glandular differentiation.

Immunohistochemistry

- Prostate cancer cells are typically positive for PSA and CK7 whilst being negative for CK20.
- Basal cell markers (e.g. p63 or cytokeratin 5, are often used to confirm a morphological diagnosis of prostate cancer by demonstrating absence of basal cells around the cancer glands).

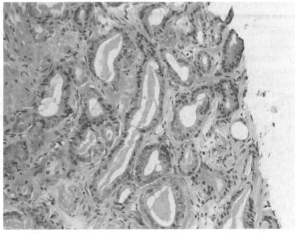

Fig 11.3 Gleason pattern 3 prostate adenocarcinoma composed of individual well-formed glandular acini (see Plate 33).

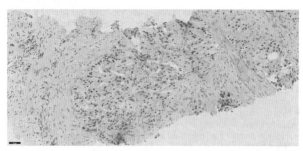

Fig. 11.4 Gleason pattern 4 prostate adenocarcinoma composed of fused poorly formed glands (see Plate 34).

Prognosis
- The Gleason score is a powerful prognostic indicator, with a higher score associated with a worse outcome.
- Other important factors include the serum PSA level and the stage of the disease.

Prostate cancer screening
- Screening using serum PSA is a controversial subject.
- At present, most countries do not operate an organized prostate screening programme.
- Current evidence suggests that screening would result in overdiagnosis and overtreatment of many men with prostate cancers that are unlikely to behave in an aggressive manner.

Prostate cancer grade groups

The WHO have adopted a new grading system for prostate cancer that simplifies the existing Gleason scoring system into a 5-point system:

Gleason score	Grade group
3 + 3 = 6	1
3 + 4 = 7	2
4 + 3 = 7	3
4 + 4 = 8	4
9 or 10	5

Testicular germ cell tumours

Definition
- A group of malignant tumours of the testis arising from germ cells.

Epidemiology
- >90% of all testicular tumours are germ cell tumours.
- Most arise in young men aged from 20 to 45.

Aetiology
- The most consistent risk factor is the presence of cryptorchidism
  (➲ Cryptorchidism, p. 251), which increases the risk by 3- to 5-fold.
- Other prenatal risk factors include low birthweight and small-for-gestational age.
- No consistent adulthood risk factors have been identified.

Carcinogenesis
- Most germ cell tumours arise from a precursor lesion known as **germ cell neoplasia *in situ*** (**GCNIS**), characterized by the presence of neoplastic germ cells confined to the seminiferous tubules.
- It is likely that the malignant process begins in foetal life and that GCNIS is present during childhood and young adulthood, during which time further genetic aberrations lead to malignant transformation.
- One consistently observed structural chromosomal aberration is gain of 12p sequences.

Presentation
- Most patients present with a painless testicular lump.
- ~10% present with symptoms related to metastatic disease, most commonly back pain from retroperitoneal lymph node metastases or cough/dyspnoea from pulmonary metastases.

Serum tumour markers
- AFP is typically associated with the presence of yolk sac elements.
- β-human chorionic gonadotrophin (HCG) is associated with the presence of syncytiotrophoblastic cells; these may be present individually within a pure seminoma or as an integral component of a choriocarcinoma.

Macroscopy
- Pure seminomas tend to produce lobulated tan lesions (Fig. 11.5).
- Teratomas often show cystic and solid areas.
- Mixed tumours tend to have a variegated appearance.

Histopathology
- **Seminoma** is composed of sheets or nests of polygonal cells with clear or eosinophilic cytoplasm and round nuclei containing one or two nucleoli. A lymphocytic infiltrate is commonly present within the tumour.
- **Teratoma** is composed of tissues resembling immature fetal-type tissues and/or mature adult-type tissues.

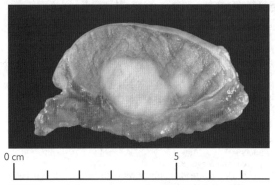

Fig 11.5 This is a testis from a young man who presented with an enlarging testicular lump. Following an ultrasound scan which was suspicious for a neoplasm, he underwent orchidectomy. The testis has been sliced in the pathology department, revealing this white solid mass in the testis. This appearance is typical of a seminoma, and microscopic examination confirmed this (see Plate 35).

Reproduced with permission from *Clinical Pathology* (Oxford Core Texts), Carton, James, Daly, Richard, and Ramani, Pramila, Oxford University Press (2006), p. 244, Figure 11.14.

- **Embryonal carcinoma** is composed of anaplastic cells with large vesicular nuclei containing large nucleoli. The tumours may grow in solid sheets or form glandular structures.
- **Yolk sac tumour** is composed of small mildly pleomorphic cells which form a wide variety of architectural patterns, of which the most common are reticular and microcystic.
- **Choriocarcinoma** is composed of a mixture of syncytiotrophoblastic and cytotrophoblastic cells. There is often extensive haemorrhage and necrosis.

▶ Germ cell tumours may be composed entirely of one subtype or a mixture of different subtypes.

Immunohistochemistry

- Seminoma: Oct3/4$^+$ CD117$^+$ CD30$^-$ AE1/AE3$^-$.
- Embryonal carcinoma: Oct3/4$^+$ CD117$^-$ CD30$^+$ AE1/AE3$^+$.
- Yolk sac tumour: Oct3/4$^-$ Glypican 3$^+$ AFP$^+$ HCG$^-$.
- Choriocarcinoma: Oct3/4$^-$ Gypican 3$^{+/-}$ AFP$^-$ HCG$^+$.

Prognosis

- Excellent 5-year survival rates of ~98% in most countries.
- This reflects the high sensitivity of germ cell tumours to modern platinum-based chemotherapeutic regimes.

Testicular non-germ cell tumours

Testicular lymphomas
- ~5% of all testicular tumours.
- Mostly seen in elderly men.
- The testis is usually replaced by a large grey/tan mass which may extend into the cord.
- Histologically, the most common type is **diffuse large B-cell lymphoma** (⊃ Diffuse large B-cell lymphoma, p. 452).
- Survival is generally poor.

Leydig cell tumour
- A sex cord stromal tumour which accounts for ~3% of all testicular tumours.
- May occur at any age.
- Prepubertally, they tend to present with signs of precocious puberty due to androgen production.
- Post-pubertally, they present with a testicular mass.
- Macroscopically, they are well-circumscribed tumours, often with a brown cut surface.
- Histologically, they are composed of sheets or nests of polygonal cells with eosinophilic cytoplasm and round nuclei with a single nucleolus. Reinke's crystals (rhomboid-shaped, intracytoplasmic crystals) may be seen.
- The majority of Leydig cell tumours behave in a benign fashion; however, ~10% show malignant behaviour.
- Histology is not always entirely reliable at predicting which tumours will behave aggressively; however, worrying findings include tumour size >5 cm, necrosis, vascular invasion, cellular pleomorphism, and raised mitotic activity.

Sertoli cell tumour
- A sex cord stromal tumour which accounts for ~1% of all testicular tumours.
- Most present as a testicular mass in young and middle-aged men.
- Macroscopically, they are usually solid yellow or white tumours.
- Histologically, they are composed of oval cells forming hollow or solid tubular structures.
- ~10% of tumours are malignant; similar histological criteria are used to predict malignant behaviour as for Leydig cell tumours.

Paratesticular diseases

Epididymal cyst
- Benign cystic lesion of the epididymis.
- Usually presents as a small paratesticular swelling which may be tender.
- Grossly appears as a thin-walled, translucent cystic lesion.
- Histologically, the cyst is lined by a thin attenuated layer of bland epithelial cells.

Epididymitis
- Usually results from an ascending infection from the lower urinary tract.
- In young men <35 y, it is usually due to a sexually transmitted infection such as *Chlamydia trachomatis* or *Neisseria gonorrhoeae*.
- In men >35 y, it is usually due to *E. coli*.

Varicocele
- A persistent abnormal dilation of the pampiniform venous plexus in the spermatic cord.
- More common on the left side where the testicular vein drains into the renal vein.
- Usually presents with nodularity on the lateral side of the scrotum.
- Some cause a dull ache, especially after prolonged standing or towards the end of the day.
- May contribute to male subfertility, as the increased blood flow raises the scrotal temperature and impairs spermatogenesis.

Hydrocele
- An abnormal accumulation of fluid in the space between the two layers of the tunica vaginalis.
- A common cause of scrotal swelling.
- Usually caused by trauma or a reaction to an underlying pathology such as epididymitis, orchitis, or a tumour.

Adenomatoid tumour
- The most common benign paratesticular neoplasm.
- Can occur in the epididymis, spermatic cord, and tunica albuginea.
- Most present in young adults.
- Grossly, they are small solid, firm, grey/white tumours which are usually <3 cm.
- Histologically, they are composed of dilated tubular structures lined by attenuated mesothelial cells.

Paratesticular sarcomas
- Rare, but well-recognized, paratesticular tumours.
- The two most common types are **well-differentiated liposarcoma** in adults and **embryonal rhabdomyosarcoma** in children/adolescents.

Urethral diseases

Urethritis

- Usually caused by sexually transmitted infections.
- Divided into gonococcal and non-gonococcal urethritis.
- Non-gonococcal urethritis is more common and most are caused by *C. trachomatis*. Patients typically describe a sensation of urethral 'itching'.
- Gonococcal urethritis is due to infection with *N. gonorrhoeae*. Patients tend to present with a more purulent discharge and dysuria.
- Gram staining of urethral discharge can detect *N. gonorrhoeae* as intracellular Gram-negative diplococci. If these organisms are not detected, but numerous neutrophils confirm a urethritis, then non-gonococcal urethritis is presumed.
- Detection of *C. trachomatis* is usually by molecular methods, as culture is slow and unreliable.

Prostatic epithelial polyp

- Lesion of the prostatic urethra containing prostatic epithelium.
- Typically presents with haematuria.
- Grossly appears as a papillary lesion projecting into the prostatic urethra.
- Histologically composed of crowded collections of prostatic-type glands covered by urothelium.

Urethral caruncle

- Relatively common polypoid lesion of the distal urethra in women.
- Presents with dysuria and spotty bleeding.
- The caruncle is visible as a polypoid mass at the urethral meatus.
- Histologically, it contains a dense inflammatory cell infiltrate rich in blood vessels and is covered by hyperplastic epithelium.

Urethral carcinomas

- These are rare, but more common in women.
- Often present at a high stage with poor prognosis.
- Most are squamous cell carcinomas (70%) and arise in the distal urethra near the meatus.
- The others are either urothelial carcinomas (20%) or adenocarcinomas (10%) and tend to arise in the proximal urethra.

Malignant melanoma

- Rare, but recognized, tumour in the urethra.
- Grossly, they appear as polypoid or ulcerated urethral masses.
- Histologically, they are composed of atypical epithelioid or spindled cells. Frequently amelanotic, which can lead to diagnostic difficulty.
- Immunohistochemical reactivity of the malignant cells for melanocytic markers (S100, HMB-45, Melan-A) helps to clinch the diagnosis.

Penile diseases

Lichen sclerosus

- Penile lichen sclerosus (balanitis xerotica obliterans) is an inflammatory disease that usually affects the foreskin or glans penis.
- Most cases present in adulthood with phimosis.
- Macroscopically, the affected areas appear white and atrophic.
- Histologically, there is a band of oedematous hyalinized fibrosis and lymphocytic inflammation beneath the surface epithelium.
- Long-standing untreated disease can lead to squamous dysplasia and squamous cell carcinoma.

Lichen planus

- Penile involvement is commonly seen in patients with generalized lichen planus (→ Lichen planus, p. 480).
- The lesions often involve the glans penis.
- Histology shows a band-like inflammatory infiltrate of lymphocytes beneath the epithelium with features of basal cell damage.

Zoon's balanitis

- Usually presents as a solitary red area in uncircumcised elderly men.
- Clinically mimics penile Bowen's disease.
- Histology shows thinning of the epidermis with spongiosis and an underlying band-like inflammatory infiltrate rich in plasma cells.

Condylomas

- Caused by human papillomavirus (HPV) infection, usually types 6 and 11. Seen mostly in sexually active young men.
- Macroscopically, condylomas appear as either flat or frond-like papillary growths.
- Histologically, they show a papillomatous squamous proliferation with koilocytes (keratinocytes showing viral cytopathic changes).

Peyronie's disease

- Also known as penile fibromatosis, but probably unrelated to other forms of fibromatosis.
- Presents between ages 40 and 60 with thickening of the corpus cavernosa, leading to penile pain and curvature on erection.
- Histological examination of excised tissue shows hypocellular collagenous scar tissue with aggregates of chronic inflammatory cells.

Penile carcinoma

- Rare malignancy, usually arising on the glans penis of elderly men.
- Risk factors include HPV infection, smoking, phimosis, and long-standing lichen sclerosus. Circumcision is associated with a reduction in risk.
- Macroscopically, they are exophytic masses which may ulcerate.
- Histologically, the majority are squamous cell carcinomas which arise from areas of squamous dysplasia (sometimes termed penile intraepithelial neoplasia).

Scrotal diseases

Epidermoid cysts

- Common cause of a scrotal skin lump.
- Macroscopically, they contain yellow keratinous debris.
- Histologically, they are lined by squamous epithelium showing epidermoid-type keratinization.

Scrotal calcinosis

- An uncommon disorder in which multiple calcified nodules develop in the scrotal skin.
- The calcification is thought to be dystrophic in type and probably represents calcification of old epidermoid cysts.

Angiokeratomas

- Benign vascular lesions which usually present as multiple small blue/red lesions of the scrotal skin.
- Histologically, they are composed of dilated vascular channels in the papillary dermis, associated with hyperplasia and hyperkeratosis of the overlying epidermis.

Fournier's gangrene

- A clinical variant of necrotizing fasciitis (➍ Necrotizing fasciitis, p. 494) which involves the penis, scrotum, perineum, and abdominal wall in men.
- Main risk factors are diabetes and immunosuppression.
- Usually, a polymicrobial infection caused by a mixture of aerobic and anaerobic bacteria.
- Histology shows a severe necrotizing inflammatory process involving the skin and deep subcutaneous tissue.
- Mortality is in the order of 15–20%.

Scrotal squamous cell carcinoma

- A very rare malignancy.
- Mostly of historical interest due to its association with occupational exposure to carcinogens in chimney workers.

Chapter 12

Gynaecological pathology

Vulval skin diseases

Inflammatory Diseases of Vulvar Skin
Human Papillomavirus Infection
Herpesvirus Infection
Varicella (Herpes Zoster)
Cytomegalovirus Infection
Epstein–Barr Virus Infection
Molluscum Contagiosum
Syphilis
Granuloma Inguinale
Lymphogranuloma Venereum
Chancroid
HIV-Associated Vulva Ulcers
Tuberculosis
Fungal Infection
Parasitic Infections

Non-infectious Papulosquamous Dermatoses
Lichen Sclerosus
Lichen Simplex Chronicus
Lichen Planus
Psoriasis
Contact Dermatitis
Atopic Dermatitis
Fixed Drug Eruption
Plasma Cell Vulvitis
Behcet Syndrome
Crohn's Disease
Necrotizing Fasciitis
Hidradenitis Suppurativa
Mites, Lice, and Spider Bite

Infectious disorders of vulva

Human Papilloma virus (HPV)
- Human papillomavirus (HPV) infection is Responsible for benign tumours, that is, condylomata acuminata and precursor lesions of certain types of vulvar carcinoma Warty lesions related to low-risk HPV infection (types 6 or 11).
- Histologically, they show papillary squamous proliferations with koilocytes.
- Widespread condylomas may be seen in the immunosuppressed.

Herpesvirus infection (HSV)
- Mainly HSV-2 involves genital mucosa but may be caused by HSV-1.
- Presentation frequently includes dysuria, urinary retention, vulvar pain/painful shallow ulcers with a mild inguinal lymphadenopathy, generalized malaise, and fever.

- Histology shows vesicles/ulcer with sharply demarcated crater characteristic of 'ground glass' nuclei, and typical eosinophilic intranuclear inclusion body are seen.
- Cytologic evaluation of the scraping of the base and edges of ulcer or vesicle (Tzank preparation), shows the multinucleated cells with viral cytopathic effects.
  - Other viruses that may cause ulcerated vulvovaginitis similar to HSV with viral cytopathic inclusions include **herpes zoster**, **CMV**, **and Epstein–Barr virus (EBV)**. Infection is more common in immunocompromised individuals. Viral cultures, immunoperoxidase studies using specific antibodies or polymerase chain reaction (PCR) may be used for establishing the diagnosis.

Molluscum contagiosum
- Pox virus infection which is highly contagious and spread by direct skin to skin contact.
- Usually asymptomatic or pruritic papule with a central umbilication.
- Cytologic identification of the typical eosinophilic intracytoplasmic inclusion bodies (Henderson–Paterson bodies) within scrapings is diagnostic.
- Histology shows acanthosis and the characteristic intracytoplasmic viral inclusions.
- Most lesions regress spontaneously.

Syphilis
- Venereal disease caused by the spirochete Treponema pallidum.
- Three stages:
  - Primary lesion is the chancre. Chancre is a painless, indurated, shallow, clean-based ulcer with raised edges.
  - Secondary lesion is the condylomata lata. These are papular/elevated plaques which mimic condylomata acuminate.
  - Tertiary gumma of syphilis is rarely seen on the vulva.
- Diagnosis is difficult from histologic material alone as the findings are non-specific. There is marked acanthosis, hyperkeratosis and inflammatory response within the dermis which is predominantly plasma cell inflammatory infiltrate with arteritis that may result in obliteration.
- Dieterle, Warthin–Starry, or Steiner stain or specific immunocytochemistry antibodies may be used to identify the organism on tissue sections.
- The fluorescent treponemal antibody-absorbed (FTA-ABS) test is the 'gold standard'.
- In diagnosis. Alternatives include Treponemal enzyme immunoassays (EIAs), PCR, and immunoblotting.
- 30% of patients with primary syphilis undergo spontaneous remission. Untreated patients may progress to tertiary syphilis with cardiovascular and central nervous system effects and is fatal in 10% of those afflicted.

Granuloma inguinale (granuloma venereum)
- Caused by Calymmatobacterium granulomatous, a Gram-negative, encapsulated bacteria.
- Primary lesions may occur on the vulva, vagina, or cervix.
- Present as painless papules or necrotizing ulcers with rolled borders.

- Chronic lymphatic infiltration and fibrosis frequently result in a massive brawny oedema of the external genitalia.
- Diagnosis is best accomplished by preparing smears or a biopsy from the edge of the ulcer demonstrating Donovan bodies. These can be highlighted by a Warthin–Starry stain or Giemsa stain.

Lymphogranuloma venereum (LGV)
- Caused by chlamydia and is more frequent in men.
- Presents as erosion of the skin which progresses to adenitis with may evolve into painful groin nodes/buboes, that may rupture with exudation of a purulent discharge. This finally leads to fibrosis and destruction with chronic lymphatic obstruction is responsible for the characteristic non-pitting oedema of the external genitalia.
- Histology of LGV is not diagnostic and reveals no characteristic identifiable organisms. There is intense superficial and deep chronic inflammatory comprising predominantly lymphocytes, plasma cells, and giant cells.
- Diagnosis is based on the typical clinical presentation, along with positive complement fixation tests. Culture and specific immunohistochemical tests, can assist in the diagnosis of LGV.

Chancroid
- Caused by Haemophilus ducreyi, a Gram-negative bacillus.
- Presents with single or multiple, small ulcers with or without tender inguinal adenopathy.
- Histologic examination shows granulomatous reaction with chronic inflammatory.
- Cells mainly lymphocytes and plasma cells, and the presence of the Gram-negative organisms, in parallel chains.
- Skin tests and biopsies are not diagnostic. Identification of the organism by culture is necessary for accurate diagnosis.

Human immunodeficiency virus (HIV)
Human immunodeficiency virus may play a local role in causation or exacerbation due to secondary infection by bacteria, cytomegalovirus, Chlamydia trachomatis, or Gardnerella vaginalis. Multiple and painful ulcers may be seen.

Tuberculosis
- Caused by Mycobacterium tuberculosis or atypical mycobacteria.
- Usually associated with tuberculosis of other genital sites, primarily the fallopian tube, and endometrium.
- Caseating granulomas with Langhans giant cells are found, and acid-fast stains usually reveal the mycobacterium.
- Confirmation of the diagnosis can be made by culture techniques/PCR.

Fungal infection
- Candida and dermatophytes are frequent pathogens.
- Histologic findings usually are not diagnostic. Silver stains for fungus may demonstrate fungal organisms within the keratin.
- diagnosis generally can be accomplished by microscopic examination of skin scrapings in 10% potassium hydroxide, or by appropriate culture methods.

Other Uncommon infections

- Erythrasma is a chronic bacterial infection, usually seen in obese diabetics. *Corynebacterium minutissimum*, the causative organism, shows a coral-red fluorescence under Wood's light.
- Eggs/larvae of parasites like *Enterobius vermicularis* (pinworm, seatworm), *Schistosoma mansoni*, and *Cutaneous myiasis* may cause pruritic vulvitis.

Non-infectious papulosquamous dermatoses

Eczema

- Commonly occurs on vulval skin.
- Seborrhoeic dermatitis and irritant contact dermatitis are the two most frequent types.
- These have similar appearances to elsewhere on the skin (❸ Eczema, p. 478).

Lichen simplex chronicus

- Thickened patches of skin which probably represent a non-specific reaction to chronic itching.
- The labium majora is the predominant site on the vulva.
- Histologically, there is epidermal thickening with overlying hyperkeratosis with mild fibrosis in the dermis.

Psoriasis

- Vulval psoriasis is typically of flexural type with marked erythema and absence of scaling.
- Typical histology shows regular psoriasiform epidermal hyperplasia with plaques of parakeratosis and loss of the granular layer. Neutrophils are present within parakeratosis.
- Vulval psoriasis may, however, show atypical histology, making the diagnosis more difficult to make.

Lichen planus

- May be found in patients with generalized disease (❸ Lichen planus, p. 480) or restricted to the genital region.
- The lesions are purple, flat-topped, shiny papules. Erosive disease may occur which can lead to scarring.
- Histologically, there is a band-like inflammatory cell infiltrate containing lymphocytes, histiocytes, and plasma cells. The overlying epidermis shows basal cell damage and may be thickened or atrophic.
- Lichen planus carries a small increased risk of development of vulval intraepithelial neoplasia (VIN) and squamous cell carcinoma.

Lichen sclerosus

- An inflammatory dermatosis of unknown cause, with a predilection for the anogenital skin of women.
- Clinically, there are white papules and plaques with a wrinkled surface. There may be areas of atrophy and haemorrhage. Itching, burning, and dyspareunia are common symptoms.
- Histologically, the epidermis is thinned and there is interface change. There is a band of hyalinization beneath the epidermis and an underlying chronic inflammatory cell infiltrate.
- Lichen sclerosus carries a small increase of development of VIN and squamous cell carcinoma.

Pigmentation disorders of vulva

Pigment Disorders of Melanocytic Origin
Lentigo Simplex
Vulvar Melanosis
Congenital and Giant Nevomelanocytic Nevi
Junctional, Compound, and Intradermal Nevi
Atypical Vulvar Nevi
Dysplastic Nevi
Acanthosis Nigricans and Pseudoacanthosis Nigricans

Depigmentation and Hypopigmented Disorders
Vitiligo
Albinism
Postinflammatory Depigmentation (Leukoderma)

These have similar appearances to elsewhere on the skin and hence the histology and detailed description is not included in this chapter. Some interesting features are listed here:

- Lentigo simplex is the most common hyperpigmented lesion occurring on the vulva. This is of clinical significance except for the rare LEOPARD syndrome, characterized by abnormalities of skin, heart, inner ears and genitalia, in which thousands of lentigines are present all over the body.
- Vulvar melanosis typically occurs in women of reproductive age and the lesions are typically larger than those of lentigo. There is slight or no increase in the number of melanocytes.
- Congenital nevi are found in approximately 10% of newborns and usually are less than 4 mm in diameter.
- Giant nevomelanocytic nevi are 20 cm or more in diameter (garment type). These have an increased risk of developing malignant melanoma in prepubertal individuals.
- Most naevi biopsied on the vulva are either compound or intradermal in type. Vulval naevi are influenced by hormonal changes and appear more active or atypical during pregnancy.
- In adults, acanthosis nigricans may be associated with adenocarcinoma of the stomach or other visceral malignancies. Its presentation should prompt the search for gastric and other tumours, especially if it occurs with sudden onset and is associated with pruritus and the appearance of multiple seborrheic keratosis (Leser–Trelet syndrome).
- Amongst the hypopigmented disorders, vitiligo and albinism are an inherited genetic disorder whilst leukoderma occurs secondary to inflammation and ulceration, usually following herpes, syphilis, burns, deep laser, or cryotherapy. Vitiligo is characterized by absence of both basilar melanocytes and melanin granules whereas in albinism there is an inability of the melanocytes to produce pigment (i.e. melanin granules. Leukoderma temporarily lack a normal population of melanocytes secondary to scarring).

Bullous disorders of vulva

Bullous Diseases
Pemphigus (Pemphigus Vulgaris)
Pemphigus Vegetans
Pemphigoid (Bullous Pemphigoid)
Herpes Gestationis
Darier Disease (Keratosis Follicularis)
Warty Dyskeratoma
Erythema Multiforme (Stevens–Johnson Syndrome)
Hailey–Hailey Disease (Familial Benign Pemphigus)
Benign Chronic Bullous Disease of Childhood (Linear IgA Disease)

Cysts of vulva

> **Cysts of Vulva**
> Bartholin's Cyst
> Keratinous Cyst (epithelial inclusion cyst)
> Mucous Cyst
> Apocrine Hidrocystoma/Cystadenoma of the Vulva
> Ciliated Cysts of the Vulvar Vestibule/Vestibular Adenosis
> Mesonephric-like Cyst
> Mammary-like Cyst
> Cyst of the Canal of Nuck (mesothelial cyst)

Bartholin's cyst

- Arise due to obstruction of the vestibular orifice of the Bartholin's gland duct and accumulation of secretions.
- Usually present as painless lumps in the lateral wall of the vaginal opening (introitus) in young women.
- Histologically, they are lined by a transitional-type epithelium with areas of squamous metaplasia.
- Treatment involves excision or permanent opening (marsupialization) of the cyst.

Keratinous cyst (epithelial inclusion cyst)

- They may occur at any age, even in newborns especially in children undergoing female circumcision.
- Usually superficial and range in size from 2 to 5 mm.
- Contain a white to pale yellow, grumous, or cheesy material without hair and are lined by stratified squamous epithelium.

Ciliated cysts of the vulvar vestibule/vestibular adenosis

- Lined with tuboendometrial epithelium resembling mullerian-type epithelium.
- Reported in women with chronic inflammation associated with Stevens–Johnson syndrome or with extensive laser or 5-FU therapy.

The other less common cysts originate in various embryological derivatives, such as mucous cyst (urogenital sinus endoderm), mesonephric-like (Wolffian duct remnants), mammary-like (anogenital mammary-like sweat glands), cyst of the canal of Nuck (inclusions of the peritoneum/mesothelium at the inferior insertion of the round ligament into the labia majora).

Benign vulval tumours

Benign Solid Tumours and Tumour-like Lesions

Benign Squamous Epithelial Tumours
Fibroepithelial Polyp (Acrochordon)
Seborrheic Keratosis

Glandular Tumours
Papillary/Nodular Hidradenoma (Hidradenoma Papilliferum)
Syringoma
Mixed Tumour of the Vulva (Pleomorphic Adenoma/Chondroid Syringoma)
Trichoepithelioma
Endometriosis
Angiokeratoma
Pyogenic Granuloma

Mesenchymal Tumours
Angiomyofibroblastoma
Cellular Angiofibroma
Deep (Aggressive) Angiomyxoma

Fibroepithelial polyp (acrochordon)

- Also known as skin tag.
- These are usually small, flesh-coloured, or hyperpigmented, papillomatous growths resembling condylomata or nevi but may be large and pedunculated.
- Lined by keratinized, stratified squamous epithelium with fibrovascular core and blood vessels.

Papillary hidradenoma

- Benign sweat gland tumour which usually presents in middle-aged women as a small, painless lump on the labia majora or minora.
- Histologically, they are well-circumscribed papillary tumours of the dermis. The epithelium covering the papillae is double-layered, with inner tall columnar cells and outer small myoepithelial cells.

Granular cell tumour

- Tumour of neural Schwann cell origin that may occur in the vulva.
- Histologically composed of nests of large polygonal cells with abundant granular cytoplasm.
- The vast majority behave in a benign fashion.

Angiomyofibroblastoma

- Benign mesenchymal neoplasm that occurs almost exclusively in the vulvovaginal region of young women.
- Presents as a small subcutaneous lump, often mistaken for a cyst.

- Histologically, they are well-circumscribed lesions composed of dilated capillary-sized ves+sels set in an oedematous stroma containing many plump epithelioid stromal cells.

Cellular angiofibroma

- Benign mesenchymal neoplasm presenting as a small, painless subcutaneous mass in the vulvovaginal area.
- Occur in reproductive and post-menopausal age groups.
- Histologically, they are well-circumscribed cellular lesions composed of bland spindle cells and small, thick-walled blood vessels.

Deep (aggressive) angiomyxoma

- Locally infiltrative, but non-metastasizing, mesenchymal neoplasm that presents as a large, deep-seated mass in the pelvis and perineum of reproductive age women.
- Histologically, they are infiltrative, paucicellular tumours composed of small numbers of bland spindle cells set in a myxoid stroma containing thick-walled blood vessels.

Vulval carcinoma

Definition

- A malignant epithelial tumour arising in the vulva.
- Almost all are squamous cell carcinoma (SCC).
- Less commonly adenocarcinoma arising from Bartholin's gland, mammary gland, sweat gland, extramammary Pagets disease, or intestinal-type adenocarcinoma is seen.

Epidemiology

- Rare with an age-standardized annual incidence of 4 per 100 000.
- 1300 cases per year; 20th most common cancer in UK females.
- Most arise in women >65 y, but it can occur in younger women.

Aetiology

- HPV-associated SCC: most cases arising in younger women are linked to high-risk HPV infection of the vulva. Cigarette smoking and immunocompromised status are associated with an increased risk.
- HPV-independent SCC: some are linked to chronic vulval inflammatory disorders such as lichen sclerosus or lichen planus.

Carcinogenesis

- The precursors of SCC are divided into HPV-associated and HPV-independent lesions.
- The **HPV-associated lesions** are designated as squamous intraepithelial lesions (SILs), in keeping with the unified lower anogenital squamous terminology (LAST) standardization project recommendations. They are divided into low-grade SIL (LSIL) and high-grade SIL (HSIL). The two-tiered LSIL/HSIL system has better reproducibility and enhanced biological relevance compared to the three-tiered VIN 1/2/3 system. In the UK, the three-tiered system is used in conjunction with LAST terminology with HSILs constituting both VIN-2 and VIN-3.
- HPV-independent precursors are termed as '**HPV-independent vulvar intraepithelial neoplasia (VIN)**'. This includes differentiated VIN and two recently described lesions known as differentiated exophytic vulvar intraepithelial lesion (DEVIL) and vulvar acanthosis with altered differentiation (VAAD).
- Despite its subtle appearance, HPV-independent VIN has a high risk and shorter course of progression to malignant transformation. *TP53* mutations are frequently identified.

Macroscopy

- Firm nodule, warty mass, or ulcerated with raised firm edges.

Histopathology

- Almost all cases are **squamous cell carcinomas**, composed of infiltrating malignant epithelial cells showing squamous differentiation.
- The squamous epithelium adjacent to the tumour often shows VIN.

Prognosis

- The most important prognostic indicators are tumour size, depth of invasion, involvement of adjacent structures, and extent of lymph node metastasis.
- Tumours with depth of invasion ≤1 mm have a very low risk of lymph node metastasis and a good chance of cure following local excision.
- The 5-year survival rates in patients with unilateral lymph node disease is 65%, whereas with bilateral disease it falls to 25%.
- FIGO staging system is usually employed for vulval carcinoma, the most recent being the 2021 update.

Metastatic tumours

- Metastasis to the vulva is rare and accounts for 5–10% of all vulvar malignancies.
- May be grossly undetectable or present as single or multiple nodules that may be ulcerated.
- Most common primary sites include breast, gastrointestinal, or bladder. Pagetoid spread of rectal or bladder carcinoma to the lower genital may mimic vulvar Paget disease.
- Immunohistochemistry may help to confirm the diagnosis and the origin of the metastasis.

Non-neoplastic vaginal disorders

Developmental Disorders of Vagina
Lesions Related to *In Utero* Exposure to DES
Vaginal Epithelial Changes: Adenosis and Squamous Metaplasia
Imperforate Hymen
Vaginal Agenesis/Transverse Vaginal Septum
Epstein–Barr Virus Infection

Infectious Inflammatory Disorders
Vaginitis, Candida, Bacterial Vaginosis, Trichomonas Vaginalis, Acquired
Immunodeficiency Syndrome, Group B Streptococcus, Actinomycetes
Malakoplakia and Xanthogranulomatous Pseudotumour
Tuberculosis
Emphysematous Vaginitis
Toxic Shock Syndrome

Non-infectious Inflammatory Diseases
Desquamative Inflammatory Vaginitis
Crohn Disease
Bullous Dermatoses
Giant Cell Arteritis and Polyarteritis

Lesions That Follow Trauma, Surgery, and Radiation
Atrophic Vaginitis
Vaginal Vault Granulation Tissue
Fistula/Radionecrosis
Vaginal Prolapse/Fallopian Tube Prolapse
Postoperative Spindle Cell Nodule

Vaginal infections

Bacterial vaginosis

- Most common cause of an abnormal vaginal discharge.
- Occurs when the normal balance of vaginal bacteria is disrupted.
- Caused by overgrowth of anaerobic bacteria such as *Gardnerella vaginalis* and *Bacteroides* species.
- The metabolic products of these bacteria include volatile amines which give the discharge a distinctive fishy odour.
- There is no actual inflammation in the vaginal wall, hence why the term vaginosis is applied, rather than vaginitis.

Vulvovaginal candidosis

- Also known as 'thrush' or 'yeast infection'.
- Very common infection in young women caused by *Candida albicans*.
- Increased risk of occurrence if pregnant, diabetic, immunosuppressed, or taking contraceptive pill or antibiotics.
- The typical presentation is vulvovaginal itching and burning, dyspareunia, and dysuria. A thick, white ('cheesy') discharge is common.
- Diagnosed by a history of typical symptoms and discharge.
- The organism can also be cultured in the microbiology laboratory but is not usually necessary.

Trichomoniasis

- Sexually transmitted infection caused by the flagellate protozoan *Trichomonas vaginalis*.
- The male partner is usually asymptomatic and half of all affected women are also asymptomatic.
- Women with symptoms usually complain of vaginal itching and a thin, thick, or frothy yellow-green offensive discharge. Dyspareunia and dysuria may also occur.
- Wet mount microscopy of the discharge shows motile trichomonads.

Vaginal tumours

Cysts of Vagina
Squamous Inclusion Cyst
Mesonephric Cyst
Mullerian Cyst
Bartholin Gland Cyst

Benign Neoplasms
Condyloma Acuminatum
Fibroepithelial Polyp
Squamous Papilloma and Mullerian Papilloma
Leiomyoma
Rhabdomyoma
Endometriosis

Malignant Neoplasms
Squamous Cell Carcinoma
Clear Cell Adenocarcinoma
Embryonal Rhabdomyosarcoma (Sarcoma Botryoides)
Melanoma
Leiomyosarcoma
Malignant Mixed Tumour
Metastatic Tumour

Fibroepithelial stromal polyp
- Benign lesion of the distal female genital tract which most commonly involves the vagina but may also arise in the vulva.
- Hormonally responsive lesions which occur in reproductive age women as a small polypoid mass.
- Histologically, they are composed of a central fibrovascular core covered by hyperplastic squamous epithelium. Stellate and multinucleate stromal cells are typically seen within the core near the epithelial surface.

Vaginal leiomyoma
- Most common mesenchymal tumour of the vagina, but relatively rare.
- Derived from smooth muscle.
- Histologically composed of bundles of bland smooth muscle.
- Treated by local excision.

Genital rhabdomyoma
- Rare benign tumour showing skeletal muscle differentiation.
- Presents in middle-aged women as a nodule and may cause dyspareunia or bleeding.
- Histologically, it is composed of a haphazard proliferation of spindle cells with abundant brightly eosinophilic cytoplasm containing cross-striations.

Vaginal carcinoma

- Uncommon in comparison to cervical and vulval carcinomas.
- Most are squamous cell carcinomas which arise from a precursor dysplastic lesion known as Squamous intraepithelial lesions (SILs), also known as **vaginal intraepithelial neoplasia** (VAIN).
- Most arise in women over 50 years of age.
- Risk factors include HPV infection, smoking, and immunosuppression.
- Prognosis is generally poor, with 5-year survival rates of ~60%.

Embryonal rhabdomyosarcoma

- Rare malignant tumour showing skeletal muscle differentiation which can arise in the vagina of children.
- Most cases present in children <5 years old with vaginal bleeding. The tumour may be seen projecting through the vaginal opening.
- Macroscopically, the tumour is composed of oedematous 'grape-like' polypoid nodules projecting from the vaginal wall.
- Histologically, the tumour is composed of small, round, and spindled tumour cells condensed beneath the squamous epithelium of the vaginal wall. Some tumour cells have brightly eosinophilic cytoplasm; cytoplasmic cross-striations may be visible.
- Prognosis following treatment is generally excellent, with 10-year survival rates of >90%.

Non-neoplastic cervical disorders

Benign Tumours
Endocervical Polyps
Leiomyoma
Adenomyoma
Mesodermal Stromal Polyp
Placental Site Trophoblastic Nodule (PSN)
Miscellaneous Tumours—Haemangioma, Lymphangioma, Lipoma, etc.

Precursor Lesions
SIL (Squamous Intraepithelial Lesions)—Almost Always HPV Associated.
- LSIL (Low-grade Squamous Intraepithelial Lesions)—Condyloma/HPV Changes/CIN-1
- HSIL (High-grade Squamous Intraepithelial Lesions)—CIN-2 and CIN-3

CGIN/AIS (Cervical Glandular Intra-Epithelial Neoplasia/Adenocarcinoma In Situ)
- HPV Associated
- HPV Independent

Malignant Neoplasms
Squamous Cell Carcinoma
- HPV Associated
- HPV Independent
- Nos (Not Otherwise Specified)

Adenocarcinoma
- HPV Associated
- HPV Independent (Gastric/Clear Cell/Mesonephric and other Subtypes)

Other Epithelial Tumours—Carcinosarcomas, Glassy Cell Carcinoma, Mucoepidermoid Carcinoma, Adenosquamous Carcinoma, etc.
Mixed Epithelial and Mesenchymal Tumours—Adenosarcoma
Germ Cell Tumours
Metastatic Tumour

Cervical tumours

Inflammatory Diseases
Atypia of Repair
Radiation-Induced Atypia
Non-infectious Cervicitis
Infectious Cervicitis

Cysts
Nabothian Cyst
Tunnel Clusters
Inclusion Cyst

Tumour-Like Lesions
Decidual Pseudopolyp
Mullerian Papilloma
Postoperative Spindle Cell Nodule and Inflammatory Pseudotumour
Pseudoneoplastic Glandular Conditions
• Microglandular Endocervical Hyperplasia
• Mesonephric Hyperplasia
• Lobular Endocervical GlandularHyperplasia (LEGH)

Endometriosis
Lymphoma-like Lesions
Heterologous Tissue—Glia, Skin, Cartilage

Cervical carcinoma

Definition

- A malignant epithelial tumour arising in the cervix.

Epidemiology

- Worldwide, cervical carcinoma is the most common malignancy of the female genital tract and the fourth most common non-cutaneous malignancy in women following breast cancer.
- In developed countries, cervical carcinoma is the third most common malignancy of the female genital tract after endometrial and ovarian carcinomas. The lower incidence is largely attributable to the success of cervical screening programmes.

Aetiology

- Virtually all are caused by high-risk HPV infection (mostly types 16 and 18).
- Other risk factors include smoking and oral contraceptive use, which probably act by enhancing HPV persistence in the cervix.
▶ HPV vaccines are highly effective in preventing infection.

Carcinogenesis

- 80% are squamous cell carcinomas which arise from a precursor lesion known as **cervical intraepithelial neoplasia** (CIN).
- 20% are adenocarcinomas which arise from a precursor lesion known as **cervical glandular intraepithelial neoplasia** (CGIN).
- HPV-mediated cervical carcinogenesis is linked to the presence of two viral genes *E6* and *E7*.
- The E6 and E7 proteins interact with the tumour suppressor proteins p53 and Rb, targeting them for degradation. Loss of function of these proteins results in uncontrolled proliferation of the infected cells.

Presentation

- Non-menstrual vaginal bleeding and discharge.

Macroscopy

- Solid tumour mass or ulcer.

Histopathology

- **Squamous cell carcinomas** are characterized by infiltrating irregular nests of malignant epithelial cells showing squamous differentiation. Residual CIN may be seen adjacent to small tumours.
- **Adenocarcinomas** are characterized by infiltrating malignant epithelial cells forming glandular structures. Residual CGIN may be seen adjacent to small tumours.

Prognosis

- Depends on a number of factors, including age, stage, and presence or absence of lymphovascular invasion.
- FIGO (2018) staging is usually employed for cervical carcinoma.

Cervical screening

▶ The main aim of cervical screening is the detection of CIN—the premalignant precursor to cervical carcinoma.

NHS cervical screening programme (NHSCSP)

- Women aged between 25 and 64 are eligible for cervical screening.
- Routine screening is performed every 3 y from 25 to 49 and every 5y from 50 to 64.
- The test is a cervical brush sample for **liquid-based cytology**.
- A special device is used to brush cells from the cervix. The head of the brush is then broken off into a small glass vial containing a fixative or rinsed directly in the fixative.
- The sample is then sent to the local laboratory where a processing machine creates a thin monolayer of cells on a glass slide for cytological examination.

Cytology

- The high-risk humanpapillomavirus (hrHPV) primary screening test is now performed on all cervical screening samples taken in the NHSCSP. In the primary hrHPV screening pathway, cytology is used as a triage test in women where hrHPV is detected to determine whether immediate referral to colposcopy is required. The majority of abnormal cytology results lead to colposcopy referral—a glandular neoplasia (non-cervical) result will normally be referred for a gynaecological opinion.
- There are three possible results of hrHPV screening pathway: HPV negative, HPV positive, Inadequate sample.
- The HPV positive samples are undergo cytology triage and are further classified as: HPV positive with no abnormal cells or HPV positive with abnormal cells.
- The abnormal **dyskaryotic squamous epithelial cells** are graded into borderline, mild, moderate, or severe, depending on how abnormal the cell appears.
- A patient with any grade of abnormal cytology is referred to colposcopy immediately.
- A patient who tests positive for hrHPV with negative cytology is recalled for a repeat test at 12 months. At this repeat test, patients testing hrHPV negative are returned to routine screening.
- Patients with a negative hrHPV result do not have cytology performed and return to the routine screening interval relevant to their age.
- Patients with inadequate result are recalled for a repeat test in no less than 3 months. Women who have inadequate cytology at the 24-month repeat test are an exception and are referred to colposcopy. Women who have two consecutive unavailable or inadequate screening tests, in any combination, are referred to colposcopy.

Colposcopy

- Colposcopy is a detailed examination of the cervix using a binocular microscopy called a colposcope and an intense light source.
- Application of acetic acid and iodine to the cervix helps identify areas of possible CIN for directed biopsy.

Histopathology

- Directed cervical biopsies are sent for histopathological examination to confirm the presence of CIN and provide a grade from 1 to 3.
- There is no evidence that HPV independent precursor lesion exist, SIL in cervix is therefore grouped as HPV-associated category. It is subclassified as LSIL (CIN-1) and HSIL (CIN-2 and CIN-3).
- CIN 1 shows squamous dysplasia, in which the abnormalities are concentrated in the basal third of the thickness of the squamous epithelium (Fig. 12.1).
- CIN 2 shows squamous dysplasia, in which the abnormalities are concentrated in the basal two-thirds of the epithelium.
- CIN 3 shows squamous dysplasia, in which the abnormalities extend into the upper one-third of the epithelium (Fig. 12.2).

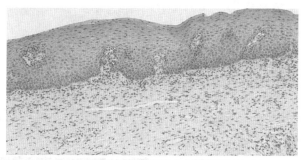

Fig. 12.1 CIN 1. Abnormalities are concentrated in the lower third of the squamous epithelium of the transformation zone (see Plate 36).

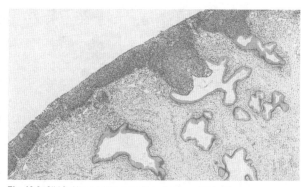

Fig. 12.2 CIN 3. Abnormalities extend into the upper third of the squamous epithelium of the transformation zone. In this example the CIN 3 also extends into an endocervical crypt (see Plate 37).

Management

- CIN 2 and 3 are high-grade lesions which are removed by excision of the transformation zone (large loop excision of the transformation zone, LLETZ).
- CIN 1 is a low-grade lesion and may be managed conservatively or excised, depending on the clinical situation.

Benign endometrial disorders

Congenital Defects
Fusion Defects of the Mullerian Ducts
Atresia of the Mullerian Ducts and Vagina

Infectious/Inflammatory Diseases
Endometritis (infective and non-infective)
- Acute
- Chronic
- Xanthogranulomatous
- Ligneous (Pseudomembranous) Endometritis

Malakoplakia
Endometrial Granulomas

Hormonal Disorders
Dysfunctional Uterine Bleeding

Administration Of Exogenous Hormones/Drugs (e.g. Oestrogen-only Hormone Replacement)
Therapy, Tamoxifen, Oral Contraceptives, Gonadotropin-Releasing Hormone Agonists

Benign Tumours
Endometrial Polyps
Adenofibroma
Adenomyoma/Atypical Polypoid Adenomyoma
Leiomyoma
Endometrial stromal nodule

Endometriosis

Definition

- The presence of endometrial tissue outside the uterine body.
- Almost all cases occur in the pelvis, most commonly the ovaries, uterosacral ligaments, peritoneum, pouch of Douglas, and sigmoid colon.
- Endometriosis is also recognized at sites outside of the pelvis, such as surgical scars and the lungs, but this is rarer.

Epidemiology

- Common, affecting up to 10% of women.

Pathogenesis

- **Implantation theory** proposes that endometrial tissue enters and implants on the peritoneal surface during menstruation. Credence to this theory is lent by experimental induction of endometriosis in animals by placing endometrial tissue in the peritoneal cavity. Changes in the immune response may prevent elimination of the endometrial tissue and promote the implantation and growth of endometrial cells.
- **Metaplastic theory** proposes that endometriosis arises due to metaplasia of the peritoneal surface epithelium into endometrial-type epithelium. Given that the peritoneum and female genital tract arise from the same embryological cells (coelomic epithelium), this seems plausible and would account for endometriotic deposits in areas in which implantation is unlikely.
- **Metastatic theory** proposes that endometriosis arises due to haematogenous spread of endometrial tissue that enters the circulation during menstruation. This would account for cases arising in locations where implantation or metaplasia are improbable (e.g. the lung).

Presentation

- Dysmenorrhoea, caused by swelling of endometriotic deposits.
- Subfertility, through unclear mechanisms, though implantation failure and/or endocrine dysfunction have been proposed. There is little evidence to support tubal distortion as a cause in most women.

Macroscopy

- Ovarian involvement typically gives rise to cysts filled with dark brown altered blood ('chocolate cysts'). Peritoneal involvement causes small nodules which often appear brown/black.

Histopathology

- Microscopy is diagnostic, demonstrating endometrial glands and endometrial stromal cells in tissues other than the uterine body.

Prognosis

- Endometriosis is chronic and progressive in 50% of cases.
- Ovarian endometriosis is thought to be a precursor to ovarian endometrioid and clear cell carcinomas (➔ Ovarian carcinomas, p. 334).

Endometrial tumours and precursors

Precursor Lesions

Endometrial Hyperplasia
- With Cytological Atypia (Atypical Hyperplasia)
- Without Cytological Atypia (Non-Atypical Hyperplasia)

Malignant Neoplasms

Epithelial Tumours
- Endometrioid Carcinoma
- Serous Carcinoma
- Clear Cell Carcinoma
- Carcinosarcoma
- Other Endometrial Carcinomas

Mesenchymal Tumours
- Leiomyosarcoma
- Endometrial Stromal Sarcoma
- Uterine Tumour Resembling Ovarian Sex Cord Tumour (Utrosct)
- Perivascular Epitheloid Cell Tumour (Pecoma)

Mixed Epithelial and Mesenchymal Tumours—Adenosarcoma
Trophoblastic Tumours (Variant of Epithelial Tumour)—Choriocarcinoma
Metastatic Tumour

Endometrial carcinoma

Definition

- A malignant epithelial tumour arising in the endometrium.

Epidemiology

- The most frequent malignant tumour of the female genital tract in developed countries.
- 80% are oestrogen-dependent, low-grade (type 1) carcinomas, occurring in women in their 50s and 60s.
- 10% are oestrogen-independent, high-grade (type 2) carcinomas, occurring in older women in their 70s and 80s.

Aetiology

- Oestrogen-dependent tumours are associated with diabetes, obesity, nulliparity, early menarche, late menopause, polycystic ovarian syndrome, oestrogen-secreting ovarian tumours, and exogenous oestrogens or tamoxifen therapy. Lynch syndrome and Cowden syndrome also increase the risk of developing endometrial carcinoma.
- The aetiology of oestrogen-independent tumours is less clear, but they are associated with multiparity and a history of breast carcinoma/tamoxifen use. *BRCA1/2* mutation carriers are more susceptible to the development of these tumours.

Genetic alterations

- Type 1 carcinomas:
  - *PTEN* (sporadic and Cowden syndrome-associated)
  - *PIK3CA*
  - *PIK3R1*
  - *ARID1A*
  - *KRAS*
  - microsatellite instability (sporadic and Lynch syndrome-associated).
- Type 2 carcinomas:
  - *TP53*
  - *PIK3CA*
  - *FBXW7*
  - *PPP2R1A*.

Carcinogenesis

- Oestrogen-dependent tumours develop from a precursor lesion called **atypical endometrial hyperplasia**. This often results from continuous unopposed oestrogenic stimulation of the endometrium and progression from endometrial hyperplasia without atypia. Loss of function of PTEN is typical.
- Most oestrogen-independent carcinomas develop from a precursor lesion called **serous endometrial intraepithelial carcinoma** on a background of endometrial atrophy. Loss of function of TP53 is typical.

Presentation

- Post-menopausal bleeding is the key symptom.

Macroscopy

- An exophytic friable mass fills the endometrial cavity and infiltrates to a varying extent into the underlying myometrium (Fig. 12.3).
- In advanced cases, the tumour may breach the serosal surface or invade the cervix.

Histopathology

- Oestrogen-dependent tumours are usually well-differentiated **endometrioid adenocarcinomas**, in which the malignant epithelial cells form complex glandular structures.
- Oestrogen-independent tumours are usually **serous carcinomas** or the uncommon **clear cell carcinomas** which look identical to their ovarian counterparts. Both are high-grade malignancies and usually have extensive spread at presentation.
- Other uncommon histological types include squamous cell carcinoma, glassy cell carcinoma, transitional cell carcinoma, choriocarcinoma, and yolk sac tumour.

Molecular subtypes

- There are four molecular subtypes that behave as biologically distinct categories of endometrial carcinoma. These can be diagnosed using surrogate markers (Immunocytochemistry for MMR, p53, and targeted POLE sequencing). Relevant prognostic information can be provided with these subtypes and it reduces both overtreatment and under treatment (PORTEC TRIAL).

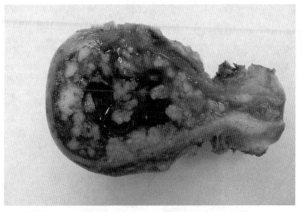

Fig. 12.3 Endometrial carcinoma filling the uterine cavity (see Plate 38).

- These subtypes are: POLE—ultramutated endometrioid carcinoma, mismatch repair—deficient endometrioid carcinoma, p53-mutant endometrioid carcinoma, and no specific molecular profile (NMSP) endometrioid carcinoma.

Prognosis

- Oestrogen-dependent tumours generally have a better outcome.
- Oestrogen-independent tumours are highly aggressive and usually fatal.
- FIGO (2023) staging is usually employed for endometrial carcinoma.

Uterine leiomyomas (fibroids)

Definition
- Benign smooth muscle tumours arising in the myometrium.

Epidemiology
- Extremely common tumours, found in up to 75% of all women.
- Symptomatic fibroids affect about 20% of women.

Aetiology
- The precise cause is unclear, but Afro-Caribbean origin, heredity, nulliparity, and obesity are risk factors.
- No single causative genetic mutation has been identified. However, the mitochondrial enzyme fumarate hydratase has been linked to rare uterine fibroid syndromes.

Pathogenesis
- Growth is driven by oestrogen, progesterone, growth factors, and angiogenesis.
- They occur almost exclusively in reproductive age women, rapidly grow in pregnancy, and regress after the menopause.
- Genetic studies show that they are clonal neoplasms with chromosomal aberrations.

Presentation
- Menorrhagia.
- Pelvic pain. This may be related to tumour infarction or twisting of a pedunculated fibroid.
- Palpable mass. Fibroids may be large enough to be felt abdominally.
- Pressure symptoms. Large fibroids may affect adjacent organs, such as the bowel or bladder, or complicate pregnancy and delivery.

Macroscopy
- Well-circumscribed, white, whorled tumours which characteristically bulge from the surrounding myometrium when cut (Fig. 12.4).
- Often multiple and may be intramural or project from the serosal surface (subserosal) or into the endometrial cavity (submucosal).
- Calcification is very common.
- Infarcted tumours appear red, rather than white ('red degeneration').

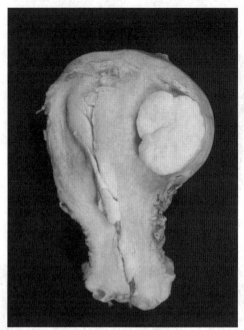

Fig. 12.4 Leiomyoma. This uterus was removed due to severe menorrhagia. On bisecting the uterus, a well-circumscribed white mass is seen in the myometrium which bulges from the cut surface. This is the typical macroscopic appearance of a leiomyoma (fibroid) and this was confirmed on microscopic examination (see Plate 39).

Reproduced with permission from *Clinical Pathology* (Oxford Core Texts), Carton, James, Daly, Richard, and Ramani, Pramila, Oxford University Press (2006), p. 269, Figure 12.9.

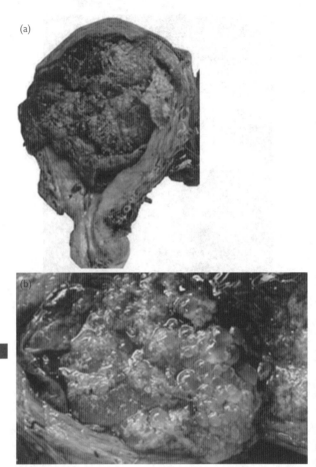

Fig. 12.5 (a) Complete mole presenting as an enlarged uterus with abnormally dilated endometrial cavity in a 55 years old female with uncontrolled vaginal bleeding. (b) Hydropic change is generalized and no fetus is present (see Plate 40).

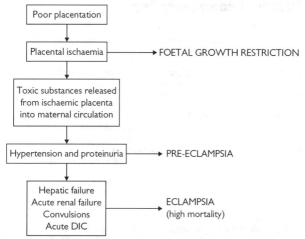

Fig. 12.6 Postulated pathogenesis of pre-eclampsia.

Reproduced with permission from *Clinical Pathology* (Oxford Core Texts), Carton, James, Daly, Richard, and Ramani, Pramila, Oxford University Press (2006), p. 282, Figure 12.18.

Histopathology

- Classical fibroids are composed of intersecting fascicles of bland smooth muscle cells with blunt-ended nuclei and eosinophilic cytoplasm. Areas of hyalinization and calcification are common.
- A number of histological variants are recognized: cellular leiomyoma, mitotically active leiomyoma, symplastic leiomyoma, hydropic leiomyoma, epithelioid leiomyoma.

Prognosis

- Benign tumours with no capacity for malignant behaviour

Uterine leiomyosarcoma

Definition
- A malignant smooth muscle tumour arising in the myometrium.

Epidemiology
- Although uncommon, representing 1–2% of uterine malignancies, it is the most common uterine sarcoma.
- Most occur in women over 50 y of age.

Aetiology and pathogenesis
- Unclear, but risk factors include history of pelvic radiation and Afro-Caribbean origin.
- Thought to arise *de novo* and not usually from leiomyomas.
- Abnormalities of the *Rb* gene commonly seen in these tumours.

Presentation
- Abnormal vaginal bleeding.
- Palpable mass.
- Pelvic pain.
- Rapid enlargement of a uterine mass may prompt suspicion for leiomyosarcoma; however, many are unsuspected preoperatively and assumed to be large fibroids.

Macroscopy
- Leiomyosarcomas are poorly circumscribed and tend not to bulge from the surrounding myometrium due to their infiltrative nature.
- They are softer than fibroids and may show evidence of necrosis.

Histopathology
- Histologically, leiomyosarcomas are composed of spindle cells and/or pleomorphic cells which demonstrate a number of atypical features such as cytological atypia, tumour cell necrosis, and high mitotic activity.

Prognosis
- Leiomyosarcomas are aggressive malignancies with a tendency to local recurrence and metastasis, particularly to the liver and lungs.

Non-neoplastic ovarian disorders

Congenital Lesions and Ectopic Tissues
Absent Ovary
Lobulated, Accessory, and Supernumerary Ovary
Adrenal Cortical Rests
Uterus-Like Ovarian Mass
Splenic–Gonadal Fusion
Prostatic Tissue

Infectious Diseases
Bacterial Infections
Parasitic Infections
Viral Infections
Fungal Infections

Non-infectious Inflammatory Disorders
Foreign Body Granulomas
Necrobiotic (Palisading) Granulomas
Granulomas Secondary to Systemic Diseases
Cortical Granulomas

Non-neoplastic Lesions of the Follicular and Stromal Elements
Follicle Cysts and Corpus Luteum Cysts
Polycystic Ovary Syndrome
Pregnancy Luteoma
Ovarian Fibromatosis
Leydig Cell Hyperplasia
Stromal Hyperplasia and Stromal Hyperthecosis/HAIR-AN Syndrome

Vascular Lesions
Ovarian Haemorrhage
Ovarian Torsion and Infarction

Endometriosis

Ovarian Pregnancy

Functional ovarian cysts

Definition
- Ovarian follicles showing pathological cystic change.
- A proposed cut-off between normal cystic follicles and follicular cysts is 2.5 cm.

Terminology
- Cysts derived from preovulatory follicles are known as **follicular cysts** and those derived from the corpus luteum are known as **corpus luteum cysts**.

Epidemiology
- Very common.

Aetiology
- Follicular cysts: disordered function of the pituitary–ovarian axis.
- Corpus luteum cysts: excessive haemorrhage in a corpus luteum.

Presentation
- Almost all are discovered incidentally, either on imaging or by a surgeon exploring the pelvis.
- Occasionally, large cysts may present as a pelvic mass.

Macroscopy
- Follicular cysts are usually single and measure from 2.5 to 10 cm in size. They are smooth-lined and contain clear fluid.
- Corpus luteum cysts usually measure from 2.5 to 5 cm in size. The cyst contains bloody fluid and the wall often is yellow.

Cytopathology
- Aspirated fluid from a follicular cyst contains many granulosa cells with round nuclei, coarse chromatin, and a small rim of cytoplasm. Nuclear grooves may be seen. Luteinized cells may also be seen.
- Aspirated fluid from a corpus luteum cyst contains blood, haemosiderin-laden macrophages, and many fully luteinized granulosa cells. These are large polyhedral cells with abundant finely granular cytoplasm. The nuclei are round to oval with finely granular chromatin and prominent nucleoli. Nuclear grooves are not present.

Histopathology
- Follicular cysts are lined by granulosa cells and theca cells which may show some luteinization.
- Corpus luteum cysts contain abundant central haemorrhage. The lining is composed of fully luteinized granulosa and theca cells.

Prognosis
- Functional ovarian cysts are entirely benign. They are predominantly of clinical importance, as large cysts may raise concern for a cystic neoplasm.

Polycystic ovarian syndrome

Definition
- A metabolic syndrome characterized by androgen excess, ovulatory failure, and, in some women, polycystic ovaries.

Epidemiology
- Common, affecting about 5% of women.

Aetiology
- Insulin resistance appears to be the key underlying cause (Fig. 12.7).

Pathogenesis
- Insulin resistance → obesity and ↑ androgen production by the ovaries.
- ↑ androgens → hirsutism, acne, and abnormal follicle maturation.
- Abnormal follicle maturation → polycystic ovaries in some women.
- Chronic anovulation → subfertility and ↑ oestrogen production.
- Prolonged oestrogen exposure → endometrial hyperplasia and risk of development of endometrial hyperplasia and endometrial carcinoma (➔ Endometrial carcinoma, p. 310).

Presentation
- Subfertility is a common presentation.
- Irregular periods or no periods.
- Weight gain.
- Some women present with hirsutism and acne.

Radiology
- Polycystic ovaries may be seen in some, but not all, women.

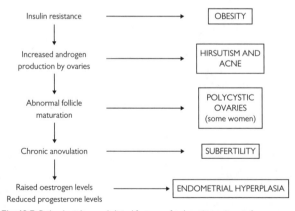

Fig. 12.7 Pathophysiology and clinical features of polycystic ovarian syndrome.
Reproduced with permission from *Clinical Pathology* (Oxford Core Texts), Carton, James, Daly, Richard, and Ramani, Pramila, Oxford University Press (2006), p. 272, Figure 12.11.

Biochemistry
- Elevated blood androgens.
- Impaired glucose tolerance or frank diabetes.

Prognosis
- The main issues are the complications associated with obesity and the risk of endometrial carcinoma.
- Weight reduction, insulin-lowering agents, and progesterone administration all act to reduce these complications.

Tumours of the ovary

Tumours of the ovary can broadly be subdivided into following categories:
- Surface epithelial tumours (80–90% of all ovarian tumours);
- Sex cord stromal tumours (5–10%);
- Germ cell tumours (5-10%);
- Miscellaneous tumours of unknown histiogenesis;
- Metastatic tumours.

Surface epithelial tumours are classified based on tumour cell type (serous, mucinous, endometrioid, clear cell, transitional) and are then further subclassified as benign borderline or malignant (carcinoma). These account for 80–90% of all ovarian tumours.

Sex cord stromal tumours and germ cell tumours are less common and are subclassified as benign and malignant. Mature teratoma is the most common tumour in this category.

Benign ovarian tumours

Surface Epithelial Tumours
Serous Cystadenoma, Adenofibroma, And Surface Papilloma of the Ovary
Mucinous Cystadenoma and Adenofibroma
Endometrioid Cystadenoma and Adenofibroma
Clear Cell Cystadenoma and Adenofibroma
Seromucinous Cystadenoma and Adenofibroma
Brenner Tumours

Sex Cord-Stromal Tumours
Fibroma
Thecoma
Sclerosing Stromal Tumour
Microcystic Stromal Tumour
Signet-Ring Stromal Tumour
Stromal Luteoma
Hilus cell tumour/Leydig Cell Tumour

Germ Cell Tumours
Mature Teratoma/Mature Cystic Teratoma

Other Rare Tumours
Tumours of Vascular and Lymphatic Differentiation—Haemangioma, Lymphangioma
Tumours of Muscle Differentiation—Leiomyoma/Rhabdomyoma
Tumours of Bone Differentiation—Osteoma
Tumours of Cartilage Differentiation—Chondroma
Tumours of Mesothelial Differentiation—Adenomatoid Tumour
Tumours of Adipose Tissue Differentiation—Adipose prosoplasia

Benign epithelial ovarian tumours

Serous cystadenoma
- Benign epithelial ovarian tumour which usually occurs in premenopausal women.
- May be picked up incidentally, with symptoms of a pelvic mass, or with an acute abdomen due to torsion.
- Macroscopically, it is cystic and may be unilocular or multilocular. The cysts contain clear, straw-coloured, or water-like fluid and have a thin wall with a smooth lining.
- Histologically, the cysts are lined by a single layer of bland columnar cells which may be ciliated or non-ciliated, similar to Fallopian tube epithelium.

Mucinous cystadenoma
- Benign epithelial ovarian tumour which usually occurs in premenopausal women.
- May be picked up incidentally, with symptoms of a pelvic mass, or with an acute abdomen due to torsion.
- Macroscopically, the tumour is usually unilateral, with a mean size of 10 cm, but massive tumours have been reported. They may be unilocular or multilocular with either a thin or thick fibrous wall. They often contain a watery mucinous fluid (Fig. 12.8).

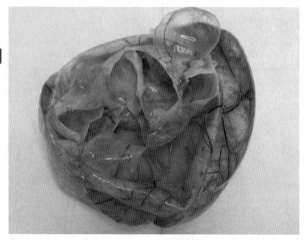

Fig. 12.8 Benign mucinous cystadenoma of the ovary (see Plate 41).

- Histologically, the tumours are composed of glands and cysts separated by varying amounts of fibrous stroma. The lining cells comprising a single layer of columnar epithelium with basal nuclei and apical mucinous cytoplasm.

Benign non-epithelial ovarian tumours

Mature cystic teratoma

- Benign germ cell ovarian tumour, also known as a 'dermoid cyst'.
- Occurs in young women, with peak incidence between 20 and 29 years old.
- Many are asymptomatic and discovered incidentally, but larger tumours may cause pelvic pain. The most serious complication is torsion or rupture, leading to an acute abdomen.
- Macroscopically, the tumour is cystic and contains greasy, soft, yellow material. Hair, cartilage, bone, and teeth may be visible (Fig. 12.9).
- Histologically, the tumour comprises mature adult-type tissues of virtually any type, including skin, brain, fat, smooth muscle, cartilage, respiratory, and gastrointestinal (GI) tissue.

▶ Note that although other ovarian germ cell tumours (e.g. dysgerminoma, immature teratoma) are much rarer, they behave in a malignant fashion.

Ovarian fibroma

- Benign sex cord stromal ovarian tumour, composed of fibroblasts and collagen.
- Occur over a wide age range, though most are found in women over 50 years old. They are often small and discovered incidentally. Large tumours may cause abdominal pain and ascites.
- Macroscopically, the tumour is firm with a solid white cut surface.
- Histologically, the tumour is composed of bland spindled cells growing in a collagenous stroma.

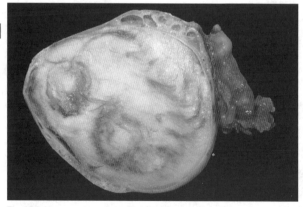

Fig. 12.9 Mature cystic teratoma. Typical appearance of a mature cystic teratoma (dermoid cyst) filled with greasy yellow material and hair (see Plate 42).

Reproduced with permission from *Clinical Pathology* (Oxford Core Texts), Carton, James, Daly, Richard, and Ramani, Pramila, Oxford University Press (2006), p. 278, Figure 12.17.

Borderline epithelial ovarian tumours

> **Borderline Surface epithelial tumours**
> Serous Borderline Tumour (SBT)/Atypical Proliferative Serous Tumour (APST);
> Atypical Proliferative Mucinous Tumour (APMT)/Serous Borderline Tumour (SBT)
> Seromucinous-type APMT (APSMT)
> Atypical Proliferative Endometrioid Tumours (APET)
> Atypical Proliferative Clear Cell Tumours (APCCT)
> Atypical Proliferative Brenner (Transitional Cell) Tumours

Borderline serous tumours

- Usually confined to the ovary at presentation but may be bilateral.
- Present with similar pressure symptoms as benign tumours but may present with ascites if extra-ovarian involvement.
- Macroscopically, these tumours show exuberant papillary growths within the cyst wall of the tumour or on the ovarian surface (Fig. 12.10).
- Histologically, the tumours show structural complexity, with complex cyst walls containing branching papillary structures. They are lined by stratified or non-stratified columnar cells, many of which are ciliated. The cells show mild to moderate cytological atypia with characteristic budding.
- There is no evidence of stromal invasion.

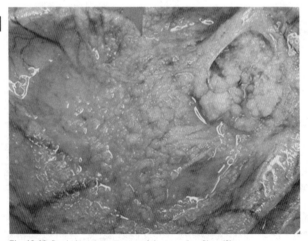

Fig. 12.10 Borderline serous tumour of the ovary (see Plate 43).

- Around 10% may have implants of similarly appearing tumours on the surface of pelvic structures that do not invade underlying tissue.
- Most are benign clinically, but a minority recur.
- Rarely may progress to low-grade serous carcinoma.

Borderline mucinous tumours

- Divided into intestinal-type and endocervical-type.
- Intestinal-type:
  - large (mean 19 cm) multiloculated tumours containing mucin;
  - usually unilateral (90%);
  - epithelial lining is enteric in type with goblet cells and forms tufts and papillae.
- Endocervical-type:
  - smaller than the intestinal type (mean 8 cm);
  - more often bilateral (40%);
  - epithelial lining is endocervical in type with mucinous columnar cells and forms papillae showing hierarchical branching.
- Both types are usually stage I at presentation and show a benign clinical course.

Malignant ovarian tumours

Surface Epithelial Tumours
Low-Grade Serous Carcinoma
High-Grade Serous Carcinoma
Invasive Mucinous Carcinomas
Endometrioid Adenocarcinoma
Clear Cell Carcinomas
Malignant Transitional Cell Tumours (Malignant Brenner Tumours and Transitional Cell Carcinomas)
Malignant Mixed Mesodermal Tumour (Carcinosarcoma)
Other Rare Types—Squamous Cell Carcinoma, Mixed Epithelial Tumours, Undifferentiated Carcinomas

Sex Cord-Stromal Tumours
Adult Granulosa Cell Tumour
Juvenile Granulosa Cell Tumour
Sertoli Cell Tumours
Sertoli–Leydig Cell Tumours
Rare types
• Gynandroblastoma
• Sex Cord Tumour with Annular Tubules (SCTAT)
• Steroid Cell Tumours

Germ Cell Tumours
Dysgerminoma
Yolk Sac Tumour
Embryonal Carcinoma
Non-gestational Choriocarcinoma
Immature Teratoma
Mixed Germ Cell Tumours

Tumours Composed of Germ Cells and Sex Cord-Stromal Derivatives
Gonadoblastoma
Mixed Germ Cell–Sex Cord-Stromal Tumour

Tumours of Uncertain Histogenesis
Small Cell Carcinoma of Hypercalcaemic Type
Malignant Melanoma
Wilms Tumour
Desmoplastic Small Round Cell Tumour

Other Rare Tumours
Sarcomas—Leiomyosarcoma, Angiosarcoma, Endometrial Stromal Sarcoma, Adenosarcoma, etc.

Metastatic Tumours
- Breast carcinoma
  - Colon carcinoma
  - Endometrioid adenocarcinoma
  - Gastric
  - carcinoma
  - Cervical adenocarcinoma
  - Ovarian neoplasms
  - Pancreatic carcinoma
  - Signet-ring cell adenocarcinoma (Krukenberg's tumour)
  - Adrenal and thyroid carcinomas rarely

Ovarian carcinomas

Definition
- A group of malignant epithelial tumours arising in the ovary.

Epidemiology
- Eight most common cause of cancer death and a leading cause of gynaecological cancer mortality due to late presentation.

Aetiology
- Multiparity, oral contraceptive use, hysterectomy, and tubal ligation are associated with a reduced risk of ovarian carcinoma.
- Family history, oestrogen replacement therapy, and obesity are associated with an increased risk.
- Hereditary factors account for up to 20% of ovarian cancers.

BRCA1 and 2 mutations
- Women with these mutations are at higher risk of developing high-grade serous carcinoma.
- The lifetime risk of developing ovarian cancer is around 50% for *BRCA1* carriers at an average age of between 49 and 53 y. For *BRCA2* mutation carriers, the lifetime risk is between 11 and 37% and tends to develop later (average age 55–58 y).
- Prophylactic bilateral salpingo-oophorectomy reduces risk.

Lynch syndrome (HNPCC)
- Most cancers associated with this syndrome are endometrioid or clear cell carcinomas.
- Nine to 12% lifetime risk of developing ovarian cancer and 40–60% of developing endometrial cancer.
- Related to mutations in DNA mismatch repair genes, especially *MLH1*, *MSH2*, and *MSH6*.

Presentation
- Abdominal pain, fatigue, abdominal distension, and diarrhoea.
- The vague and non-specific nature of the symptoms often cause women to dismiss the symptoms as stress or menopause related.
- Women who do seek medical attention are easily misdiagnosed with benign GI or urinary conditions.
- Raised serum Ca125.

Staging
- FIGO staging is usually employed for ovarian carcinoma.

High-grade serous carcinoma
- Most common ovarian cancer.
- Associated with inactivation of *BRCA1/2* and *TP53* mutations.
- Arises from a precursor lesion known as **serous tubal intraepithelial carcinoma** (STIC).
- STIC is now thought to originate in most cases within the Fallopian tube fimbrial epithelium, with subsequent spread to the ovary.
- Histologically comprises high-grade malignant epithelial cells showing papillary and micropapillary growth with slit-like glandular spaces (Fig. 12.11).

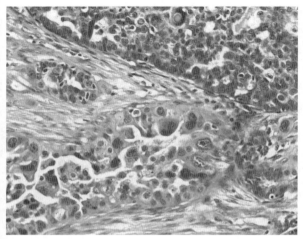

Fig. 12.11 High-grade serous carcinoma of the ovary (see Plate 44).

- Immunohistochemistry showxs CK7, WT-1, and Pax-8 positivity.

▶ Usually advanced stage at presentation, rapidly growing, and aggressive with poor survival.

Low grade serous carcinoma

- *KRAS* and *BRAF* mutations, but no *TP53* mutations and few chromosomal abnormalities.
- Arises through progression from serous cystadenoma → borderline tumour → low-grade serous carcinoma.
- Histologically comprise low-grade malignant epithelial cells growing in papillae. Psammoma bodies may be seen. Necrosis is not usually a feature.
- Prognosis excellent if confined to the ovary.

Endometrioid carcinoma

- Many are associated with endometriosis.
- Show *PTEN*, *PIK3CA*, and *ARID1A* mutations, as well as microsatellite instability in some.
- Soft solid or partly cystic mass with haemorrhage and necrosis.
- May appear as polypoid mass projecting into the endometriotic cyst.
- Usually unilateral.
- Histologically comprise malignant epithelial cells forming round or oval glands resembling endometrial carcinomas. Areas of squamous differentiation are common (Fig. 12.12).
- Survival dependent on stage, with 5-year survival rates of 78% for stage 1 cancers and 6% for stage 4.

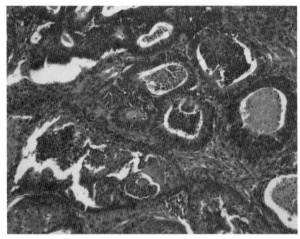

Fig. 12.12 Endometrioid carcinoma of the ovary (see Plate 45).

Mucinous carcinoma
- Large, solid, and cystic tumour.
- Histologically comprise adenocarcinomas of intestinal type, growing in complex, crowded, fused glands.
- Immunohistochemistry shows CK7, CK20, and CDX2 positivity.
- 50% are stage I, with 83% 5-year survival.
- The 5-year survival for stages II, III, and IV are 55, 21, and 9%, respectively.

Clear cell carcinoma
- Arise in most cases within endometriosis.
- They are composed of malignant epithelial cells with clear cytoplasm and hobnailing which grow in small tubules and papillae (Fig. 12.13).
- Survival for early stage 1a tumours is excellent, but high-stage disease survival is poor due to resistance to platinum-based chemotherapy.

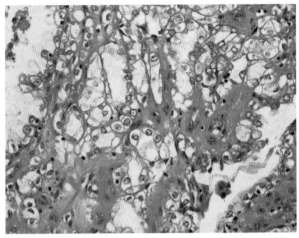

Fig. 12.13 Clear cell carcinoma of the ovary (see Plate 46).

Non-neoplastic fallopian tube disorders

Congenital Anomalies
In Utero Exposure To DES
Tubal Duplication
Accessory Fallopian Tubes

Salpingitis
Acute Salpingitis—Pathologic Correlate of the Clinical Entity Pelvic Inflammatory
Disease (PID)
Chronic Salpingitis
Granulomatous Salpingitis
• Infectious
  • Tuberculous Salpingitis
  • Parasitic Salpingitis (Pinworm, Schistosomiasis, Echinococcus Granulosus, Cysticercosis, etc.)
  • Fungal Salpingitis
• Non-infectious
  • Pseudoxanthomatous Salpingitis
  • Sarcoidosis
  • Crohn's Disease
  • Malakoplakia
  • Vasculitides
  • Foreign Body Granulomasdue to Starch and Talc/Pulse Granulomas

Fungal Infections
Torsion, Prolapse, and Intussusception
Endometriosis and Endosalpingiosis
Ectopic Pregnancy and Gestational Trophoblastic Disease of the Fallopian
Tube
Tubal Hydatidiform Mole

Pelvic inflammatory disease

Definition
- An infection of the upper female genital tract.

Epidemiology
- Most cases are seen in young sexually active women aged 15–25.
- True incidence is difficult to estimate, as many cases go undiagnosed.

Aetiology
- Most cases are caused by ascending infection by either *Chlamydia trachomatis* or *Neisseria gonorrhoeae*. Both organisms are sexually transmitted bacteria.
- Cases unrelated to a sexually transmitted infection are often associated with intrauterine devices or retained products of conception postpartum or post-miscarriage.

Presentation
- Usually there are persistent symptoms of pelvic pain, dyspareunia, and post-coital or intermenstrual bleeding.
- Severe cases may cause an acute illness with fever, abdominal pain, and peritonism.
- ▶ Note that many women are asymptomatic and go undiagnosed.

Complications
- Infertility. The risk of infertility increases with each episode of infection. Women with three or more episodes of pelvic inflammatory disease (PID) have a 40% chance of being infertile.
- Ectopic pregnancy. There is a sixfold increased risk, presumably due to tubal distortion and scarring.
- Chronic pelvic pain and dyspareunia.

Fallopian tube neoplasms

Benign Tumours
Adenomatoid Tumour
Cystadenoma
Papilloma
Leiomyoma and Adenomyoma
Teratoma

Precursor Lesions
Serous tubal intraepithelial carcinoma (STIC)

Malignant Neoplasms
Carcinoma
- serous (80%)
- adenocarcinoma, not otherwise specified (10%)
- endometrioid (7%)
- clear cell (2%)
- mucinous (2%)
- mixed serous-mucinous (1%)
Sarcomas and Mixed Epithelial–Mesenchymal
Metastatic Tumours/Secondary Involvement
- Most Commonly—Ovarian, Endometxrial, Endocervix, Peritoneal Adenomucinosis
Lymphoma
Trophoblastic Tumours—Choriocarcinoma

Ectopic pregnancy

Definition
- Abnormal implantation of a fertilized ovum outside the uterine cavity. Nearly all occur in the Fallopian tubes, usually in the ampullary region. Other sites include the ovaries and abdominal cavity, but these are rare.

Epidemiology
- Annual incidence is 12 per 1000 pregnancies and rising.

Aetiology
- Tubal scarring from previous episodes of PID is the most common predisposing factor.
- Other risk factors include previous tubal surgery and endometriosis.
- About half occur for no apparent underlying reason.

Pathogenesis
- Trophoblast implanting within the Fallopian tube causes intense haemorrhage into the tube.
- The embryo may be dislodged and shed, or absorbed into the tubal wall.
- Rupture of the tubal wall may be sudden or gradual.

Presentation
- The typical presentation is gradually increasing abdominal pain and vaginal bleeding.
- Sudden rupture causes an acute abdomen with peritonism and shock.

▶ Consider the diagnosis in any woman of reproductive age with abdominal pain.

Macroscopy
- The involved Fallopian tube is markedly dilated and congested.
- The tubal lumen is filled with blood and friable material.

Histopathology
- Chorionic villi and infiltrating extravillous trophoblast are seen within the Fallopian tube.

Prognosis
- Prognosis is good, provided the diagnosis is made and appropriate management follows.
- Having one ectopic pregnancy is associated with a higher risk of future ectopics.

Hydatidiform moles

Definition

- A type of gestational trophoblastic disease characterized by abnormal trophoblastic proliferation.
- Also known as 'molar pregnancy'.
- Two types are recognized: **complete moles** and **partial moles**.

Epidemiology

- About 1 in 1000 pregnancies in the western world are molar.
- For unknown reasons, they are much more common in areas of the Far East where incidence rates are as high as 1 in 80.

Genetics

- Complete moles are usually diploid (46 XX or 46 XY), with all chromosomes being paternally derived. They arise from fertilization of an anucleate ovum by a haploid sperm which then duplicates its genetic material.
- Partial moles are triploid (69 XXY, 69 XXX, or 69 XYY), with one set of maternal chromosomes and two sets of paternal chromosomes. They arise from fertilization of an ovum by two sperm.

Presentation

- Most present with early miscarriage. Usually there is no clinical suspicion of molar pregnancy, the diagnosis being made following histopathological examination of the evacuated products of conception.

Macroscopy

- Most molar products of conception are grossly unremarkable.
- Cases presenting late may contain visibly hydropic villi (Fig. 12.5).

Histopathology

- Complete moles show villi with a characteristic lobulated 'budding' architecture. The villi have a myxoid stroma containing collapsed empty blood vessels and karyorrhectic debris. There is abnormal non-polar trophoblastic hyperplasia and sheets of pleomorphic extravillous trophoblast may be present. A prominent implantation site reaction is often seen, but with absence of the normal trophoblast plugging of decidual blood vessels.
- Partial moles show villi with irregular, 'dentate', or 'geographic' outlines. The villi are often fibrotic and contain prominent villous pseudoinclusions and villous blood vessels with nucleated fetal red cells. Abnormal non-polar trophoblastic hyperplasia is present, though this is usually focal and less marked than in complete moles. The implantation site is usually unremarkable with normal trophoblast plugging of decidual blood vessels.
- P57 immunocytochemistry can be used to confirm the diagnosis of complete mole (p57 negative). Partial moles and non-molar miscarriages, however are p57 positive.

Prognosis

- In most cases, evacuation of molar tissue is curative and β-HCG levels rapidly fall to normal.
- Persistence of β-HCG levels is indicative of persistent gestational trophoblastic disease; this complicates ~15% of complete moles and ~1% of partial moles, and requires chemotherapy to cure.

Gestational choriocarcinoma

One other type of gestational trophoblastic disease is **choriocarcinoma**, a rare, but highly malignant, trophoblastic tumour. About half develop from a preceding hydatidiform mole, with the remainder following a normal pregnancy or non-molar miscarriage.

Histologically, choriocarcinomas are composed of a mixture of cytotrophoblast and syncytiotrophoblast, typically forming bilaminar structures. By definition, chorionic villi are absent.

Choriocarcinomas have a great propensity for vascular invasion, leading to early dissemination to multiple distant sites. Fortunately, gestational choriocarcinomas respond extremely well to chemotherapy, and the prognosis for most women is very good.

Pre-eclampsia

Definition
- Pregnancy-induced hypertension with proteinuria.

Epidemiology
- Complicates about 6% of pregnancies.
- More frequent in women carrying their first child.

Aetiology
- Exact cause unknown, but abnormal placentation is key (Fig. 12.6).

Pathogenesis
- Abnormally shallow invasion of the trophoblast, with failure of physiological conversion of intradecidual spiral arteries and basal arteries into large low-resistance vessels.
- Maternal blood pressure rises in an attempt to compensate, but the net result is placental ischaemia.
- Toxic substances released from the ischaemic placenta enter the maternal circulation and cause endothelial damage.
- Progression to eclampsia is heralded by widespread formation of fibrin thrombi within the microcirculation and risk of renal failure, hepatic failure, cardiac failure, and cerebral haemorrhage.

Presentation
- Usually routine antenatal surveillance picks up hypertension after 20 weeks' gestation, together with proteinuria.

Macroscopy
- Placentas tend to be smaller than those from normal pregnancies.
- The incidence of placental infarcts is much higher.

Histopathology
- Placental villi show increased number and prominence of villous cytotrophoblast with irregular thickening of the basement membrane. Villous blood vessels are often small and inconspicuous. Maternal decidual arteries show failure of physiological conversion by the trophoblast. A minority also show fibrinoid necrosis of the arterial wall, together with intramural accumulation of lipid-laden macrophages ('atherosis').
- The kidneys show enlarged 'bloodless' glomeruli containing swollen endothelial cells. Fibrin microthrombi may be seen within glomerular capillary loops in more severe cases.
- The liver may show fibrin thrombi in hepatic sinusoids, with hepatic necrosis and haemorrhage in severe cases.

Prognosis
▶▶ Delivery is the only cure. The danger to the foetus from premature delivery must be weighed against the risks to the mother. The disease behaves very unpredictably and can progress very rapidly, so patients must be closely monitored for signs of deterioration.

Syndromes associated with female genital tract neoplasms

Lynch syndrome (LS)

- Autosomal dominant disorder with mutations, affecting the DNA mismatch repair genes *MLH1*, *MSH2*, *MSH6*, and *PMS2*.
- Increased risk for carcinomas of endometrium, ovary, colorectum, stomach, small bowel, gallbladder, hepatobiliary tract, pancreas, renal pelvis, and/or ureter, bladder, kidney, brain, or prostate.
- Most frequent histological subtype in the female genital tract includes endometrioid and non-endometrioid subtypes, such as clear cell, undifferentiated carcinomas and carcinosarcoma.

BRCA1/2-associated hereditary breast and ovarian cancer syndrome

- Autosomal dominant syndrome with inherited germline mutations of the *BRCA1* (17q21) or *BRCA2* (13q13) gene resulting in defective repair of DNA breaks (homologous recombination repair pathway).
- Increased risk for breast, ovary, fallopian tube, and peritoneal cancer.
- Patients may also develop prostatic, pancreatic, and endometrial carcinomas as well as other types of cancer.
- Most frequent histological subtype in the female genital tract is high-grade serous carcinoma and carcinosarcomas.

Li-Fraumeni syndrome (LFS)

- Autosomal dominant cancer caused by germline mutations of the *TP53* gene.
- Increased risk for carcinomas of cancers of the breast, soft tissue, bone, brain, adrenal glands, female genital tract, and leukaemia.
- Involvement of the female genital tract (ovary, uterus, cervix, and vagina) occurs infrequently.

DICER1 syndrome

- Autosomal dominant disorder with pathogenic mutations in *DICER1* resulting in aberrant posttranscriptional regulation of multiple cancer gene networks.
- Characterized by pleuropulmonary blastoma, thyroid cancers, paediatric cystic nephroma, embryonal rhabdomyosarcoma of the uterine cervix, and ovarian Sertoli–Leydig cell tumour.

Hereditary leiomyomatosis and renal cell carcinoma (HLRCC).

- Autosomal dominant inherited germline mutation of the fumarate hydratase gene (*1q*).
- Cutaneous and uterine leiomyomas, as well as aggressive renal cell carcinomas.

Peutz–Jeghers syndrome (PJS)

- Autosomal dominant syndrome associated with *STK11* mutation.
- Characterized by mucocutaneous melanin pigmentation, gastrointestinal polyposis, and an increased risk for carcinomas of cervix and ovary, gastrointestinal tract, breast, skin, and lung.

- Cervical tumours are usually gastric-type mucinous adenocarcinomas and sex cord tumour with annular tubules (SCTAT), and much less commonly Sertoli cell tumours are seen in the ovary.

Cowden syndrome

- Autosomal dominant syndrome with germline mutation of the *PTEN* gene.
- Affects various organs, including the uterus (endometrial carcinomas and uterine leiomyomas), skin (trichilemmomas, storiform collagenomas), breast (carcinoma, fibrocystic breast disease), gastrointestinal tract (gastrointestinal hamartoma or ganglioneuroma), brain, thyroid, kidney, and soft tissue.
- Endometrial carcinomas are mainly endometrioid and less commonly serous subtype.

Breast pathology

Duct ectasia

Definition
- Inflammation and dilation of large breast ducts.

Epidemiology
- Common in adult women of all ages.

Aetiology
- Unclear.
- Whilst infection may complicate duct ectasia, it does not seem to be the underlying cause.

Presentation
- Nipple discharge is the most common presenting symptom. The discharge may be clear, creamy, or bloodstained.
- More florid cases may cause pain, a breast mass, and nipple retraction.

Macroscopy
- Subareolar ducts are visibly dilated and contain thick secretions.

Cytopathology
- Smears prepared from a sample of nipple discharge contain proteinaceous debris and macrophages.
- Ductal epithelial cells are usually not seen.

Histopathology
- Subareolar ducts are dilated and filled with proteinaceous material and macrophages.
- Periductal chronic inflammation and fibrosis are also seen.

Prognosis
- Duct ectasia is a benign condition with no increased risk of malignancy.

Granulomatous mastitis

Definition
- Two types; idiopathic granulomatous mastitis a.k.a cystic neutrophilic granulomatous mastitis and others occurring as a complication of a variety of granulomatous inflammations.
- Appears after pregnancy (2–6 years).
- Could be seen in drug induced hyperprolactineamia.

Presentation
- Hard lump without signs of systemic disease.
- Pain, nipple retraction, fistula, and/or abscess.
- Linked to hormone therapy, or infection (*Corynebacterium*-linked).
- Presents as a hard mass, may mimic carcinoma but is completely benign.

Microbiology
- *Corynebacterium* has been recently implicated.
- Staphylococci and streptococci in lactating women.

Pathogenesis
- *Corynebacterium* is a resident of normal skin. Likely bacterial access to the breast and lowered immunity promotes infection.

Macroscopy
- A firm to hard breast mass with a nodular pattern.
- Purulent material may be present with abscess formation.

Histopathology
- Granulomatous inflammation in the perilobular region.
- Inflammatory reaction comprises granulomas, multinucleate giant cells, and eosinophils; small lipogranuloma with a central degenerate vacuole.
- Fat necrosis and abscess formation.
- Special stains (Gram) show *Corynebacterium* bacteria, thought to be the source of abscess.

Histologic mimics
- Plasma cell mastitis.
- Tuberculous mastitis.
- Breast abscess.
- Sarcoidosis.
- Drainage and appropriate antibiotic treatment usually result in resolution.

Treatment and prognosis
- No relationship to carcinoma.
- Usually responds to extending antibiotic and steroid therapy.
- Rarely resistant cases treated with methotrexate.

Fat necrosis

Definition
- An inflammatory reaction to damaged adipose tissue.

Epidemiology
- Common.

Aetiology
- Related to trauma, breast surgery, radiation, infection; idiopathic.

Pathogenesis
- Damaged adipocytes spill their lipid contents, resulting in an inflammatory reaction which gives rise to a palpable mass.

Presentation
- Palpable breast mass.
- Clinically mimics carcinoma.

Macroscopy
- The breast tissue shows yellow-white flecks of discoloration.

Cytopathology
- Fine needle aspiration cytology shows foamy macrophages, multinucleated giant cells, and background debris.

Histopathology
- Degenerating adipocytes are present, surrounded by foamy macrophages, multinucleated giant cells, lymphocytes, and plasma cells.
- Scar and calcifications are common in late lesions.
- Later changes include fibrosis and calcification.

Differential diagnosis
- Ductal carcinoma.

Prognosis
- Benign with no increased risk of breast cancer.

Fibrocystic change

Definition
- A number of alterations within the breast, which reflect normal, albeit exaggerated, responses to hormonal influences.

Epidemiology
- Very common.
- Found in more than one-third of premenopausal adult women.

Aetiology
- A hormonally driven condition in response to oestrogens.

Pathogenesis
- Somewhat unclear, though some workers speculate that the initial event is apocrine metaplasia of breast ducts.
- Secretions produced by these cells lead to duct dilation and formation of cysts.

Presentation
- Breast nodularity and lumpiness are the main features.
- There may also be cyclical tenderness.

Macroscopy
- The breast tissue has a firm, rubbery texture.
- Visible cysts are usually evident with a brown or bluish hue.

Cytopathology
- Aspirates of cysts show debris, foamy macrophages, and apocrine cells.
- Aspirates of non-cystic areas contain cohesive fragments of bland ductal epithelial cells and many background bare bipolar nuclei.

Histopathology
- Associated with a number of histological changes, including cystic change, apocrine metaplasia, adenosis, mild epithelial hyperplasia, and stromal hyperplasia.

Prognosis
- Benign with no increased risk for subsequent invasive breast carcinoma.

Fibroadenoma

Definition
- A benign fibroepithelial lesion of the breast.
- Variants include myxoid fibroadenoma, juvenile fibroadenoma, complex fibroadenoma.
- Comprises proliferation of the ducts and the stroma of the breast tissue.

Epidemiology
- Most common type of breast lump, occurs mostly in adolescent and young women.

Genetics
- MED12 exon 2 mutations described in usual type.
- Myxoid variants lack MED12 mutations.
- Juvenile fibroadenomas can occur in women < 20 years.

Pathogenesis
- Neoplastic fibroblasts proliferate within intralobular stroma, entrapping, and compressing terminal duct lobular units and interlobular stroma to form well-circumscribed nodular masses.
- Clinically painless, mobile breast lump ('breast mouse').
- May increase in size during pregnancy or when taking oral contraceptives.

Macroscopy
- Well-circumscribed mobile breast masses; usually measure 3 cm or less.
- The cut surface is usually solid, whorled, and grey-white in colour.

Cytopathology
- Fine needle aspirates are cellular, containing many branching sheets of cohesive bland ductal epithelial cells and abundant bare bipolar nuclei in the background.
- Fragments of stromal material may also be seen.

Histopathology
- Histology shows a multinodular mass well demarcated from the surrounding breast tissue surrounded by a fibrous capsule.
- Each nodule contains an expanded myxoid intralobular stroma containing bland spindled fibroblastic cells. Ducts often compressed into slit-like channels (intracanalicular pattern).
- Narrow strands of fibrous tissue separate nodules.
- Older lesions often show fibrosis and calcification.

Prognosis
- Benign lesions, no risk for malignancy.
- Surgical excision includes simple 'shelling out' and is curative.
- Recurrences are rare.

Phyllodes tumour

Definition
- Rare fibroepithelial tumour of the breast composed of a hypercellular proliferative stromal component wrapping around ducts in a leaf-like pattern (phyllodes = leaf like).

Epidemiology
- Account for only 1% of all breast tumours.
- Usually affects adults (fifth/sixth decades).
- Rapidly growing, discrete, palpable breast mass.

Genetics
- MED12 and RARA (retinoic acid receptor alpha) is seen in most grade of phyllodes tumour.

Pathogenesis
- Neoplastic stromal cells proliferate and induce gland formation.
- Loss of epithelial/glandular interaction believed to responsible for malignant transformation.

Macroscopy
- Well-circumscribed, bulging masses.
- Cut surface is fleshy.
- Whorled pattern with curved clefts.
- May show myxoid areas, haemorrhage, or necrosis.

Histopathology
- Circumscribed pushing border, stromal hypercellularity, and overgrowth.
- Stroma typically overgrows the glandular component.
- Stromal nodules project into the lumen, producing the characteristic leaf-like fronds.
- Pleomorphism of stromal cells and mitotic counts per high power field (hpf) important for distinction between benign, borderline, and malignant tumours (0–4 mitoses/hpf = benign, 5–10 mitoses/hpf = borderline, and >10 mitoses/hpf = malignant).

Treatment
- In recent studies simple excision usually suffices for benign lesions.
- In borderline lesions, wide local excision is suggested, with follow-up due to risk of local recurrence (10–20%).
- Malignant lesions should be treated as sarcomas and managed at specialized sarcoma units.

Prognosis
- Benign tumours have a very low risk of recurrence regardless of margin status.
- Borderline tumours show a higher risk of local recurrence and a small risk of metastasis.

- Malignant tumours show a 25–30% risk of local recurrence and up to 10% risk of distant metastasis.
- Positive margins increases risk of local recurrence in borderline and malignant tumours.

Intraductal papilloma

Definition
- A benign papillary tumour arising within the duct system of the breast.
- Papillomas can develop anywhere in the ductal system but show a predilection for either small terminal ductules (peripheral papillomas) or large lactiferous ducts (central papillomas).

Epidemiology
- Common.
- Seen mostly in women in their 40s and 50s.

Aetiology
- Believed to be neoplastic growths of glandular and stromal breast tissue but show a frond-like, papillary architectural pattern.

Presentation
- Most women with central papillomas present with nipple discharge.
- Small peripheral papillomas usually present with a breast mass.

Macroscopy
- Large papillomas present with central ducts are visible as friable masses within a dilated duct.

Cytopathology
- Smears prepared from nipple discharge may contain branching papillary groups of benign appearing epithelial cells.

Histopathology
- Cystically dilated space with a frond of papillae lined by epithelial cells.
- The papillae are broad and rounded, such that the fronds fit neatly around each other.
- Each frond contains abundant stroma composed of blood vessels and fibrous tissue.
- The epithelium covering the fronds is double-layered, composed of inner columnar epithelial cells and outer myoepithelial cells.

Prognosis
- Benign papillomas, particularly those involving a single duct, have little risk of carcinoma, particularly when there is no associated atypia.
- Excision is often curative with a low risk of upgrade to malignancy.
- When multiple papillomas are present, there is a twofold increased risk of subsequent invasive breast carcinoma.

Radial scar

Definition

- A benign sclerosing breast lesion, characterized by a central zone of scarring surrounded by a radiating rim of proliferating glandular tissue.
- Radial scars range in size from tiny microscopic lesions to larger clinically apparent masses.
- Large lesions >1 cm in size are sometimes called 'complex sclerosing lesions'.

Aetiology

- Little is known about the aetiology or pathogenesis of radial scars.
- One hypothesis is that they represent a reparative phenomenon in response to areas of tissue damage in the breast.

Presentation

- Large radial scars are usually detected on mammography as stellate or spiculated masses.
- ▶ They can closely mimic the appearance of a carcinoma.

Macroscopy

- Grossly, radial scars are stellate, firm masses which appear to infiltrate the surrounding parenchyma.

Histopathology

- Symmetrical stellate breast lesion with a characteristic zonal architecture.
- The centre of the lesion (nidus) comprises fibroelastotic collagen tissue, within which are entrapped haphazardly arranged tubules.
- Surrounding the nidus are radially arranged clusters of ducts and lobules, each of which points towards the centre of the lesion. The ducts and lobules within this zone typically exhibit florid benign changes, including fibrocystic change, sclerosing adenosis, and marked usual epithelial hyperplasia.

Prognosis

- Benign lesions.
- Any relationship to cancer is still debated.
- Reports suggest a mildly increased risk, about twofold although in the absence of atypia, this is considered lower.

Proliferative breast diseases with/ without atypia

Definition
- A diverse group of intraductal proliferative lesions of the breast, associated with a variably increased risk for subsequent development of invasive breast carcinoma.

Epidemiology
- Commonly seen in the breast.
- Increasingly identified since the introduction of breast screening programme.

Aetiology
- Similar to invasive breast carcinoma.

Genetics
- Most cases of flat epithelial atypia and *in situ* lobular neoplasia show genetic abnormalities, most notably the loss of heterozygosity of chromosome 16p.
- Only a minority of cases of usual epithelial hyperplasia show genetic abnormalities.

Macroscopy
- The vast majority are picked up either on screening mammography or incidentally in breast tissue removed for other reasons.

Histopathology
- **Usual epithelial hyperplasia (UEH)** is a benign proliferation of ductal epithelial cells expanding ducts in a haphazard pattern forming fenestrations and irregular slit-like spaces. It shows a good mix of luminal ductal cells and abluminal myoepithelial cells.
- **Flat epithelial atypia (FEA)** represents cyto-architectural atypia seen within the acini, comprising flattened epithelial cells, usually single but occasionally more than one layer of cells thick. The cells are mildly atypical with nucleoli. This pattern is thought to be the precursor of flat-type low-grade ductal carcinoma *in situ* (DCIS).
- **Atypical ductal hyperplasia (ADH)** or atypical intraductal proliferation (AIDP) is a high-risk lesion comprising atypical ductal cells showing cytological and architectural atypia falling short of DCIS. Lesions are usually occupy less than two duct spaces and measure less than 2 mm in size.
- ***In situ* lobular neoplasia (ISLN)** is a proliferation of small, poorly cohesive epithelial cells arising in the terminal duct lobular system and characterized by a monomorphic population of small cells showing loss of E-cadherin expression immunohistochemically. Morphologically, lesion of atypical lobular hyperplasia (ALH) and lobular carcinoma *in situ* (LCIS) are included in this category.

Prognosis

- UEH is not considered a direct precursor lesion to invasive breast carcinoma but is a marker for a slightly increased risk for subsequent invasive carcinoma (1.5–2 times that of the general population).
- Large series on relative risk of FEA are lacking, but current evidence suggests it carries a relative risk of about four times for subsequent invasive carcinoma.
- ADH carries an increased risk of invasive breast carcinoma 4–5 times that of the general population. This risk is further increased if the patient has a first-degree relative with breast cancer.
- ISLN is closely related to ADH but is more likely to be bilateral and multifocal. Relative risk for invasive breast carcinoma is similar to ADH (i.e. 4–5 times that of the general population).

Ductal carcinoma *in situ*

Definition

- A heterogeneous group of neoplastic intraductal epithelial proliferations arising from the terminal duct lobular unit.
- The clonal proliferation is limited to the duct system which they distend and distort.
- There is no extension into surrounding breast stromal tissue.
- They carry a risk of progression to invasive breast carcinoma.

Epidemiology

- Common.
- Incidence has markedly increased since the introduction of breast screening programmes.

Aetiology

- Risks similar to invasive breast carcinoma.

Genetics

- Microarray and laser capture microdissection have shown that gene expression signatures of DCIS may be similar to invasive carcinoma.
- Low-grade DCIS often is associated with loss of 16q.
- High-grade DCIS is genetically distinct with a more complex karyotype with gains of 17q, 8q, and 5p with losses of 11q, 13q, and 14q.

Presentation

- 85% are detected on mammography as areas of microcalcification.
- 10% produce clinical findings such as a lump, nipple discharge, or eczematous change of the nipple (**Paget's disease of the nipple**).
- 5% are diagnosed incidentally in breast specimens removed for other reasons.

Macroscopy

- DCIS is often macroscopically invisible, even to an experienced pathologist.
- Extensive high-grade DCIS may be visible as gritty, yellow flecks due to calcified necrotic debris in the involved ducts.

Histopathology

- DCIS is subclassified into low, intermediate, and high nuclear grade.
- **Low-grade DCIS** has small monotonous cells growing in cribriform, solid, or micropapillary patterns with good cellular polarization (cells have basally positioned nuclei and apical cytoplasm directed towards the duct lumen). Necrosis in the centre of the duct is unusual.
- **Intermediate grade DCIS** has cells with moderately sized nuclei and coarse chromatin growing in solid, cribriform, or micropapillary patterns with a moderate degree of cellular polarization. Central necrosis may be present.
- **High-grade DCIS** has cells with large, markedly pleomorphic nuclei with clumped chromatin, prominent nucleoli, and poor cellular polarization. Central necrosis is common.

Prognosis

- Complete surgical excision with clear margins is curative.
- Current evidence points towards low-grade DCIS being a risk lesion similar to ISLN. While the standard of care is surgical excision, other management options including 'wait-and-watch' or hormonal manipulation using anti-oestrogen receptors for pure DCIS are also being considered for low-grade DCIS.
- For high-grade DCIS, surgical excision is the recommendation with or without radiotherapy depending upon the extent of the disease.
- Prognosis depends on the persistence of *in situ* disease and grade. Recurrence is more likely with extensive disease and high nuclear grade.
- Van Nuy's prognostic index uses tumour size, margin width, and grade of DCIS to prognosticate pure DCIS lesions, dividing this into low, intermediate, and high-risk categories for local recurrence that may benefit from radiation therapy.

Invasive breast carcinomas

Definition

- A group of malignant epithelial tumours of the breast arising from the terminal duct lobular unit with the capacity to invade the stroma and spread to distant sites.

Epidemiology

- The most common cancer in women, with a lifetime risk of 1 in 8.
- Incidence rates rise rapidly with increasing age, such that most cases occur in older women.
- Rarely occur in 20s and 30s with a family history of breast carcinoma.
- Can occur anywhere in the breast.

Aetiology

- Early menarche, late menopause, increased weight, high alcohol consumption, oral contraceptive use, and a positive family history are all associated with increased risk.
- 5% of cases show evidence of inheritance. *BRCA* mutations cause a lifetime risk of invasive breast carcinoma of up to 85% and tend to occur at an early age.

Carcinogenesis

- Recent genetic studies have led to the hypothesis that breast cancer evolution is broadly classified into two groups: luminal and basal. These are also defined by differential expression of hormone receptors.
- The luminal group (which includes low-grade invasive ductal carcinoma, lobular carcinoma, mucinous carcinoma, tubular carcinoma) classically expresses oestrogen (ER) and progesterone (PR) receptors with lack of HER2 overexpression. These are thought to arise within luminal ductal cells and do not express basal markers. Genetically, they have simple diploid or near diploid karyotypes and, as a hallmark, show deletion of 16q and gains of 1q.
- The basal group typically lack ER and PR expression and may or may not overexpress HER2. Tumours that do not express ER, PR, or HER2 are also known as triple negative breast cancers (TNBC). Genetically, they have complex karyotypes with many unbalanced chromosomal aberrations showing frequent gains of 1q, 2q and 1p and losses of 1p, 12q, 17q, 8p, and 17p.

Presentation

- Most cases present symptomatically with a breast lump, usually an ill-defined mass, sometimes adherent to the skin or the underlying pectoralis muscle.
- An increasing proportion of asymptomatic cases are detected on screening mammography.

Macroscopy

- Most breast carcinomas produce a firm, solitary, stellate mass in the breast. Certain types of cancers may show multifocal bilateral involvement.
- Axillary lymph nodes may be involved.

Cytopathology

- FNA from breast carcinomas are typically highly cellular, containing a poorly cohesive population of malignant epithelial cells. Background bare bipolar nuclei are absent.

Histopathology

- **Invasive ductal carcinomas** (80%) are composed of nests of atypical epithelial cells with variable degrees of tubule formation.
- **Invasive lobular carcinomas** (15%) are composed of small, poorly cohesive cells with scant cytoplasm, which characteristically grow in linear cords and encircle pre-existing normal ducts.
- **Tubular carcinomas** (5%) are composed of well-formed tubular structures lined by a single layer of epithelial cells with low-grade atypia.
- **Mucinous carcinomas** (5%) are characterized by the production of abundant quantities of mucin within which the tumour cells float.
- **Basal-like carcinomas** are composed of sheets of atypical cells surrounded by a prominent lymphocytic inflammatory reaction. On immunohistochemistry they are typically positive for basal-type keratins (e.g. cytokeratins 5 and 14).

Grading

- All invasive breast cancers are graded histologically by assessing nuclear pleomorphism, tubule formation, and mitotic activity.
- Each parameter is scored from 1 to 3, and the three values are added together to produce total scores from 3 to 9.
- 3–5 points = grade 1 (well differentiated).
- 6–7 points = grade 2 (moderately differentiated).
- 8–9 points = grade 3 (poorly differentiated).

Prognosis

- The single most important prognostic factor is the status of the axillary lymph nodes.
- Other important factors include tumour size, histological type, and histological grade.

Treatment

- Based on prognostic factors that include tumour size, histological grade, nodal stage, and hormone receptor status, invasive cancers are treated with a combination regimen that includes surgery (localized or radical), chemotherapy, hormone manipulation, and local radiotherapy.
- Frequent expression of programmed death-ligand 1 (PD-L1) in TNBC has led to the development of PD-L1 inhibitors for these tumours which are resistant to other common breast cancer therapies.

Genomic tests

- These are predictive tests that analyse a group of genes that can affect how a cancer is likely to behave and respond to treatment. The test include Oncotype DX® and EndoPredict®.
- **EndoPredict®** testing is a multigene test used to predict the risk of distant recurrence of early-stage, ER-positive, HER2-negative invasive breast cancer that is either node-negative (pN0) or has up to three

positive nodes (pN1). The EndoPredict® clinical score (EP clinscore) categorizes patients into low- and high-risk groups. The low-risk group is less likely to develop recurrences, compared with high-risk groups, and hence can be spared the side effects of chemotherapy.
- **Oncotype DX®** testing is done for low-stage (1 and 2), ER-positive, and lymph-node-negative (pN0) invasive breast cancers. A recurrence score (RI) is generated by testing for the activity of 21 genes.
- Invasive cancer with a low score (<18) is deemed to have a low chance of recurrence and less likely to derive benefit from chemotherapy.
- Invasive cancer with a high score (≥31) have a higher risk of recurrence and likely to derive benefit from chemotherapy.
- Invasive cancer with intermediate score (18–30): risk is unclear.

Current/recent clinical trials in breast cancer
- PRIME TIME: investigating radiotherapy for women with a very small risk of breast cancer recurrence
- Add ASPIRIN: investigating if aspirin can prevent cancer from coming back after treatment
- BC-PReDICT: investigating breast cancer risk at the time of breast cancer screening
- HERPET: investigating if PET scans can assess HER2 protein in breast cancer
- OPTIMA: investigating a test to predict which cohort of patients could benefit from chemotherapy

Breast screening

▶The aim of screening is to pick up DCIS or early invasive carcinoma.

NHS breast screening programme

- Anyone registered with a GP as female is invited for screening every 3 years between the ages of 50 and 71.
- The screening test is a set of four mammograms (two for each breast) which looks for abnormal areas of calcification or a mass within the breast.

Assessment clinic

- ~5% of women have an abnormal mammogram and are recalled to an assessment clinic for further investigation.
- This may include more mammograms or an ultrasound, followed by sampling of the abnormal area, usually by core biopsy.

Histopathology

- Core biopsies taken from breast screening patients are given a B code from 1 to 5.
- B1 is normal breast tissue. This usually implies the biopsy missed the area of interest.
- B2 is a core containing a benign abnormality. This is appropriate for a range of lesions, including fibroadenomas, fibrocystic change, sclerosing adenosis, and fat necrosis.
- B3 is a lesion of uncertain malignant potential. This category mainly consists of lesions which may be benign in the core but are known to show heterogeneity or to have an increased risk (albeit low) of an adjacent malignancy. This is appropriate for cores showing FEA, ISLN, ADH, partly sampled papillomas, phyllodes tumours, and radial scars.
- B4 is a core showing features suspicious of malignancy, but in which unequivocal diagnosis is not possible due to reasons such as insufficient abnormal tissue or crushing of the biopsy.
- B5 is a core biopsy showing unequivocal features of malignancy. This is subdivided into B5a for DCIS or B5b for invasive carcinoma.

Management

- B1: rebiopsy.
- B2: reassure and return to normal recall.
- B3: excision of the abnormal area.
- B4: rebiopsy or excision of the abnormal area.
- B5: surgical excision with wide local excision or mastectomy.

Effectiveness

- Published figures state that the NHS breast screening programme saves about 1250 lives each year.

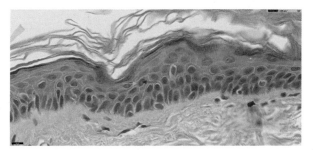

Plate 1. Haematoxylin and eosin (H&E) stained section of normal skin. Haematoxylin stains the nucleus of cells purple (red arrow). Eosin stains the cytoplasm of cells pink (green arrow).

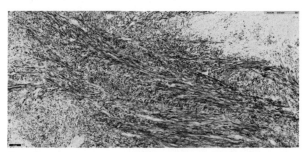

Plate 2. An example of a leiomyosarcoma demonstrating positive brown staining for desmin by immunohistochemistry, indicating muscle phenotype.

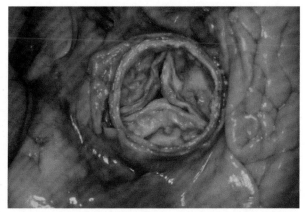

Plate 3. Calcific aortic stenosis. This aortic valve is studded with nodules of calcium causing significant narrowing of the valve orifice.

Reproduced with permission from *Clinical Pathology* (Oxford Core Texts), Carton, James, Daly, Richard, and Ramani, Pramila, Oxford University Press (2006), p.96, Figure 6.18.

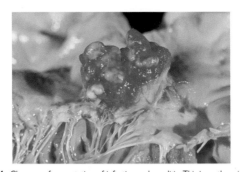

Plate 4. Close-up of a vegetation of infective endocarditis. This is on the mitral valve; you can see the chordae tendinae attached to the valve leaflets.

Reproduced with permission from *Clinical Pathology* (Oxford Core Texts), Carton, James, Daly, Richard, and Ramani, Pramila, Oxford University Press (2006), p.97, Figure 6.19.

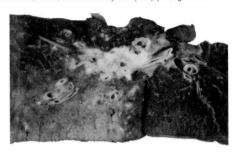

Plate 5. A central lung carcinoma. Note how the lung tissue distal to the tumour shows flecks of yellow consolidation due to an obstructive pneumonia. The tumour was found to be a squamous cell carcinoma when examined microscopically.

Reproduced with permission from *Clinical Pathology* (Oxford Core Texts), Carton, James, Daly, Richard, and Ramani, Pramila, Oxford University Press (2006), p.131, Figure 7.13.

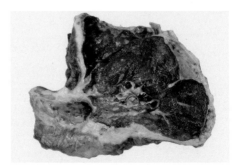

Plate 6. Typical macroscopic appearance of malignant mesothelioma. Note how the tumour encases and compresses the lung.

Reproduced with permission from *Clinical Pathology* (Oxford Core Texts), Carton, James, Daly, Richard, and Ramani, Pramila, Oxford University Press (2006), p. 136, Figure 7.15.

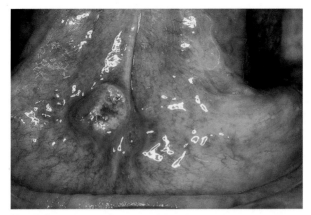

Plate 7. Early squamous cell carcinoma of the oral cavity, presenting as a persistent ulcerated lesion on the undersurface of the tongue.

Reproduced with permission from *Clinical Pathology* (Oxford Core Texts), Carton, James, Daly, Richard, and Ramani, Pramila, Oxford University Press (2006), p.452, Figure 19.4.

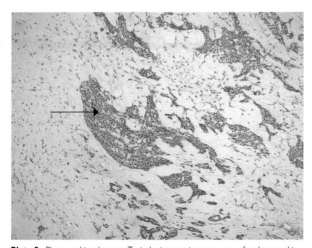

Plate 8. Pleomorphic adenoma. Typical microscopic appearance of a pleomorphic adenoma with an intermingling of epithelial elements (arrow) set within a mesenchymal component.

Reproduced with permission from *Clinical Pathology* (Oxford Core Texts), Carton, James, Daly, Richard, and Ramani, Pramila, Oxford University Press (2006), p.456, Figure 19.7.

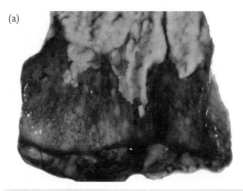

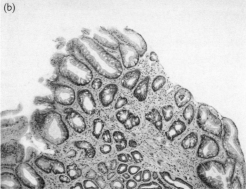

Plate 9. Barrett's oesophagus. (a) This segment from the lower oesophagus shows the white keratinized squamous epithelium at the top. The red area at the bottom represents an area of Barrett's oesophagus. (b) An oesophageal biopsy taken from an area of endoscopic Barrett's oesophagus, confirming the presence of glandular epithelium.

Reproduced with permission from *Clinical Pathology* (Oxford Core Texts), Carton, James, Daly, Richard, and Ramani, Pramila, Oxford University Press (2006), p.139, Figure 8.1.

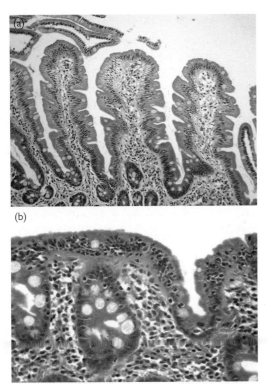

Plate 10. (a) Normal duodenal mucosa. The villi have a normal height and shape, and there is no increase in intraepithelial lymphocytes. (b) Duodenal biopsy from a patient with gluten-sensitive enteropathy. The villi have completely disappeared and the surface epithelium contains many intraepithelial lymphocytes.

Reproduced with permission from *Clinical Pathology* (Oxford Core Texts), Carton, James, Daly, Richard, and Ramani, Pramila, Oxford University Press (2006), p.154, Figure 8.8.

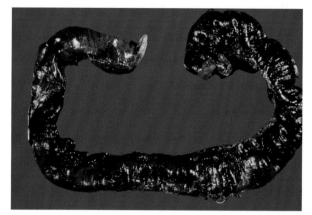

Plate 11. Small bowel infarction. Typical appearance of an infarcted segment of the small bowel. The dark colour is due to the intense congestion and haemorrhage within the intestine as a result of blockage to venous outflow.

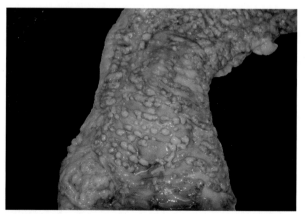

Plate 12. *Clostridium difficile* colitis. This is a freshly opened colon from a patient with profuse diarrhoea, following broad-spectrum antibiotic treatment. Note the large number of cream-coloured plaques studded across the mucosal surface, representing collections of neutrophils, fibrin, and cell debris.

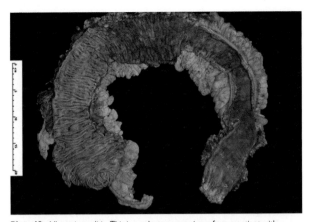

Plate 13. Ulcerative colitis. This is a colectomy specimen from a patient with ulcerative colitis. The right colon is on the left of the picture (note the appendix), and the left colon and rectum are on the right side of the picture. The inflamed mucosa, which looks red, begins at the rectum and continuously affects the left colon until the transverse colon where there is a sharp transition into normal mucosa.

Reproduced with permission from *Clinical Pathology* (Oxford Core Texts), Carton, James, Daly, Richard, and Ramani, Pramila, Oxford University Press (2006), p. 163, Figure 8.15.

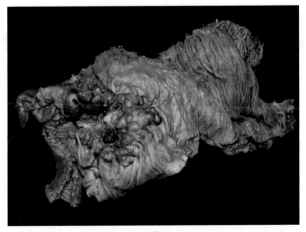

Plate 14. Adenocarcinoma of the caecum. This is a right hemicolectomy specimen, in which a small piece of the terminal ileum, the caecum, the appendix, and the ascending colon have been removed. A large tumour is seen in the caecum, which was confirmed on microscopy to be an adenocarcinoma. This tumour was picked up at colonoscopy performed because the patient was found to have an unexplained iron deficiency anaemia.

Reproduced with permission from Clinical Pathology (Oxford Core Texts), Carton, James, Daly, Richard, and Ramani, Pramila, Oxford University Press (2006), p.168, figure 8.20.

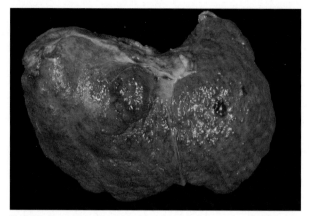

Plate 15. The cirrhotic liver. This liver was removed at post-mortem from a patient known to abuse alcohol. The whole of the liver is studded with nodules. Microscopically, the liver showed nodules of regenerating hepatocytes separated by dense bands of fibrosis, confirming established cirrhosis.

Reproduced with permission from *Clinical Pathology* (Oxford Core Texts), Carton, James, Daly, Richard, and Ramani, Pramila, Oxford University Press (2006), p. 168, Figure 9.9.

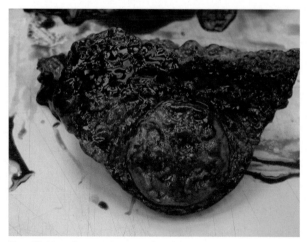

Plate 16. Liver cell cancer arising in a cirrhotic liver.

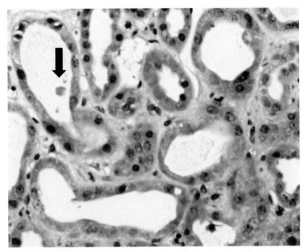

Plate 17. Acute tubular injury. Haematoxylin and eosin stain. The epithelial cells are flattened and the tubular lumen is widened. Arrow indicates a sloughed tubular epithelial cell in the lumen of a tubule.

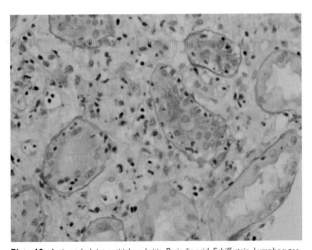

Plate 18. Active tubulointerstitial nephritis. Periodic acid–Schiff stain. Lymphocytes and cells of monocytic lineage appear as small dark nuclei amongst the tubular epithelial cells, which have larger nuclei with more dispersed chromatin. Tubulitis is defined by inflammatory cells within the spaces delimited by the tubular basement membranes, seen on this PAS stain as bright pink lines around individual tubular profiles.

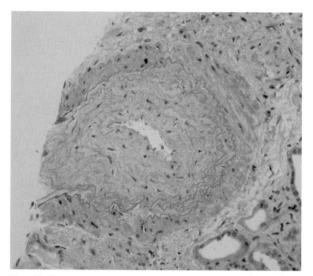

Plate 19. Fibrous arterial intimal thickening. Hematoxylin and eosin stain. A thick layer of fibrous tissue is present under the endothelium and above the duplicated layers of elastic lamina, which appear as thin wavy dark pink lines. In a normal artery, the endothelium is much more closely apposed to the elastic lamina, with only a thin intervening layer of matrix.

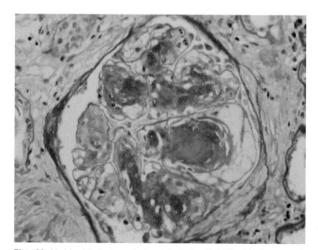

Plate 20. Nodular diabetic glomerulosclerosis (periodic acid–Schiff stain). The mesangial matrix is expanded by nodules of matrix referred to as Kimmelstiel–Wilson nodules.

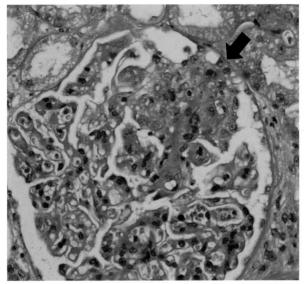

Plate 21. Focal and segmental glomerulosclerosis, not otherwise specified (NOS). Haematoxylin and eosin. A portion of the tuft between 1 and 2 o'clock is replaced by fibrous stroma, with closure of the capillary lumens. This part of the glomerulus also adheres to Bowman's capsule (arrow).

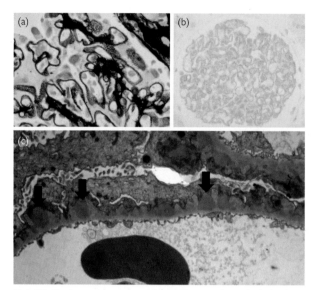

Plate 22. Membranous glomerulonephritis. (a) Silver stain showing 'spikes' and 'holes' (irregularities) along the glomerular capillary walls. (b) Immunoperoxidase staining for IgG showing granular capillary wall staining in brown (c) Electron microscopy showing subepithelial 'electron-dense deposits' (arrows) corresponding to the immune complex deposition.

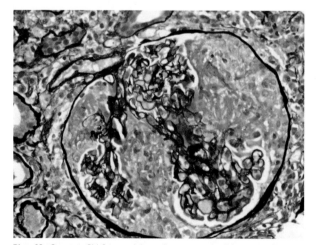

Plate 23. Crescentic GN: Segmental glomerular necrosis with cellular crescent (Jones silver stain). Bowman's space is filled with/obliterated by cells and fibrin strands.

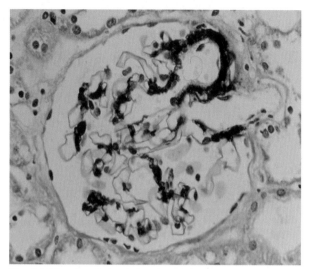

Plate 24. IgA nephropathy. Immunohistochemistry for IgA showing mesangial positivity in a case of IgA nephropathy.

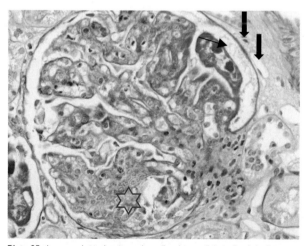

Plate 25. Lupus nephritis showing endocapillary hypercellularity (star), hyaline thrombi within capillary loops (thick arrows) and 'wireloops' (thin arrow) along a capillary wall.

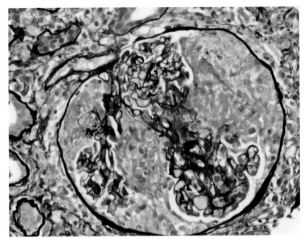

Plate 26. ANCA vasculitis affecting a glomerulus. There is a large cellular crescent (arrows) and there is fibrinoid necrosis (star) of the glomerular tuft.

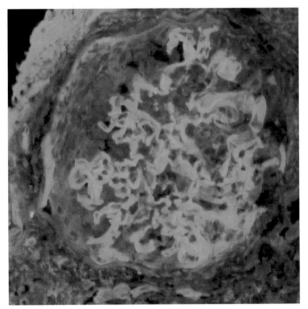

Plate 27. Anti-GBM disease on immunofluorescence for IgG: there is bright linear positivity along the glomerular basement membrane.

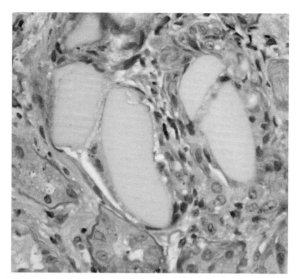

Plate 28. Light chain cast nephropathy (PAS stain). The casts stain weakly with PAS in contrast to usual hyaline casts or granular casts. They often have angular edges, 'cracks' and a border of cells around the edge.

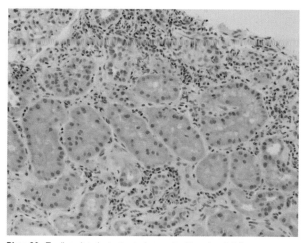

Plate 29. T-cell-mediated rejection is characterized by a chronic inflammatory infiltrate (predominantly T lymphocytes and monocytes) in the interstitium, with tubulitis.

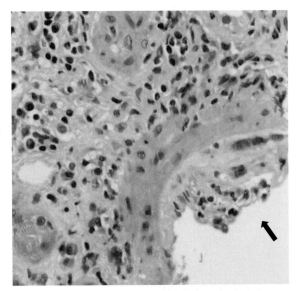

Plate 30. In both T-cell-mediated rejection and antibody-mediated rejection, endarteritis can be seen. This is characterized by inflammatory cells beneath the endothelium, within the intima (arrow)

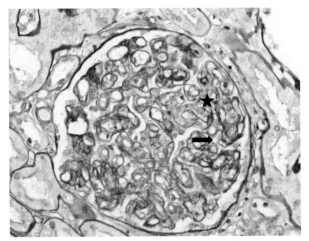

Plate 31. In chronic active antibody-mediated rejection, a 'transplant glomerulopathy' develops in response to fixation of an antibody against donor HLA antigens on the endothelium: there is endocapillary hypercellularity (star) and double contours along capillary wall (two parallel lines instead of one, arrow).

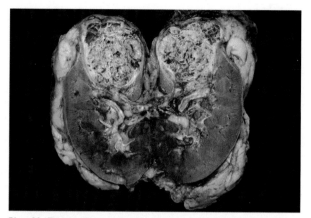

Plate 32. This patient presented with macroscopic haematuria and was found to have a solid renal mass on CT imaging. A nephrectomy was performed and sent to pathology. The kidney has been sliced open by the pathologist to reveal a large tumour in the upper pole of the kidney. Subsequent microscopic examination of samples of the tumour revealed this to be a clear cell renal cell carcinoma.

Reproduced with permission from *Clinical Pathology* (Oxford Core Texts), Carton, James, Daly, Richard, and Ramani, Pramila, Oxford University Press (2006), p.233, Figure 11.6.

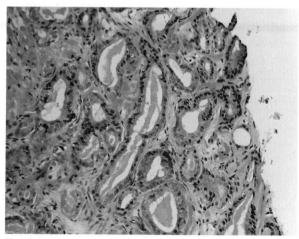

Plate 33. Gleason pattern 3 prostate adenocarcinoma composed of individual well-formed glandular acini.

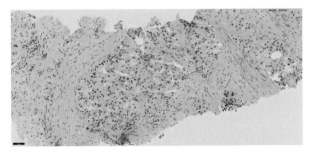

Plate 34. Gleason pattern 4 prostate adenocarcinoma composed of fused poorly formed glands.

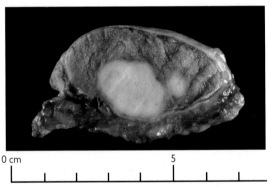

0 cm   5

Plate 35. This is a testis from a young man who presented with an enlarging testicular lump. Following an ultrasound scan which was suspicious for a neoplasm, he underwent orchidectomy. The testis has been sliced in the pathology department, revealing this white solid mass in the testis. This appearance is typical of a seminoma, and microscopic examination confirmed this.

Reproduced with permission from *Clinical Pathology* (Oxford Core Texts), Carton, James, Daly, Richard, and Ramani, Pramila, Oxford University Press (2006), p. 244, Figure 11.14.

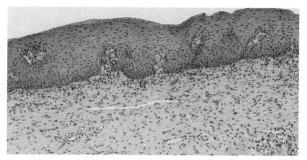

Plate 36. CIN 1. Abnormalities are concentrated in the lower third of the squamous epithelium of the transformation zone.

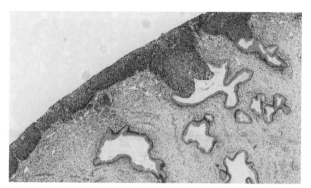

Plate 37. CIN 3. Abnormalities extend into the upper third of the squamous epithelium of the transformation zone. In this example the CIN 3 also extends into an endocervical crypt.

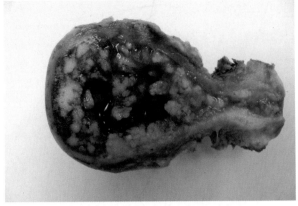

Plate 38. Endometrial carcinoma filling the uterine cavity.

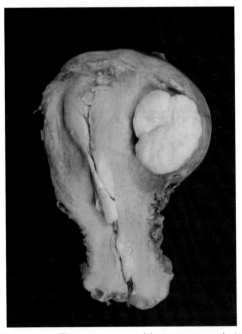

Plate 39. Leiomyoma. This uterus was removed due to severe menorrhagia. On bisecting the uterus, a well-circumscribed white mass is seen in the myometrium which bulges from the cut surface. This is the typical macroscopic appearance of a leiomyoma (fibroid) and this was confirmed on microscopic examination.

Reproduced with permission from *Clinical Pathology* (Oxford Core Texts), Carton, James, Daly, Richard, and Ramani, Pramila, Oxford University Press (2006), p. 269, Figure 12.9.

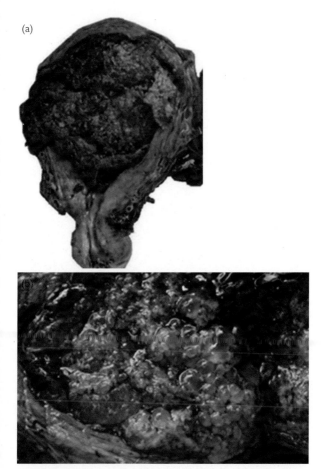

Plate 40. (a) Complete mole presenting as an enlarged uterus with abnormally dilated endometrial cavity in a 55 years old female with uncontrolled vaginal bleeding. (b) Hydropic change is generalized and no fetus is present.

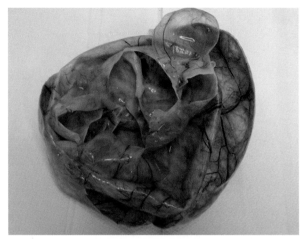

Plate 41. Benign mucinous cystadenoma of the ovary.

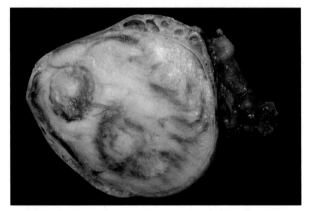

Plate 42. Mature cystic teratoma. Typical appearance of a mature cystic teratoma (dermoid cyst) filled with greasy yellow material and hair.

Reproduced with permission from *Clinical Pathology* (Oxford Core Texts), Carton, James, Daly, Richard, and Ramani, Pramila, Oxford University Press (2006), p. 278, Figure 12.17.

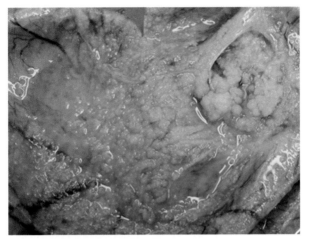

Plate 43. Borderline serous tumour of the ovary.

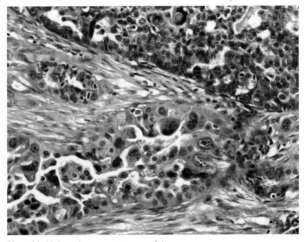

Plate 44. High-grade serous carcinoma of the ovary.

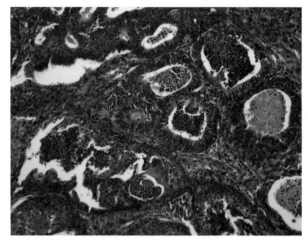

Plate 45. Endometrioid carcinoma of the ovary.

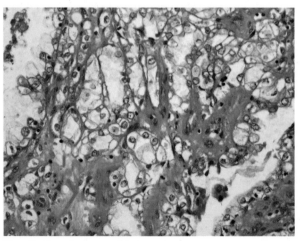

Plate 46. Clear cell carcinoma of the ovary.

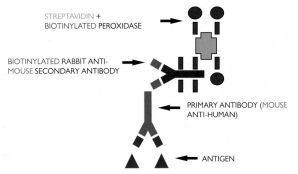

STREPTAVIDIN +
BIOTINYLATED PEROXIDASE

BIOTINYLATED RABBIT ANTI-
MOUSE SECONDARY ANTIBODY

PRIMARY ANTIBODY (MOUSE
ANTI-HUMAN)

ANTIGEN

Plate 47. Immunohistochemistry. There are different detection methods, the avidin/biotin complex (ABC) is the most extended. The primary antibody is detected with a biotic-labelled antibody that then interacts with an avidin/biotin complex containing many labels.

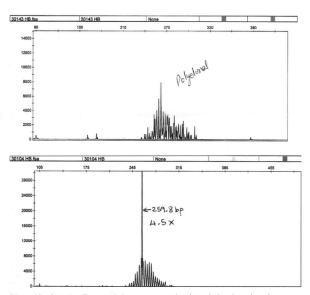

Plate 48. Clonality. Top panel shows an example of a polyclonal result with a variety of different peaks. Bottom panel shows an example of a mononclonal result with a strong peak (arrowed) on a polyclonal background.

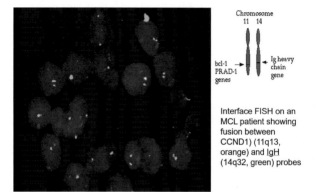

Interface FISH on an MCL patient showing fusion between CCND1 (11q13, orange) and IgH (14q32, green) probes

Plate 49. Fluorescence in situ hybridisation (FISH) result in a case of mantle cell lymphoma (MCL). Tumour cells show abnormal juxtaposition of the orange and green probes due to a t(11;14) chromosomal translocation.

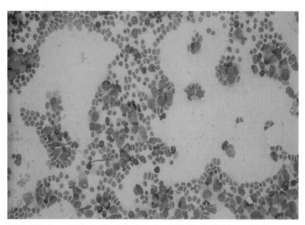

Plate 50. Acute B-lymphoblastic leukaemia. >20% of cells in this preparation are lymphoid blasts characterized by medium to large cells with a high nuclear to cytoplasmic ratio and finely dispersed chromatin.

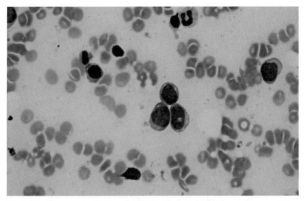

Plate 51. Acute myeloid leukaemia. >20% of cells in this preparation are myeloid blasts characterized by medium to large cells with a high nuclear to cytoplasmic ratio. Some myeloid blasts contain cytoplasmic granules or Auer rods.

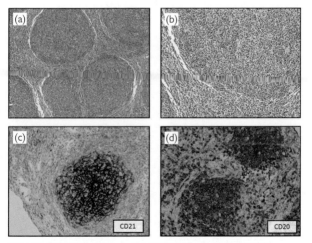

Plate 52. Follicular lymphoma. (a, b) Lymphoma characterized by a nodular pattern. The nodules are well defined and lack mantle areas (haematoxylin and eosin). (c) Follicular pattern highlighted with CD21 (staining follicular dendritic cells). (d) The cells in the follicle centres are CD20-positive (B-cell marker).

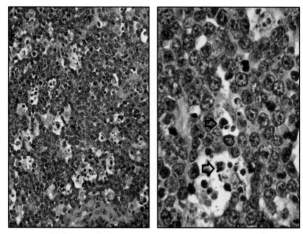

Plate 53. Burkitt's lymphoma. Lymphoma characterized by monomorphic medium-sized lymphoid cells with a 'starry sky' pattern. Detail of tingible body macrophages containing apoptotic tumour cells (arrows).

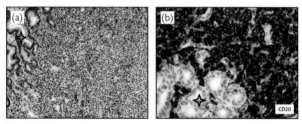

Plate 54. Extranodal marginal zone lymphoma involving the stomach. (a) Gastric mucosa (asterisk indicates gastric glands) infiltrated by a lymphoma composed of small centrocyte-like lymphocytes (haematoxylin and eosin). (b) The lymphoma cells are CD20 diffuse-positive.

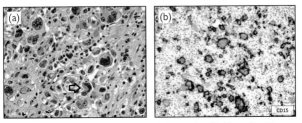

Plate 55. Classical Hodgkin's lymphoma. (a) Mononuclear Hodgkin cells and large atypical Reed–Sternberg cells (arrow), multinucleated with prominent nucleoli. (b) The cells are positive with CD15 (membrane staining).

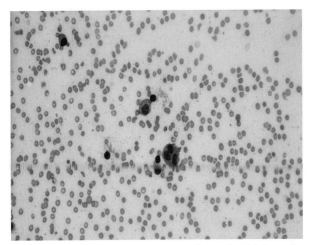

Plate 56. Multiple myeloma bone marrow aspirate. Groups of atypical plasma cells are present.

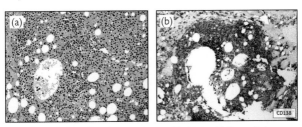

Plate 57. Multiple myeloma bone marrow trephine biopsy. (a) Sheets of plasma cells infiltrate the bone marrow. The plasma cells have a round eccentric nucleus and abundant basophilic cytoplasm (haematoxylin and eosin staining). (b) The plasma cells are diffusely and strongly positive with CD138 (plasma cell marker).

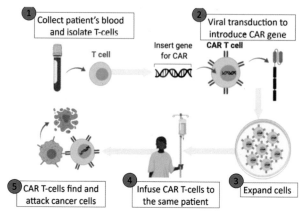

Plate 58. CAR T immunotherapy.

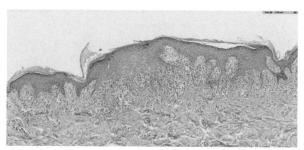

Plate 59. Lichen planus. Histology shows a lichenoid tissue reaction pattern characterized by an irregularly acanthotic squamatised epidermis and an obscuring band of lymphocytic inflammation at the dermo-epidermal junction.

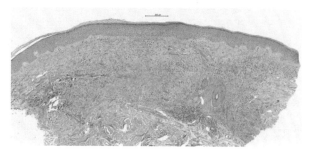

Plate 60. Granuloma annulare. Histology shows a necrobiotic granulomatous inflammation in the dermis characterized by a zone of degenerate collagen surrounded by a palisade of histiocytes and perivascular lymphocytic inflammation.

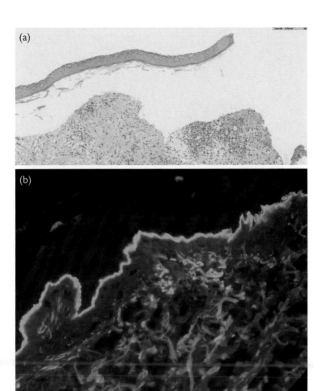

Plate 61. Bullous pemphigoid. (a) Histology of blistered skin shows a subepidermal blister with inflammation in dermis rich in eosinophils. (b) Direct immunofluorescence performed on perilesional skin shows linear deposition of C3 along the basement membrane zone.

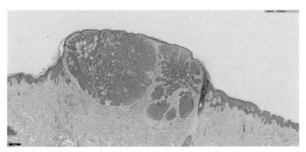

Plate 62. Basal cell carcinoma, nodular subtype. Histology shows well circumscribed nests of basaloid epithelial cells with peripheral palisading and mucinous stroma.

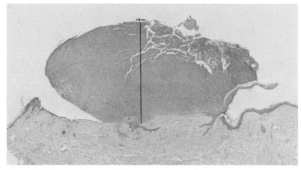

Plate 63. Melanoma Breslow thickness

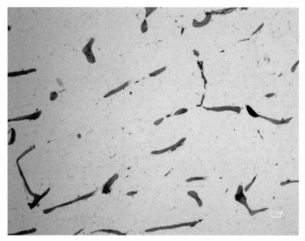

Plate 64. Osteoporosis characterized by thin, disconnected trabeculae of lamellar bone within fatty marrow.

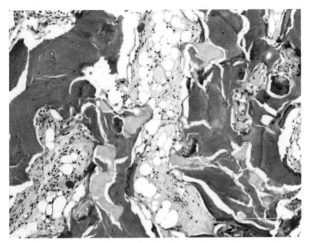

Plate 65. Osteopetrosis is characterized by a distorted bony architecture, with thick trabecular and compact bone largely obliterating the bone marrow space.

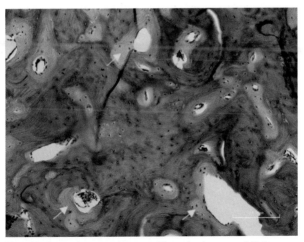

Plate 66. Osteomalacia, as seen in compact bone, showing mature viable bone covered by a thick layer of unmineralized matrix (osteoid)—pale pink (arrows). Similar features are seen in rickets.

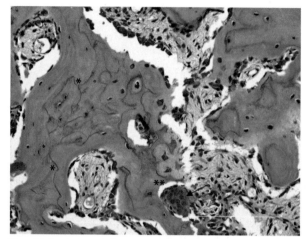

Plate 67. Paget's disease. Diffuse remodelled cancellous bone with prominent cement lines* and deep Howship's lacunae** which, in areas, are associated with osteoclasts, containing very large numbers of nuclei (arrow).

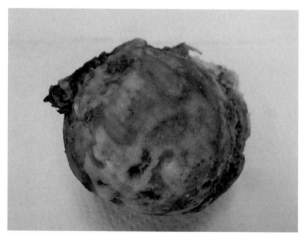

Plate 68. Osteoarthritis. Femoral head shows an eroded and irregular articular surface.

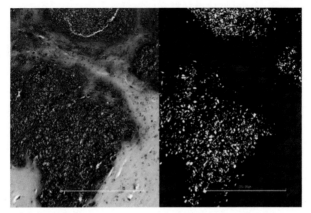

Plate 69. Pseudogout. Rhomboid/rod-shaped crystals under polarized light showing positive birefringence.

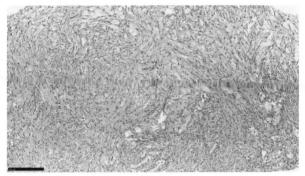

Plate 70. Nodular fasciitis. Myofibroblastic proliferation with a "tissue culture" appearance.

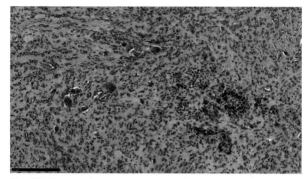

Plate 71. Tenosynovial giant cell tumour. Mononuclear cells in a collagenous background associated with associated with osteoclast-like multinucleated cells and haemosiderin-laden macrophages.

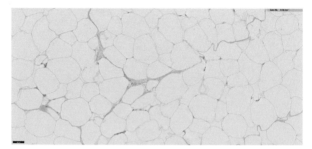

Plate 72. Lipoma. Mature adipocytes with mild variation in size and no atypical stromal cells.

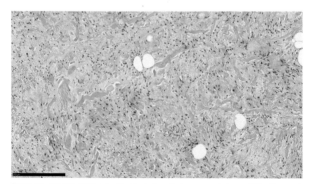

Plate 73. Spindle cell lipoma. Bland spindle cells in a somewhat myxoid background associated with ropey collagen bundles. Occasional mature adipocytes in this example.

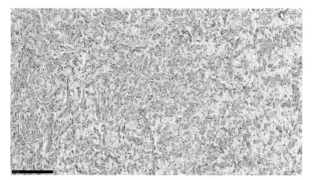

Plate 74. Neurofibroma. Haphazardly arranged, cytologically-bland spindle cells in a variably collagenous and myxoid stroma.

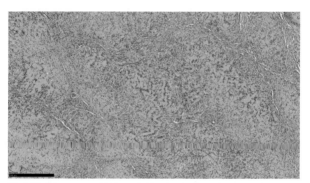

Plate 75. Schwanomma. Nuclear palisading (Verocay bodies) in a schwanomma.

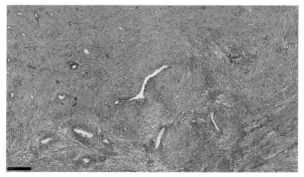

Plate 76. Angioleiomyoma. Spindle cells with eosinophilic cytoplasm asociated with a population of muscularised blood vessels.

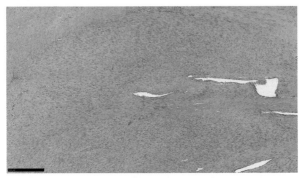

Plate 77. Plantar fibromatosis. Sweeping fascicles in a collagenous background.

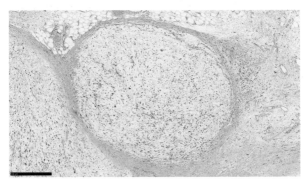

Plate 78. Myxofibrosarcoma. Lobular architecture with myxoid stroma, curvilinear vessels and hyperchromatic tumour cells.

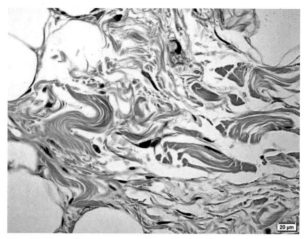

Plate 79. Atypical lipomatous tumour. Mature adipocytes with scattered hyperchromatic spindled stromal cells.

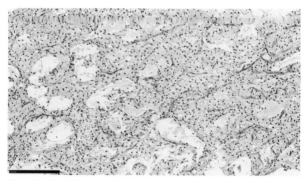

Plate 80. Myxoid liposaroma. Small oval shaped cells set within a myxoid stroma containing a delicate, abororising capillary network.

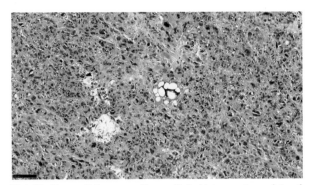

Plate 81. Pleomorphic liposarcoma. Pleomorphic lipoblast amongst a population of pleomorphic cells with eosinophilic cytoplasm.

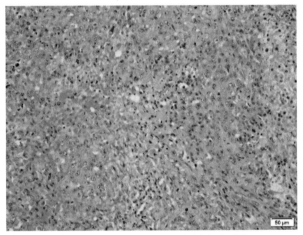

Plate 82. Epithelioid sarcoma, classic-type. Atypical epithelioid cells forming aggregates and surrounding necrotic areas in a granuloma-like pattern. This could be mistaken for a carcinoma.

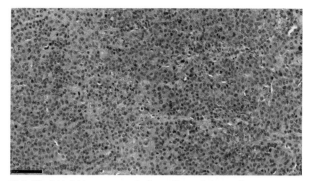

Plate 83. Epithelioid sarcoma, proximal-type. Sheets of pleomorphic epithelioid cells.

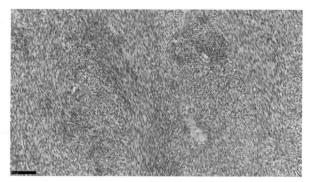

Plate 84. Synovial sarcoma, monophasic-type. Cellular fascicles of monomorphic, blue-appearing spindle cells.

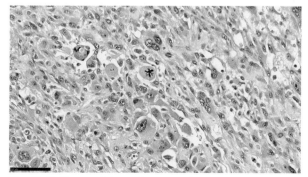

Plate 85. Undifferentiated pleomorphic sarcoma. Sheets of markedly pleomorphic cells with atypical mitotic figures.

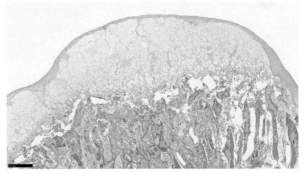

Plate 86. Osteochondroma. Cartilaginous cap showing enchondral ossification merging with trabecular bone.

Plate 87. Non ossifying fibroma. Fibroblastic cells in a storiform arrangement with scattered osteoclast-type giant cells.

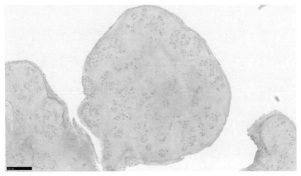

Plate 88. Synovial chondromatosis. Multiple nodules of hyaline cartilage with clustering of chondrocytes.

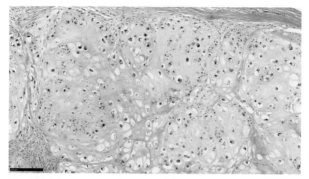

Plate 89. Grade III chondrosarcoma. Cartilaginous tumour displaying markedly atypical chondrocytes.

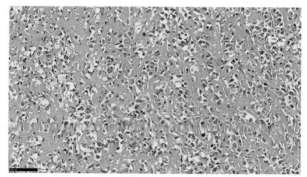

Plate 90. Conventional (osteoblastic) osteosarcoma. Atypical cells associated with abundant osteoid formation.

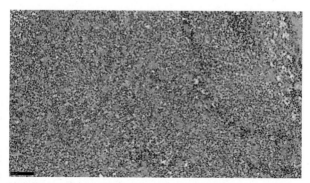

Plate 91. Ewing Sarcoma. Sheets of monotonous small round cells.

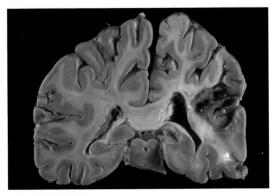

Plate 92. Cerebral infarction.

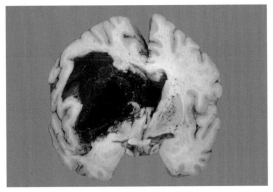

Plate 93. Intracerebral haemorrhage. This is a slice of brain taken at post-mortem from a patient who suddenly collapsed and died. There is a massive intracerebral haematoma which led to a huge rise in intracranial pressure and herniation. The cause in this case was hypertension, and other changes of hypertension at post-mortem included left ventricular hypertrophy and nephrosclerosis of both kidneys.

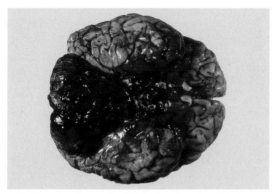

Plate 94. Subarachnoid haemorrhage. This is the undersurface of the brain removed at post-mortem from a patient who suddenly cried out, collapsed, and died. Blood is seen filling the subarachnoid space. When the blood clot was cleared away, a ruptured berry aneurysm was found in the circle of Willis.

Reproduced with permission from *Clinical Pathology* (Oxford Core Texts), Carton, James, Daly, Richard, and Ramani, Pramila, Oxford University Press (2006).

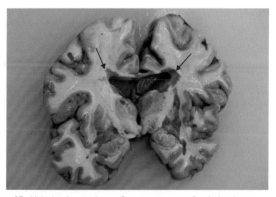

Plate 95. Multiple sclerosis plaques. Brown appearance of multiple sclerosis plaques, seen here in a characteristic location around the lateral ventricles (arrows).

Reproduced with permission from *Clinical Pathology* (Oxford Core Texts), Carton, James, Daly, Richard, and Ramani, Pramila, Oxford University Press (2006).

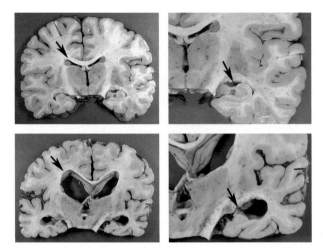

Plate 96. Alzheimer's disease. The top images are from a normal patient aged 70, whilst the bottom images are from a patient with Alzheimer's disease. Note the ventricular dilation (left- hand side) and cortical atrophy in the brain from the patient with Alzheimer's disease, particularly marked in the hippocampus (right- hand side).

Reproduced with permission from *Clinical Pathology* (Oxford Core Texts), Carton, James, Daly, Richard, and Ramani, Pramila, Oxford University Press (2006).

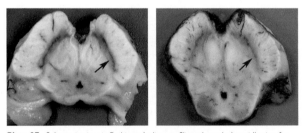

Plate 97. Substantia nigra in Parkinson's disease. Slices through the midbrain of a normal person (left) and a patient with Parkinson's disease (right) showing loss of pigmentation in the substantia nigra in Parkinson's disease (arrows).

Reproduced with permission from *Clinical Pathology* (Oxford Core Texts), Carton, James, Daly, Richard, and Ramani, Pramila, Oxford University Press (2006).

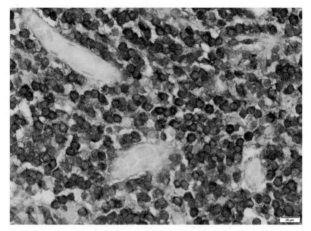

Plate 98. Astrocytoma demonstrating IDH mutation by immunohistochemistry.

Reproduced with permission *from Clinical Pathology* (Oxford Core Texts), Carton, James, Daly, Richard, and Ramani, Pramila, Oxford University Press (2006).

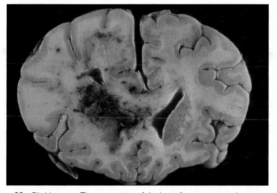

Plate 99. Glioblastoma. This is a section of the brain from a patient who presented with signs of raised intracranial pressure, rapidly deteriorated, and died. There is an ill-defined tumour with areas of haemorrhage. Microscopy revealed this to be a glioblastoma which was much more extensive than was apparent macroscopically.

Reproduced with permission from *Clinical Pathology* (Oxford Core Texts), Carton, James, Daly, Richard, and Ramani, Pramila, Oxford University Press (2006).

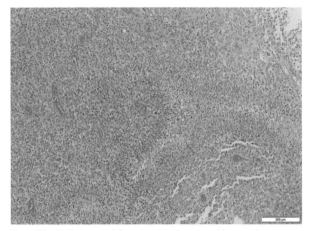

Plate 100. Glioblastoma multiforme histology characterized by atypical astrocytes showing areas of palisading necrosis.

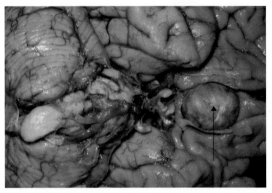

Plate 101. Meningioma. this very well- circumscribed tumour (arrow) has the typical macroscopic appearance of a meningioma, a suspicion that was confirmed microscopically (Plate 58).

Reproduced with permission from *Clinical Pathology* (Oxford Core texts), Carton, James, Daly, richard, and ramani, Pramila, Oxford University Press (2006).

Male breast diseases

Gynaecomastia

- Refers to the enlargement of the male breast.
- Usually seen in boys around puberty and older men aged >50.
- Most cases are either idiopathic or associated with drugs (both therapeutic and recreational).
- Histologically, the breast ducts show epithelial hyperplasia with typical finger-like projections extending into the duct lumen. The periductal stroma is often cellular and oedematous.
- The condition is benign, with no increased risk of malignancy.

Male breast cancer

- Carcinoma of the male breast is rare (0.2% of all cancers).
- The median age at diagnosis is 65 y.
- Most patients present with a palpable lump.
- Grossly, the tumours are firm, irregular masses.
- Histologically, the tumours show similar features to female breast cancers.

Endocrine pathology

Diabetes mellitus

Definition

- A metabolic disorder characterized by chronic hyperglycaemia due to a relative or complete lack of insulin and/or insulin resistance.

Epidemiology

- Very common, affecting ~2% of the population.
- Rising in incidence.
- Major cause of morbidity and mortality.

Aetiology

- Type 1 diabetes is due to the autoimmune destruction of insulin-producing beta-cells by CD4+ and CD8+ T-lymphocytes. Autoantibodies against beta-cell components and insulin may be detectable.
- Type 2 diabetes is associated with obesity and insulin resistance. Initially, the pancreas compensates for insulin resistance by increasing insulin secretion, but eventually beta-cell failure ensues and insulin secretion becomes inappropriately low.

Pathogenesis and genetics

- Lack of insulin drives the mobilization of energy stores from muscle, fat, and the liver (Fig. 14.1).
- Glucose accumulates in the blood, causing hyperglycaemia.
- In the kidneys, the glucose reabsorption mechanism becomes saturated and glucose appears in the urine.
- Glucose within renal tubules draws water in by osmosis, leading to osmotic diuresis.
- The raised plasma osmolality stimulates the thirst centre.
- Over time, diabetes damages capillaries and markedly accelerates atherosclerosis.

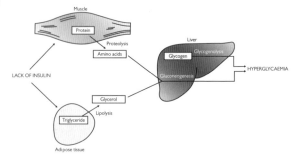

Fig. 14.1 Mechanism of hyperglycaemia in diabetes mellitus. Lack of insulin causes the breakdown of protein in muscle and of triglyceride in fat, providing substrates for gluconeogenesis in the liver. This, together with glucose formed from glycogen in the liver, causes hyperglycaemia.

Presentation

- Polyuria and polydipsia are the classic signs of diabetes mellitus.
- Hyperglycaemia also predisposes to recurrent skin and urinary tract infections.
- Type 1 diabetics may present acutely in diabetic ketoacidosis and/or rapid weight loss.

Biochemistry

- Fasting plasma glucose >7.0 mmol/L or a random plasma glucose >11.1 mmol/L.
- For Type 2 diabetes, HbA1c >=48 mmol/mol in presence of symptoms of hyperglycaemia.
- Patients with borderline values should have an oral glucose tolerance test.

Complications

- A number of organ systems are at risk in diabetes (Fig. 14.2).
- Ischaemic heart disease due to coronary artery atherosclerosis.

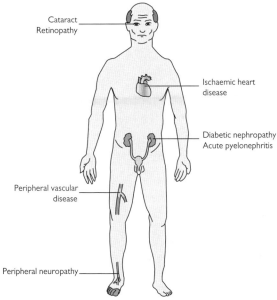

Fig. 14.2 Long-term complications of diabetes mellitus.

Reproduced with permission from *Clinical Pathology*, Carton, Daly, and Ramani, Oxford University Press, p. 326, Figure 14.14.

- Chronic kidney disease due to diabetic nephropathy (p. 208).
- Visual impairment due to cataract and diabetic retinopathy.
- Peripheral vascular disease due to athcrosclerosis.
- Foot ulceration due to peripheral neuropathy and ischaemia.

Hashimoto's thyroiditis

Definition
- An autoimmune thyroid disease characterized by diffuse enlargement of the thyroid and high titres of thyroid autoantibodies.

Epidemiology
- Common, affecting ~1% of the population.
- Predominantly occurs in middle-aged women.

Aetiology
- Poorly understood. Combination of genetic susceptibility (as with other autoimmune conditions) and environmental factors/precipitating factors.

Pathogenesis
- Activated CD4+ helper T-cells recruit CD8+ cytotoxic T-cells which destroy thyroid follicular epithelial cells.
- Anti-thyroid autoantibodies produced by activated B-cells may also contribute.

Presentation
- Diffuse firm goitre and features of hypothyroidism.

Biochemistry
- Increased thyroid-stimulating hormone (TSH) and decreased T4.
- Autoantibodies against thyroglobulin, thyroid peroxidase, and TSH receptor are usually present. Note the latter antibody is different from that seen in Graves' disease as it blocks the TSH receptor rather than activates it.

Macroscopy
- The thyroid is diffusely enlarged and nodular.
- The cut surface is often soft and white, resembling lymphoid tissue.

Cytopathology
- Aspirates are cellular, containing abundant lymphoid cells and scanty follicular epithelial cells showing Hurthle cell change.
- Hurthle cells have abundant granular cytoplasm and enlarged nuclei with vesicular chromatin.

Histopathology
- The thyroid shows diffuse heavy lymphoid infiltration with the formation of germinal centres.
- Often widespread fibrosis confined to thyroid parenchyma (c/w Riedel's thyroiditis).
- Thyroid follicles are atrophic and show widespread Hurthle cell change (sometimes called Askanazy cells in Hashimoto's thyroiditis) characterized by abundant eosinophilic granular cytoplasm and nuclear enlargement.

Prognosis

- Good with thyroxine replacement therapy.
- There is an increased incidence of thyroid lymphoma, usually extranodal marginal zone B-cell lymphoma however this is rare (p. 450).

Graves' thyrotoxicosis

Definition
- An autoimmune thyroid disease characterized by thyrotoxicosis and diffuse hyperplasia of the thyroid.

Epidemiology
- Common, affecting up to 1% of the population.
- Peak incidence is in young adults in their 30s and 40s.
- Women are affected much more frequently than men.

Aetiology
- A poorly understood combination of genetic and environmental factors but with dominant production of TSH receptor-stimulating antibodies.

Pathogenesis
- TSH receptor-stimulating antibodies bind to the TSH receptor and activate it, stimulating hyperplasia of the thyroid follicular epithelium and unregulated secretion of thyroid hormones.

Presentation
- Patients present with thyrotoxicosis and a diffuse goitre.
- Some patients may also develop a form of orbital disease known as Graves' ophthalmopathy (more common in smokers).
- Rarely also a dermopathy called pre-tibial myxoedema and a periosteal reaction of the digits (similar to clubbing) called thyroid acropachy.

Macroscopy
- The thyroid is diffusely enlarged with a firm red cut surface.
- If treatment has been administered, the thyroid may show a nodular appearance.

Cytopathology
- Aspirates are highly cellular with little colloid and many follicular epithelial cells showing hyperplastic changes.
- In practice, aspiration is rarely performed in cases of active Graves' disease as the diagnosis is usually straightforward clinically. This is fortunate as the highly cellular aspirates can easily be mistaken for a neoplastic process by the unwary.

Histopathology
- The thyroid shows diffuse hyperplasia with loss of colloid which shows 'scalloped' edges and marked hyperplastic and hypertrophic changes of the follicular epithelium. Colloid tincture is notably variable between follicles.
- A patchy lymphoid infiltrate, with or without germinal centres, is usually present.

Prognosis
- Excellent with medical anti-thyroid medication (thionamides), surgery, or radio-iodine ablative therapy.

Multi-nodular hyperplasia

Definition
- Multi-nodular enlargement of the thyroid gland.
- Also termed 'nodular goitre', though as goitre can refer to any clinical enlargement of the thyroid, hyperplasia is preferred.

Epidemiology
- Very common.
- Clinically apparent nodular hyperplasia affects up to 5% of the population.
- Significantly more common in women.

Aetiology
- Endemic goitre occurs due to dietary iodine deficiency in geographic areas of the world with low levels of iodine in soil and water. This remains the commonest cause of goitre worldwide and is initially diffuse, progressing to nodularity with time.
- For non-endemic goitre a combination of genetic and environmental factors are thought to play a part with increasing incidence with age.
- Sporadic hyperplasia may rarely be due to ingestion of substances that interfere with thyroid hormone synthesis or due to genetic variations in components of the thyroid hormone synthetic apparatus.

Pathogenesis
- For endemic hyperplasias, reduced levels of thyroid hormones stimulate the release of TSH from the anterior pituitary causing growth of the thyroid.
- Less certain for non-endemic hyperplasias within which different nodules may develop differing degrees of autonomy.

Presentation
- A palpably enlarged, nodular goitre.
- Most patients are euthyroid but increasing autonomy or an iodine load (e.g. CT contrast) may precipitate thyrotoxicoisis in non-endemic multi-nodular hyperplasias.

Macroscopy
- See Fig. 14.3.
- The thyroid gland is enlarged and multinodular.
- Slicing reveals numerous unencapsulated nodules of varying size, usually containing abundant colloid.
- Areas of cystic change, haemorrhage, and calcification are common.

Cytopathology
- Aspirates contain abundant colloid with scanty thyroid follicular epithelium.
- Haemosiderin-laden macrophages may be present due to previous haemorrhage.
- Foamy macrophages often indicate cystic change within a nodule.

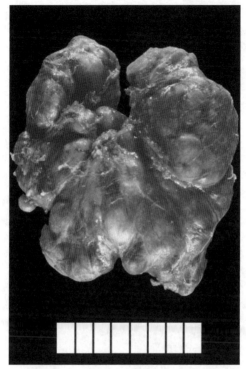

Fig. 14.3 Multinodular goitre. This massive multinodular goitre was removed from an elderly lady because it was compressing her trachea.

Reproduced with permission from *Clinical Pathology* (Oxford Core Texts), Carton, James, Daly, Richard, and Ramani, Pramila, Oxford University Press (2006), p. 269, Figure 12.9.

Histopathology

- The thyroid contains numerous nodules of varying sizes with areas of cystic change and haemorrhage.
- The follicles within the nodules are heterogeneous in appearance. Some are markedly distended with colloid, some appear hyperplastic, whilst others are small and tightly packed, forming nodules which resemble adenomas: cellular 'adenomatoid' nodules.

Prognosis

- Multi nodular hyperplasia is a benign condition with no reported increased risk of development of thyroid carcinoma. On microscopy, occasional carcinomas may be found. The vast majority of these are of no clinical significance.

- The main potential complication is compression of nearby structures such as the trachea by a markedly enlarged nodular goitre. Thyrotoxicosis may also occur.
- Treatment may be conservative, surgical, or radioactive iodine.

Follicular adenoma

Definition
- A benign fully encapsulated thyroid tumour showing follicular differentiation.

Epidemiology
- Most common thyroid neoplasm.
- True incidence is difficult to ascertain due to a lack of consistent diagnostic criteria in distinguishing follicular adenomas from cellular adenomatoid nodules in nodular hyperplasias.

Aetiology
- Associated with radiation exposure.

Genetics
- Chromosomal trisomies (particularly trisomy 7) are the most frequent type of genetic aberration.

Presentation
- Most present with a solitary thyroid nodule, either palpated by the patient or picked up incidentally on imaging.
- Spontaneous haemorrhage into an adenoma may cause acute pain and enlargement of the nodule.

Macroscopy
- The thyroid contains a well-demarcated thinly encapsulated solid nodule with a grey, tan, or brown cut surface.

Cytopathology
- Aspirates are cellular, containing numerous follicular cells and little colloid.
- The follicular cells are both dissociated and present in small microfollicular arrangements.
- Note that it is not possible to distinguish between follicular adenoma and follicular carcinoma on cytology. This can only be done histologically.

Histopathology
- Follicular adenomas are encapsulated epithelial tumours showing follicular differentiation. Microscopic examination of the capsule should always be thorough to exclude Follicular carcinoma.
- By definition, there is no capsular or vascular invasion.
- Some completely encapsulated tumours may show nuclear clearing similar to that seen in papillary carcinoma (see below) but lacking other diagnostic features. Formerly termed 'encapsulated follicular variant of papillary carcinoma' they were overtreated in some centres. However, a hemithyroidectomy is curative and in both genetics (RET mutations) and behaviour they are akin to follicular adenomas. The term 'non-invasive follicular thyroid neoplasm with papillary-like nuclear features (NIFTP)' is used to describe them.

Prognosis

- Follicular adenomas and NIFTP are benign lesions. As it is not possible to differentiate them from follicular carcinomas without excision they are treated by hemithyroidectomy. Once excised they require no further treatment.

Thyroid carcinomas

Definition

- A group of malignant epithelial tumours arising in the thyroid.

Types

- Papillary carcinoma. Many subtypes described including:
  - Usual type
  - Follicular variant
  - Encapsulated
  - Diffuse sclerosing
  - Tall cell
  - Columnar cell
  - Cribriform morular (this subtype may soon be regarded as a distinct type separate from papillary)
- Follicular carcinoma
  - Minimally invasive
  - Encapsulated angioinvasive
  - Widely invasive
- Medullary carcinoma.
- High grade differentiated thyroid carcinoma.
- Poorly differentiated carcinoma.
- Anaplastic carcinoma.

Epidemiology

- Uncommon, accounting for ~1% of all malignancies.
- Mean age at diagnosis mid-40s to early 50s for papillary, 50s for follicular and medullary, and 60s for anaplastic carcinoma.

Aetiology

- Radiation exposure is a well-documented risk factor for differentiated thyroid carcinoma.
- Iodine deficiency, particularly for follicular carcinomas.
- ~25% of medullary carcinomas are linked to the inherited syndromes, multiple endocrine neoplasia (MEN) 2A, MEN 2B, and familial medullary thyroid cancer (FMTC).
- Familial percutaneous transhepatic cholangiogram (PTC) is rare, but mist described in Japan.
- There are associations with a number of other cancer syndromes (Cowden's, familial adenomatous polyposis, etc.)

Presentation

- Well differentiated thyroid carcinomas may present with a solitary thyroid nodule or cervical lymphadenopathy but increasingly they are being detected as incidental findings on imaging. Thyroid function is usually normal.
- Anaplastic carcinoma usually presents with a rapidly enlarging neck mass; involvement of nearby structures causes hoarseness, dysphagia, and dyspnoea.

Papillary carcinoma

- Cytology aspirates contain papillaroid fragments of follicular epithelial cells with the characteristic nuclear features of papillary carcinoma (i.e. powdery chromatin, thick nuclear membranes, nuclear grooves, and nuclear pseudoinclusions). Multinucleated giant cells, psammoma bodies, and thick colloid may be present.

- Histology shows an epithelial tumour, usually with a papillary architecture, showing characteristic nuclear features: oval shape, overlapping, clearing of the nuclear chromatin, nuclear grooves, and pseudoinclusions (Fig 14.4). Laminated calcified concretions (psammoma bodies) are also a common feature. However, no single feature is entirely sensitive and specific and a constellation of the features is required for diagnosis.

- Numerous variants are reported. These include encapsulated papillary carcinoma which has an exceptionally good prognosis. Follicular variant papillary may be misleading on pathology, as it lacks papillae but shows nuclear features. Diffuse sclerosing variant occurs in young women and shows numerous psammoma bodies. Both tall cell and columnar cell more commonly are advanced in stage. Cribriform morular variant occurs more commonly in people with familial adenomatous polyposis. Subtype therefore affects behaviour and treatment options.

- Genetically they demonstrate gain of function mutations in *RET/TRK* or *BRAF*.

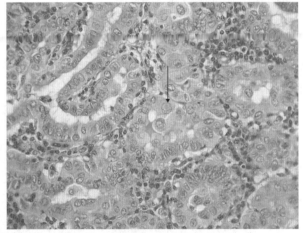

Fig. 14.4 Papillary carcinoma. This histological image from a papillary carcinoma of the thyroid shows the diagnostic nuclear features of nuclear clearing, nuclear grooving, and intranuclear inclusions (arrow).

Reproduced with permission from *Clinical Pathology* (Oxford Core Texts), Carton, James, Daly, Richard, and Ramani, Pramila, Oxford University Press (2006), p. 269, Figure 12.9.

Follicular carcinoma

- Cytology aspirates are cellular, containing follicular epithelial cells present singly and in microfollicular arrangements. Note these appearances are identical to follicular adenomas; cytology cannot distinguish between these entities.
- Histology shows an invasive follicular neoplasm that lacks the nuclear features of papillary thyroid carcinoma.
- *Minimally invasive* tumours show limited capsular invasion alone.
- *Encapsulated angioinvasive* tumours show vascular invasion as well as capsular invasion.
- *Widely invasive* tumours show widespread infiltration of the thyroid.
- Genetically they demonstrate gain of function mutations in RAS or PI-3K.

Medullary carcinoma

- Cytology aspirates are cellular, containing loosely cohesive epithelial cells which may be round or spindled. Some cells may have eccentric nuclei with a plasmacytoid appearance. The nuclei contain coarsely granular chromatin. Fragments of amyloid may be seen.
- This is a neuroendocrine carcinoma derived from parafollicular C cells, whose normal function is secretion of calcitonin (which may be used as a tumour marker).
- Histology shows sheets, nests, or trabeculae of round or spindled neoplastic epithelial cells with granular cytoplasm and nuclei with coarse chromatin. Amyloid deposits may be seen. The diagnosis can be confirmed by immunoreactivity for calcitonin.
- Medullary carcinomas may be sporadic or associated with inherited conditions, notably MEN type 2. In inherited cases, there may be background C cell hyperplasia.

Poorly differentiated carcinoma

- Tumours intermediate in behaviour between the differentiated thyroid cancers and anaplastic carcinoma and defined by the 'Turin criteria' which include:
  - Solid/trabecular/insular growth pattern.
  - No papillary nuclear features.
  - Presence of at least one of convoluted nuclei/mitotic count greater or equal to 3 per 10 high power fields or necrosis.
- Poorer outcome

Anaplastic carcinoma

- Cytology aspirates are highly cellular, containing markedly atypical malignant cells.
- Histology shows highly pleomorphic epithelioid and spindled cells with extensive necrosis and vascular invasion.
- Demonstrate inactivating mutations in TP53 in addition to mutations seen in follicular or papillary carcinomas.
- May loose markers of thyroid differentiation such as thyroglobulin and TTF-1.

Prognosis

- Papillary carcinomas and most follicular carcinomas are low-grade malignancies with excellent prognosis. Even after metastasis, due to treatment with radioactive iodine, they have a high cure rate. Some smaller tumours are treated by lobectomy alone.
- Tumours showing extensive strap muscle invasion are sometimes given external beam radiotherapy to the neck.
- Tumours which fail to take up iodine have a worse prognosis and need to be treated by alternative means. A small number show mutations in kinase pathways which can be targeted.
- Medullary carcinomas are NETS on a spectrum of behaviour depending on their proliferation rate, usually assessed by immunochemistry for the proliferation marker Ki-67. They may progress slowly with a protracted natural history if cure is not achieved by surgery.
- Anaplastic carcinomas are highly malignant and almost always fatal.

Staging

- Staging by UICC TNM 8th edition is important for treatment and based on tumour size and invasion into other structures (oesophagus, trachea, skeletal muscle, carotid vessels). Gross invasion of skeletal muscle, often best assessed by the surgeon is also important in defining high-risk cases.

The parathyroid

The parathyroids secrete parathyroid hormone (PTH) and play a vital role in calcium homeostasis. PTH may be increased in physiological or pathological conditions:

- Primary hyperparathyroidism: Autonomous secretion of PTH.
- Secondary hyperparathyroidism: Increase in PTH production secondary to calcium loss, usually in renal failure.
- Tertiary hyperparathyroidism: Autonomous secretion of PTH following longstanding hyperplastic stimulation secondary to a calcium loss (often apparent after renal transplant).

Parathyroid adenoma

Definition
- A benign epithelial neoplasm of the parathyroid.

Epidemiology
- Common, accounting for ~90–95% of primary hyperparathyroidism.
- Peak incidence 50–60 years old.
- Women are affected more than men (2:1).

Aetiology
- Poorly understood although prior irradiation of the neck appears to increase the risk.

Pathogenesis
- Autonomous production of PTH from the adenoma causes hypercalcaemia due to an unregulated mobilization of calcium from the bone and enhanced absorption of calcium from the kidneys and gut.

Presentation
- Patients present with symptoms of hypercalcaemia, or incidentally discovered raised PTH level.
- Some may present with vague symptoms of fatigue, nausea, constipation, polyuria, and arthralgias.

Macroscopy
- A single parathyroid gland is enlarged in size (>6 mm) and weight (>60 mg).
- The adenoma is usually smooth, solid, soft, and light brown in colour.

Histopathology
- The parathyroid gland contains a well-circumscribed, usually delicately encapsulated, mass composed of parathyroid epithelial cells usually without fat. A compressed rim of normal parathyroid tissue is often present at one edge.
- Chief cells usually predominate, though an intermingling of oxyphil cells is common, and less commonly pure oxyphil adenomas. The cells may be arranged in solid sheets, trabeculae, or follicles.
- Stromal oedema, fibrosis, and haemorrhage are sometimes present.

Prognosis
- Parathyroid adenomas are benign lesions which are cured by excision.

Parathyroid hyperplasia (primary hyperparathyroidism associated)

Definition
- An autonomous and multifocal increase in parathyroid cell mass not secondary to hypocalcaemia.

Epidemiology
- Uncommon, accounting for ~10% of primary hyperparathyroidism.
- Women are affected more than men (3:1).

Aetiology
- Most patients have sporadic hyperplasia with no clear underlying cause.
- ~20% of cases have familial disease, most commonly one of the MEN syndromes (p. 400).

Pathogenesis
- Parathyroid hyperplasia leads to overproduction of PTH.
- Raised PTH levels cause hypercalcaemia by stimulating increased bone resorption, increased absorption of calcium from the kidneys and increasing activation/hydroxylation of Vitamin D to increase gut absorption of calcium.

Presentation
- Patients present with primary hyperparathyroidism, a biochemical syndrome defined by the presence of hypercalcaemia and an inappropriately normal or raised PTH level.
- Many patients are asymptomatic when this is discovered.
- Some may present with vague symptoms of fatigue, nausea, constipation, polyuria, and arthralgias.

Macroscopy
- All of the parathyroid glands are increased in weight (>60 mg) and size (>6 mm), though this may be to varying degrees between the glands.

Histopathology
- The key feature is an increase in cell mass within the gland, associated with a decrease in fat content.
- Usually the gland shows multiple nodules of parathyroid tissue.
- Generally, both chief and oncocytic cell types are increased.
- Secondary fibrosis and haemorrhage are common findings.

Prognosis
- The success rate for surgery for parathyroid hyperplasia is lower than that for parathyroid adenoma. Persistent or recurrent hypercalcaemia occurs about 20% of the time and medical treatment preferred.

Parathyroid carcinoma

Definition
- A malignant epithelial neoplasm of the parathyroid.

Epidemiology
- Rare, accounting for ~1% of cases of primary hyperparathyroidism.
- Peak incidence 40–50 years old with no gender predilection.

Aetiology
- Unknown though anecdotal reports have linked it with secondary hyperparathyroidism and prior neck irradiation.
- Parathyroid carcinoma has only rarely been linked with MEN 1.

Pathogenesis
- Mutation of the *HRP2* gene is the most frequently reported somatic and germline association.

Presentation
- Unlike patients with parathyroid hyperplasia or adenoma, patients usually present with symptomatic primary hyperparathyroidism.
- Calcium levels are usually very high (>3 mmol/L) as are PTH levels with associated symptoms of polyuria, polydipsia, weakness, renal colic, and bone pain.

Macroscopy
- Parathyroid carcinomas are generally much larger than adenomas, weighing on average 12 g.
- They may be well-circumscribed or have clearly infiltrative borders.

Histopathology
- Parathyroid carcinomas are composed of sheets of epithelial cells which are often deceptively bland. Follicle formation is unusual.
- They often have a thick capsule and are traversed by thick bands of fibrous tissue which divide the tumour into multiple expansile nodules.
- Capsular invasion, vascular invasion, tumour necrosis, and a high mitotic index are all very suggestive of malignancy.
- Cases which are intermediate in features are termed 'atypical adenomas' and usually behave as parathyroid adenomas.

Prognosis
- 10-year survival rates are ~65%, but hard to assess given the difficulty making the pathological diagnosis in some cases.
- Management of metastatic disease focuses on controlling the metabolic effects of severe hyperparathyroidism.

Addison's disease

Definition

- Primary adrenocortical insufficiency.

Epidemiology

- Rare with an estimated annual incidence of 1 in 100 000 people.
- Most cases present in young to middle-aged adults.
- Women are affected more than men.

Aetiology

- Autoimmune destruction in developed countries.
- Disseminated tuberculosis in developing countries.
- Other causes such as adrenal metastases, haemorrhagic infarction, and other infections.

Pathogenesis

- Addison's disease leads to a lack of glucocorticoid and mineralocorticoid production from the adrenal cortex. Clinical features do not become manifest until ~90% of the gland has been destroyed.

Presentation

- Tiredness, lethargy, and weakness.
- Anorexia, nausea, vomiting, and diarrhoea.
- Loss of weight may be prominent.
- Increased pigmentation due to raised adrenocorticotropic hormone (ACTH).

▶ The clinical presentation is often insidious and non-specific, making the diagnosis challenging.

Biochemistry

- ↓ Sodium and ↑ potassium.
- <u>Acute renal failure and shock.</u>
- Low cortisol for illness with high ACTH.
- Low aldosterone and high renin.
- Anti-adrenal autoantibodies if autoimmune.

Prognosis

- Good once diagnosis is made and lifelong replacement therapy is started with a synthetic glucocorticoid and mineralocorticoid (fludrocortisone).
- However standardized mortality rate remains high and steroid sick day rules are vital, increasing the dose of hydrocortisone during any intercurrent illness.
- N.B. Untreated or undertreated Addison's disease can cause acute adrenal failure ('Addisonian crisis') with hypovolaemic shock and renal failure.

Adrenocortical hyperplasia

Definition
- Diffuse or multinodular hyperplasia of the adrenal cortex, usually bilateral.

Epidemiology
- Unknown due to the inability to distinguish nodular adrenal hyperplasia from true neoplastic adenomas.

Aetiology
- Numerous causes: ACTH producing pituitary adenoma, CRH producing tumours, ectopic ACTH from a non-pituitary tumour, and also associated with hyperaldosteronism, congenital adrenal hyperplasia, ACTH independent macronodular adrenal hyperplasia and primary pigmented nodular adrenocortical disease (PPNAD).

Genetics
- Primary macronodular hyperplasia causing Cushing disease is associated with *ARMC5* mutation.
- PPNAD associated with *PRKAR1A* gene and Carney complex.
- Congenital adrenal hyperplasia usually secondary to 21-hydroxylase deficiency.

Macroscopy
- Removal of both adrenals for hyperplasia usually limited to uncontrolled Cushing's disease. Glands increased in weight and cortical thickness. Pigmented nodules are marked in PPNAD (Carney complex).

Histopathology
- Diffuse or nodular increase in adrenocortical cells with lipid rich or depleted cells. Pigment common in PPNAD.

Prognosis
- Dependent on underlying condition.

Adrenal cortical adenoma

Definition
- A benign epithelial neoplasm of the adrenal cortex.

Epidemiology
- Most cases occur in adults with no gender predilection.
- True incidence figures are unknown, largely due to the inability to distinguish nodular adrenal hyperplasia from true neoplastic adenomas.

Aetiology
- Unknown in most cases.

Genetics
- Hyperaldosteronism associated with mutations in many ion transporter genes such as *KCNJ5*.

Presentation
- Most non-functional tumours are diagnosed incidentally when the abdomen is imaged for unrelated reasons (up to 4% of adults having a CT will have an adrenal 'incidentaloma').
- Aldosterone-producing adenomas present with primary hyperaldosteronism (Conn's syndrome) characterized by hypertension and, in some patients, hypokalaemia. Hyperaldosteronism secondary to either hyperplasia or an adenoma is a much more common cause of hypertension than previously thought and lead to significant morbidity.
- Cortisol-producing adenomas may present with Cushing's syndrome. However, cortisol production may be sub-clinical so all incidentalomas should be assessed for function.
- Hyperaldosteronism almost always a sign of a benign tumour.
- Hypercortisolaemia may be present in malignant tumours.
- Sex steroid production almost inevitably a sign of malignancy.

Macroscopy
- The adrenal gland contains a well-circumscribed tumour which may be encapsulated.
- The median tumour weight is 40 g.
- Aldosterone-producing adenomas may be bright yellow while those associated with Cushing's syndrome may be yellow to tan.
- A small number of adenomas have a black colour ('black adenoma') secondary to pigment deposition.

Histopathology
- The tumours are composed of large polygonal cells arranged in nests and trabeculae separated by a fine vascular network.
- The cells have cytoplasm which is either clear and microvesicular or compact and eosinophilic. Nuclei are round to oval and usually bland.
- Spironolactone pre-treatment of Conn's adenomas reveals laminated concretions called spironolactone bodies.
- Rarely, striking nuclear pleomorphism may be seen, though this does not equate with malignant behaviour.

- IHC now allows relation of structure to function with the availability of CYP11B1 (surrogate for cortisol secretion) and CYP11B2 (surrogate for aldosterone secretion).
- Adrenal away from the tumour is normal or is compressed in larger tumours.

Prognosis

- Adrenal cortical adenomas are benign tumours with no capacity for malignant behaviour.
- Prognosis is largely determined by the severity of the endocrine effects of functional tumours.

Adrenal cortical carcinoma

Definition

- A malignant epithelial neoplasm arising in the adrenal cortex.

Epidemiology

- Rare tumours with an annual incidence of 1 per million population.
- Most occur in adults aged >60 y old.
- F:M approx. 2:1.

Aetiology

- Unknown in most cases. >50% of childhood cases associated with germline TP53 mutation in Li-Fraumeni syndrome (25% of which occur de novo).
- More rarely associated with Beckwith-Wiedemann syndrome, Lynch syndrome, MEN type 1, familial adenomatous polyposis, neurofibromatosis type 1.

Carcinogenesis

- The most frequent genetic aberrations are overexpression of IGF2 and estimated glomerular filtration rate (EGFR) and loss of function of p21 and p16.

Presentation

- 40–60% are functioning tumours which present with endocrine manifestations related to hormone overproduction. Most frequently this is cortisol excess causing Cushing's syndrome but may also be androgen excess (virilization in women).
- Flank pain may be present if the adrenal mass is large.
- The investigation (imaging criteria and functional assessment) of frequently found adrenal incidentalomas is directed towards excluding adrenocortical carcinoma as these may now be detected incidentally.
- Overproduction of mineralocorticoids is extremely rare.

Macroscopy

- A large bulky tumour mass replaces the adrenal gland.
- Most tumours weigh >100 g. The mean size is 12 cm.
- The cut surface of the tumour appears lobulated and heterogeneous with areas of necrosis and haemorrhage.
- Invasion into adjacent structures may be seen in some cases.

Histopathology

- Most tumours show obvious invasive growth with extension beyond the capsule and vascular invasion.
- Broad fibrous bands are often present which divide the tumour into expansile nodules.
- The tumour cells are highly pleomorphic and arranged in sheets, nests, and trabeculae.
- Areas of necrosis may be seen.
- Scoring systems (Weiss and modified Weiss) may help define malignancy in borderline cases.

- Separate scoring systems are available for paediatric and oncocytic tumours, where prognosis tends to be more favourable.

Prognosis
- 5-year survival is 50–70%.
- The most important prognostic factors are age and stage.
- Weiss and modified Weiss histologic scoring systems are prognostic.
- Ki-67 also a helpful prognostic marker.

Phaeochromocytoma and paraganglioma

Definition

- A neoplasm of the chromaffin cells of the adrenal medulla or paraganglia, respectively.

Epidemiology

- Rare with an annual incidence of 8 per million, although many remain undiagnosed in life.

Aetiology

- This is the most heritable tumour.
- ~40% are associated with a germline mutation. Historically 10% of cases were associated with MEN type 2, von Hippel-Lindau disease, and neurofibromatosis type 1. Now more than 15 other associated genes have been described, most commonly are the subunits (A, B, C & D) of the succinate dehydrogenase gene, a critical enzyme in the Krebs cycle.

Genetics

- All patients should be considered for genetic testing.

Presentation

- Most tumours secrete catecholamines which may lead to sustained or paroxysmal hypertension. Classically associated symptoms include headaches, sweating, and palpitations, although the complete triad is rarely present. Numerous other symptoms may be reported.
- A significant proportion of tumours may be non-secretory (including the majority of head and neck paragangliomas) and therefore present with mass effect or as incidental findings on imaging.

Biochemistry

- Assessment of plasma or 24-hour urine metanephrine levels are the most sensitive and specific tests for the secretory tumours.

Macroscopy

- A well-circumscribed tumour with a firm grey cut surface.
- Mean size of 6 cm and weight of 200 g.

Histopathology

- The tumour cells form characteristic balls of cells ('zellballen') separated by a delicate vascular network.
- The cells are polygonal with granular basophilic cytoplasm.
- Nuclei have a typical stippled chromatin pattern.
- Scattered pleomorphic nuclei may be seen.
- Immunohistochemical loss of SDH-B predicts germline mutation of any one of the 4 SDH subunits (A-D) but most commonly, B.

Prognosis

- WHO defines all tumours as potentially malignant.
- Local or metastatic recurrence may occur many years (5–20 years) after initial presentation and surgery.

- Unfortunately, histology is not reliable at predicting which will be malignant. Size (>4–5 cm), Ki-67 (>5%) and certain gene associations (e.g. *SDHB*, *FH*) should all be considered as worrying features. Attempted histological based scoring systems to predict behaviour have proven insensitive.

Neuroblastoma

Definition
- A malignant childhood tumour arising from neural crest-derived cells of the sympathetic nervous system.
- Most arise in the adrenal medulla or paraspinal sympathetic ganglia.

Epidemiology
- Third most common malignant childhood tumour.
- Incidence of 1 in 10 000 live births per year.
- Most arise in the first 4 years of life.

Aetiology
- Unknown.

Genetics
- Tumour genetics have important prognostic implications.
- Amplification of *MYCN*, diploidy, and deletions at chromosome 1p are all associated with poorer prognosis.

Presentation
- Most children present unwell with weight loss, fever, watery diarrhoea, and a palpable abdominal mass.

Biochemistry
- High urinary concentrations of catecholamines and their metabolites, vanillylmandelic acid (VMA) and homovanilic acid (HMA), are an important diagnostic aid.

Macroscopy
- A lobulated soft grey tumour mass averaging 6–8 cm in size, which is intimately related to the adrenal gland or sympathetic chain.

Histopathology
- **Undifferentiated neuroblastoma** is composed of undifferentiated neuroblasts with no evidence of ganglionic differentiation. They appear identical to a number of other 'small round blue cell tumours' of childhood and so require ancillary techniques to confirm the diagnosis (e.g. immunoreactivity for CD56 and synaptophysin).
- **Poorly differentiated neuroblastoma** shows limited evidence of ganglionic differentiation (<5% cells) with neurofibrillary stroma.
- **Differentiating neuroblastoma** contains many ganglionic cells (>5%, but <50% cells) and plentiful neurofibrillary stroma.
- **Ganglioneuroma** is composed almost entirely of ganglionic cells (>50% cells) and neurofibrillary stroma.

Prognosis
- Depends on several factors including stage, age, histology, and genetics.
- Cure rates are >90% for low-risk disease, 70–90% for intermediate-risk disease, but only 10–40% for high-risk disease.

Neuroendocrine tumours (NETS) at other sites

- Many other sites outside the formal endocrine organs may develop neuroendocrine tumours which show variable differentiation and behaviour.
- Most common sites include gastrointestinal tract, lung, and the pancreas.
- Although most NETS are non-functional, a minority secrete serotonin or other vasoactive polypeptides. Poorly differentiated NETS may secrete other hormones such as ACTH.
- At some sites, well differentiated NETS were referred to as carcinoid tumours, though NET is now preferred.
- When very poorly differentiated they are termed neuroendocrine carcinomas.
- NETS are often graded based on mitotic activity or Ki-67 dependent on site.
- Staging is based on specific criteria at each site.
- NETS may be mixed with other tumour types (e.g. mixed NET and adenocarcinoma).

Pituitary adenoma

Definition

- A benign epithelial neoplasm of the anterior pituitary.
- 60–70% are functioning tumours which overproduce prolactin, growth hormone (GH), ACTH, or TSH (extremely rare), in descending order of frequency.
- Functional adenomas producing TSH, follicle-stimulating hormone (FSH), or luteinizing hormone (LH) are very rare.

Epidemiology

- Uncommon with an incidence of 1 in 100 000 per year.
- Most arise in middle-aged adults.
- Women are affected more than men.

Aetiology

- Unknown in the majority of cases.
- A small proportion is seen in association with inherited tumour syndromes (e.g. MEN 1).

Genetics

- The two best characterized gene aberrations are MEN 1 and *gsp*, a mutation in the G-protein alpha subunit.

Presentation

- Features of endocrine hyperfunction, depending on the hormone produced (e.g. galactorrhoea and sexual dysfunction; prolactin-secreting), acromegaly (Fig. 14.5) if GH-secreting, or Cushing's syndrome (Fig. 14.6) if ACTH-secreting.

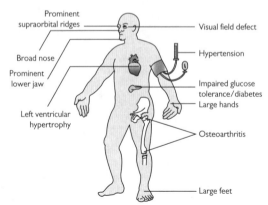

Fig. 14.5 Clinical features of acromegaly.

Reproduced with permission from *Clinical Pathology* (Oxford Core Texts), Carton, James, Daly, Richard, and Ramani, Pramila, Oxford University Press (2006), p. 303, Figure 14.5.

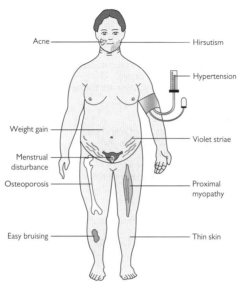

Fig. 14.6 Clinical features of Cushing's syndrome.

Reproduced with permission from *Clinical Pathology* (Oxford Core Texts), Carton, James, Daly, Richard, and Ramani, Pramila, Oxford University Press (2006), p. 303, Figure 14.5.

- Large adenomas may also produce symptoms of mass effect such as headache, nausea, and visual field disturbance due to compression of the overlying optic chiasm.
- Many patients will also have symptoms and signs of hypopituitarism, though rarely present with these.

Macroscopy

- Soft tumours which may be very small microadenomas (<10 mm in size) or larger macroadenomas (>10 mm in size).

Histopathology

- Composed of solid nests or trabeculae of neoplastic cells with uniform round nuclei, stippled chromatin, and inconspicuous nucleoli.
- Immunohistochemistry using antibodies against prolactin, GH, and ACTH can be used to identify the hormone produced by the tumour.

Prognosis

- Generally good following appropriate medical or surgical treatment, though some patients may suffer recurrences.
- The endocrine effects of these tumours may, however, have significant consequences (e.g. cardiovascular disease in acromegaly).

Multiple endocrine neoplasia (MEN) syndromes

Definition

- A group of inherited conditions characterized by proliferative lesions arising in multiple endocrine organs.
- Lesions typically occur at a younger age than sporadic lesions and may be multifocal.

MEN type 1

- Caused by germline mutation of *MEN1* gene.
- Prevalence of 2 per 100,00 people.
- Common lesions include:
  - Multiple parathyroid adenomas;
  - Pancreatic and duodenal endocrine tumours;
  - Pituitary tumours.

MEN type 2A

- Caused by activating germline mutation of *RET* gene.
- Characterized by:
  - Medullary thyroid carcinoma (virtually 100%).
  - Multiple parathyroid adenomas in 10–20%.

MEN type 2B

- Caused by germline mutation of *RET* gene.
- Characterized by:
  - Medullary thyroid carcinoma
  - Phaeochromocytomas
  - Neuromas/ganglioneuromas of skin, mouth, gut
  - Marfanoid habitus

MEN type 4

- Caused by germline mutation of the *CDKN1B* gene.
- Propensity to develop the same spectrum of endocrine tumours as patients with MEN type 1.
- Hyperparathyroidism is usually the earliest manifestation of the syndrome.

Haematopathology

Iron deficiency anaemia

Definition
- A reduction in haemoglobin (Hb) concentration due to inadequate iron supply.

Epidemiology
- The most common cause of anaemia.

Aetiology
- Chronic blood loss from the gut is the most common cause.
- Worldwide, this is usually related to hookworm infection.
- Common causes in developed countries include peptic ulcers (non-steroidal anti-inflammatory drug (NSAID) intake), gastric carcinoma, sigmoid diverticular disease, and colorectal carcinoma.
- Heavy menstrual loss in women (menorrhagia) can also lead to iron deficiency.
- Gastrointestinal (GI) diseases causing malabsorption of iron can also cause iron deficiency (e.g. coeliac disease, atrophic gastritis, and history of partial gastrectomy).

▶ Ruling out a GI tract malignancy is mandatory in any adult patient with unexplained iron deficiency anaemia.

Pathogenesis
- Iron is an essential constituent of the haem group of Hb.
- Chronic iron deficiency interrupts the final step in haem synthesis.

Presentation
- May be asymptomatic and diagnosed on routine full blood count.
- Pallor of mucous membranes, palms, and nail beds is common (usually when Hb is <9 g/dL).
- Symptoms include tiredness and breathlessness on exertion.
- Some cases may cause additional features such as koilonychia, angular cheilitis, and glossitis.

Full blood count
- ↓ Hb.
- ↓ Mean corpuscular volume (MCV).
- ↓ Serum ferritin, ↓ serum iron, ↓ transferrin saturation, ↑ total iron binding capacity.
- Platelet count might be raised, particularly if haemorrhagic episodes.

Peripheral blood film
- Small red cells (microcytic).
- Pale red cells (hypochromic).
- Variability in red cell size (anisocytosis) and shape (poikilocytosis).
- Long elliptical red cells are often seen ('pencil cells').

Bone marrow
- Mild to moderate erythroid hyperplasia (normoblastic).
- Absence of stainable iron (Perl's staining).

Anaemia of chronic disease

Definition

- A reduction in haemoglobin concentration related to chronic inflammatory disorders, chronic infections, and malignancy.

Epidemiology

- Second most common cause of anaemia.

Aetiology

- Any chronic inflammatory disease, chronic infection, or malignancy.
- Most frequent causes include: autoimmune disorders (e.g. inflammatory bowel disease, rheumatoid arthritis, lupus, vasculitis, sarcoidosis), long-term infections (e.g. hepatitis, HIV), cancer, and chronic kidney disease.

Pathogenesis

- The underlying mechanisms are complex and multifactorial.
- Micro-organisms, malignant cells or autoimmune dysregulation lead to activation of CD3+ T cells and monocytes, with subsequent production of cytokines (IFN-gamma, TNF-α, IL-1, IL-6, and IL-10).
- IL-6 stimulates the hepatic expression of the acute phase protein hepcidin, which inhibits the duodenal absorption of iron. TNF-α, IL-1, IL-6, and IL-10 induce ferritin expression and stimulate the storage and retention of iron within macrophages, leading to a decreased iron concentration in the circulation.
- TNF-α and IFN-gamma inhibit the production of erythropoietin in the kidney.
- The end result is a reduction in erythropoiesis which is often ineffective.

Presentation

- Tiredness and breathlessness.

Full blood count

- ↓ Hb which is usually mild to moderate (8–9.5 g/dL).
- MCV is usually normal but may be low.
- ↓ Iron; normal/low transferrin; ↓ transferrin saturation; normal/increased ferritin; ↓ ratio of soluble transferrin receptor to log ferritin; ↑ cytokine levels.

Peripheral blood film

- Red cells usually normochromic and normocytic but can be small.
- There is no noticeable variation in size or shape.

Bone marrow

- The marrow is usually of normal cellularity.
- Decreased bone marrow sideroblasts, but stainable iron is present.

Megaloblastic anaemias

Definition
- A reduction in haemoglobin concentration due to impaired erythroid DNA synthesis.
- Most cases are related to either vitamin B_{12} or folate deficiency.

Aetiology
- Autoimmune gastritis (➲ Autoimmune gastritis, p. 114) is the most common cause of vitamin B12 deficiency. Megaloblastic anaemia due to autoimmune gastritis is also known as **pernicious anaemia**. This affects about 1 in 1000 people, with a female predilection.
- Poor diet is the most common cause of folate deficiency. The main dietary sources of folate are leafy green vegetables. Deficiency is typically seen in the elderly and alcoholics.
- Some cases might be secondary to medication: antifolate drugs (methotrexate) or drugs interfering with DNA synthesis (e.g. mercaptopurine, hydroxyurea).

Pathogenesis
- Vitamin B12 and folate are both required to convert deoxyuridine monophosphate into deoxythymidine monophosphate, a molecule required for DNA synthesis.
- Developing red cells are unable to divide because they cannot make enough DNA to form two nuclei.
- Therefore, red blood cells (RBCs) become arrested in their development as large immature cells (megaloblasts), many of which die in the bone marrow.
- Some megaloblasts survive and develop into abnormally large red cells (macrocytes) which are released into the circulation.

Presentation
- Usually insidious onset with symptoms not appearing until anaemia is severe.
- Mild jaundice may be present due to haemolysis and ineffective erythropoiesis. Lactate dehydrogenase (LDH) might be also increased.
- Vitamin B_{12} deficiency may also cause neurological symptoms, including cognitive impairment, peripheral neuropathy, and subacute combined degeneration of the spinal cord.
- Glossitis and angular cheilosis are also present.

Full blood count
- Hb concentration is typically very low (approaching only 2 g/dL).
- MCV is typically very high.

Peripheral blood film
- Prominent anisocytosis and poikilocytosis with large oval macrocytes.
- Nucleated RBCs may be seen.
- Hypersegmented neutrophils (>5 lobes).

Bone marrow

- The marrow is hypercellular, containing many immature large erythroid blasts (megaloblasts) and large metamyelocytes.
- The myeloid:erythroid ratio is reversed due to an increase in erythroid precursors.
- Megakaryocytes might be hypersegmented and show open chromatin.

Hereditary spherocytosis

Definition
- An inherited (dominant pattern) haemolytic condition caused by mutations in genes encoding proteins involved in maintaining the integrity of the red cell membrane.

Epidemiology
- Common with an incidence of up to 1 in 2000.

Aetiology
- Mutations in genes encoding red cell membrane proteins (ankyrin, band 3, and β-spectrin), leading to protein deficiency.

Pathogenesis
- Mutations cause destabilization of the red cell membrane, with loss of lipid from the membrane.
- Reduction in the surface area of the membrane forces red cells to assume a spherical shape (spherocyte).
- Spherocytes are less deformable than normal red cells and are susceptible to becoming trapped in the spleen and destroyed by splenic macrophages.

Presentation
- Clinically, findings vary from asymptomatic patients to severe haemolysis. Diagnosis is usually made in childhood or young adult life.
- Most patients have mild to moderate anaemia (Hb 8–12 g/dL).
- Jaundice and splenomegaly are common. However, some patients have normal bilirubin values.

Full blood count
- Mild to moderate anaemia (Hb 8–12 g/dL).
- Raised reticulocyte count.
- Raised mean corpuscular haemoglobin concentration (MCHC).

Peripheral blood film
- Spherocytes are readily identifiable.
- Reticulocytes are also present.

Ancillary tests
- The **direct antiglobulin test** is negative, distinguishing spherocytosis from immune haemolytic anaemia, which has similar blood film findings but is rare in children.
- The recommended laboratory tests are the eosin-5-maleimide (EMA) binding test or the cryohaemolysis test.

Prognosis
- Most patients have well-compensated disease and only require folate supplements to avoid megaloblastic anaemia.
- Splenectomy might be beneficial in children with severe disease, but not to be performed in those with mild disease as splenectomy is associated with an increased risk of infection.

- Recognized complications include gallstone disease (from pigment gallstones) and aplastic crisis due to parvovirus B19 infection. The latter is potentially fatal.

Glucose-6-phosphate dehydrogenase deficiency

Definition
- An inherited haemolytic condition caused by a mutation in the glucose-6-phosphate dehydrogenase (G6PD) gene.
- Several variants have been proposed, based on the extent of enzyme deficiency and on the severity of haemolysis: (a) class I: severe, associated with non-spherocytic haemolytic anaemia; (b) class II: <10% activity; (c) class III: 10–60% activity; (d) class IV: normal activity; and (e) class V: increased activity.

Epidemiology
- Common, affecting up to 10% of the population worldwide.
- There is much geographical variability, with the highest rates in Africans (prevalence 28% in Nigeria), Asians, Italians, and Greeks.

Genetics
- The *G6PD* gene is located on the long arm of the X chromosome (Xq28).
- A single mutated copy therefore causes G6PD deficiency in men.
- Homozygous women are also affected, but such individuals are not often seen.
- Heterozygous women do not have clinical manifestations, as the other normal copy produces enough enzyme activity.
- Polymorphisms of the G6PD gene are common and ~200 variant alleles are described.

Pathogenesis
- G6PD is one of the enzymes of the hexose monophosphate pathway, a metabolic process necessary for generating reduced glutathione.
- Reduced glutathione protects the red cell membrane from oxidative damage.
- Individuals with G6PD deficiency suffer from episodes of haemolysis following oxidant stress.

Presentation
- Most individuals are asymptomatic with normal Hb levels.
- If exposed to oxidants, however, they suffer from an acute haemolytic episode with fever, jaundice, and dark urine, due to haemoglobinuria.
- Common precipitants include drugs (especially antimalarials), fava beans (a common food in Mediterranean countries), severe infection, and diabetic ketoacidosis.
- Haemoglobinuria and neonatal jaundice can also occur.

Full blood count
- ↓ Hb during an acute haemolytic episode.

Peripheral blood film
- Variation in red cell shape (poikilocytosis).

- Red cells with punched-out defects in their contours ('bite cells') are characteristic.
- Spherocytes may also be seen.

Ancillary tests

- Screening tests for G6PD deficiency are available which indirectly assess G6PD activity by testing the ability of red cells to reduce dyes.
- The NADPH fluorescence test is a qualitative test and is the gold standard for G6PD deficiency screening.
- Definitive diagnosis requires direct assay of the enzyme.

Thalassaemias

Definition

- A group of inherited red cell disorders caused by the underproduction of α- or β-globin chains.

Pathogenesis and genetics

- Underproduction of either α- or β-globin chains causes accumulation of excess unpaired chains.
- This leads to the destruction of developing red cells and premature removal of circulating red cells in the spleen.
- The anaemia in thalassaemia is therefore a combination of ineffective erythropoiesis and haemolysis in the spleen.
- Point mutations in or near the globin gene are responsible for the majority of the β-thalassaemias. More than 400 genetic alterations have been documented in β-thalassaemias.

Beta-thalassaemia major

- Caused by mutations in both β-globin genes.
- Problems begin in the first few months of life (usually <6 months of age), as HbF levels decline and excess α-chains begin to accumulate in red cells.
- Worsening anaemia leads to intense erythropoietic drive, with expansion of the bone marrow compartment and resumption of extramedullary haematopoiesis. Osteoporosis is frequent, even in well-transfused patients, and spontaneous fractures might occur.
- Presents in infancy with pallor, poor feeding, and failure to thrive.
- Full blood count shows a hypochromic, microcytic anaemia.
- Bone marrow shows red cell hyperplasia with precipitated α-chains in the cytoplasm of erythroblasts.
- Diagnosis is confirmed by the near absence of HbA on Hb electrophoresis.
- Regular transfusions from the age of onset is the standard treatment, but this results in iron overload, and splenectomy might be needed to reduce transfusion requirements.

Beta-thalassaemia minor

- Caused by mutations in only one β-globin gene.
- Silent carriers who have an asymptomatic mild microcytic anaemia with a high red cell count.
- A raised HbA2 level on Hb electrophoresis is a key diagnostic feature.

Alpha-thalassaemia

- Alpha-chains are required for both adult and foetal Hb.
- In the foetus, excess γ-chains form tetramers known as Hb Bart's.
- In adults, excess β-chains form tetramers known as HbH.
- Alpha-thalassaemias are classified according to the number of genes affected.
- Deletion of all four α-globin genes (the more severe form) causes severe foetal anaemia, generalized oedema, massive

hepatosplenomegaly, and foetal demise between 28 and 40 weeks' gestation.
• Deletion of three α-globin genes causes HbH disease with variable levels of chronic haemolysis. Most patients have a moderate chronic haemolytic anaemia throughout life (Hb 7–10 g/dL) and splenomegaly.
• Deletion of one or two α-globin genes leads to α-thalassaemia minor or α-thalassaemia trait which is usually asymptomatic. There may be a very mild microcytic anaemia.

Sickle-cell disorders

Definition
- A group of inherited red cell disorders caused by HbS (sickle Hb)

Epidemiology
- Seen most frequently in people of African descent and other areas of current or previous malaria endemicity.
- The mutant gene has survived because heterozygote carriers are protected against the effects of severe *Plasmodium falciparum* malaria.

Genetics
- HbS is caused by a point mutation in the β-globin gene on chromosome 11, which causes a replacement of valine for glutamic acid in the sixth position of the β-chain.
- Heterozygotes are said to have the **sickle-cell trait**.
- Homozygotes suffer from **sickle-cell disease** (SCD) or **sickle-cell anaemia**.

Pathogenesis
- HbS is 50 times less soluble than HbA.
- Under conditions of low oxygen tension, HbS polymerizes into rod-like aggregates which cause the red cell to adopt a sickled shape.

Presentation
- Individuals with the sickle-cell trait do not suffer from sickling because the normal HbA protein reduces the formation of HbS aggregates. Patients are usually asymptomatic and have normal Hb levels. They are nevertheless genetically important as carriers of the sickle-cell gene.
- Typically, patients present with asthenia, jaundice, and ulcers around the ankles. Bone deformities and infections can also occur.
- Individuals with SCD present at around 2 y of age once they have lost most of their HbF, and virtually all their Hb is HbS. Their red cells sickle in venous blood, causing persistent haemolysis and episodes of vascular crises.

Full blood count
- ↓ Hb, typically between 7 and 9 g/dL.

Peripheral blood film
- Sickled red cells and their variants are present.
- In adults, there is also evidence of hyposplenism/splenic atrophy (target cells, Howell–Jolly bodies, Pappenheimer bodies).
- In the marrow, the myeloid:erythroid ratio is preserved.

Diagnosis
- The **sickle-cell solubility test** is a useful screening test in which a reducing agent is added to Hb extracted from red cells. HbS readily precipitates and the solution goes cloudy.
- Definitive diagnosis requires **Hb electrophoresis** which shows a single major HbS band and no normal HbA.

Prognosis
- Patients with SCD have a significantly decreased lifespan.
- The median age of death is ~42y in men and 48y in women.
- Multiple trials are currently evaluating the therapeutic use of haematopoietic stem cell transplant (HSCT) in patients with SCD. However, graft versus host disease (GvHD) remains the main complication in patients receiving HSCT.

Complications of sickle-cell disease

Childhood
- Hand and foot syndrome (unequal growth of small bones of the hands and feet).
- Splenic sequestration crisis.
- Stroke (usually as a result of embolism from fractured bones and stenosis of vessels in the circle of Willis).

Later life
- Bacterial infections, including osteomyelitis from *Salmonella* species.
- CKD.
- Priapism.
- Lower limb ulceration.
- Pigment gallstones.
- Avascular necrosis of the femoral head.
- Pulmonary syndrome.

Idiopathic thrombocytopenic purpura

Definition

- A reduction in platelet number due to platelet autoantibodies, which contributes to accelerate platelet destruction and inhibit their production.

Epidemiology

- Uncommon with an incidence of 1.6–3.9 per 100 000 persons per year.
- Occurs in adults and children.
- The female-to-male ratio ranges from 1.2 to 1.9.
- Adult idiopathic thrombocytopenic purpura (ITP) is more common in women (3:1).
- Childhood ITP has a peak incidence between ages 5 and 6, with no gender predilection.
- 20% of cases are secondary.

Aetiology

- Platelet autoantibodies are formed for unknown reasons.
- The majority are idiopathic, but some forms are secondary (e.g. lupus, antiphospholipid syndrome, common variable immunodeficiency (CVID), chronic lymphocytic leukaemia (CLL), infection, drugs).

Pathogenesis

- Platelets become coated with autoantibodies and are destroyed in the spleen. However, platelet antibodies are only detected in ~60% of patients.

Presentation

- Sudden onset of cutaneous petechiae, nosebleeds (epistaxis), and gum bleeding.
- A preceding viral infection is often noted in childhood cases.
- Annual risk of fatal haemorrhage is 1.6–3.9 cases per 100 patient years.

Full blood count

- Severe thrombocytopenia (platelet count <100 × 10^9/L).
- Normal Hb and white cell count (WCC).
- Anaemia may exist if there is concomitant immune haemolytic anaemia (Evan syndrome).

Peripheral blood film

- A mixture of normal and large platelets is present.
- Platelet counts are reduced.

Bone marrow findings

- Normal or increased numbers of megakaryocytes.
- Normal megakaryocyte morphology.
- Normal haematopoiesis.

▶ Note that ITP is a diagnosis of exclusion once other causes of thrombocytopenia have been ruled out.

Prognosis
- Childhood cases usually resolve within 1–2 months.
- Adult cases are more likely to persist with a chronic mild to moderate bleeding tendency.
- Risk of thrombosis.
- B-lymphocyte depletion with anti-CD20 (rituximab) has proved to be useful in some patients with chronic ITP.

Thrombotic thrombocytopenic purpura

Definition

- A thrombotic microangiopathy associated with haemolytic anaemia due to lack of *ADAMTS13*.

Epidemiology

- Rare; annual incidence of 6–11.3 per 10^6 population.

Aetiology

- Inherited cases are due to genetic mutations of *ADAMTS13* (von Willebrand factor (vWF) cleaving protein).
- Sporadic cases are due to autoantibodies against *ADAMTS13* (incidence of 6 per 10^6 population per year).

Pathogenesis

- *ADAMTS13* is a metalloproteinase which cleaves vWF into small fragments.
- Deficiency of *ADAMTS13* leads to the accumulation of ultra-high molecular-weight forms of vWF which attach to endothelial cells and stimulate microthrombus formation in small vessels.
- Microthrombi cause organ impairment, most notably affecting the brain and kidneys.
- Platelets are rapidly consumed in the microthrombi, causing thrombocytopenia.
- RBCs passing through the microthrombi are sheared apart, causing anaemia.

Presentation

- Fever, petechiae, jaundice, and bleeding (epistaxis, gingival bleeding, GI bleeding).
- Neurological symptoms are typically prominent, including confusion, headache, aphasia, and visual problems.
- Acute renal failure may also occur (proteinuria and microhaematuria).

Haematology

- ↓ Hb with normal MCV.
- ↑ reticulocyte count.
- ↓ platelets.
- Normal clotting (prothrombin time (PT), fibrinogen).
- Troponin T levels are raised (50% cases).
- LDH raised due to haemolysis.

Blood film

- Red cell anisocytosis.
- Prominent schistocytes (fragmented red cells).

Prognosis

- If untreated, the mortality is 90%, but survival rates are 80–90% with early diagnosis and plasma exchange.
- Around one-third of patients suffer from relapses within 2 y.

- Patients with refractory or relapsing immune-mediated thrombotic thrombocytopenic purpura (TTP) might benefit from rituximab therapy.
- Caplacizumab, a monoclonal antibody that binds to vWF, has been approved for treatment of TTP, and has proved to be particularly useful in the first phases of the disease.

von Willebrand disease

Definition

- An inherited bleeding tendency caused by a quantitative or qualitative deficiency of vWF.

Epidemiology

- The most common inherited bleeding disorder.
- Incidence varies from 23 to 100 per 10^6 population.
- Type 1 (75%) is a quantitative defect.
- Type 2 (20%) is a qualitative defect and includes four subtypes (2A, 2B, 2M, and 2N) on the basis of the phenotype.
- Type 3, although rarer, is the most severe form of the disease (virtually complete deficiency of vWF).
- Acquired forms of von Willebrand disease also exist probably due related to autoimmune disorders or medications.

Genetics

- The vWF gene is located on the short arm of chromosome 12 (12p13.3).
- Type 1 is autosomal dominant, and type 2 can be autosomal dominant or recessive depending on the type (2A: dominant or recessive, 2B dominant, 2M dominant or recessive, and 2N recessive).
- Type 3 is an autosomal recessive trait.

Pathogenesis

- vWF acts as an adhesion molecule which allows platelets to bind to subendothelial tissues and it also acts as a carrier for factor VIII.
- Lack of vWF activity leads to a bleeding tendency due to a combination of failure of platelet adhesion and factor VIII deficiency.

Presentation

- Mucosal bleeding, particularly nosebleeds, and bleeding after injury or surgery are the main manifestations.
- Joint and muscle bleeds are rare and only occur in type 3 disease.

Clotting studies

- Prolonged activated partial thromboplastin time (APTT).
- Prolonged bleeding time.
- Normal PT.
- Formal diagnosis requires the measurement of plasma vWF (VWF:Ag) and testing of vWF functionality (e.g. ristocetin-induced platelet agglutination assay or VWF:RCo which measures the ability of vWF to bind to platelets).

Prognosis

- Most patients require no regular treatment.
- Prophylactic treatment is given before surgery.

Haemophilia

Definition

- An inherited disorder of haemostasis characterized by bleeding tendency due to a deficiency of either factor VIII (haemophilia A) or factor IX (haemophilia B).

Epidemiology

- Prevalence of 10 in 100 000 people.
- Haemophilia A occurs in about 1 in 5–10 000 male births.
- Haemophilia B, also called Christmas disease, is less common with an incidence of about 1 in 20–30 000 male births.

Genetics

- The factor VIII and factor IX genes are both located on the X chromosome, so haemophilia demonstrates sex-linked inheritance, with males being predominantly affected. Both disorders are X-linked recessive disorders.
- Numerous mutations have been described, leading to a wide variation in the severity of haemophilia. Other alterations (deletions, insertions, inversions) are also associated with haemophilia in some patients.

Pathogenesis

- Factors VIII and IX together form the factor VIII–factor IX complex which activates factor X in the clotting cascade.
- Lack of these factors impairs clotting.

Presentation

- Easy bruising and massive bleeding after trauma or surgery.
- Spontaneous haemorrhages into large weight-bearing joints, such as the knee, elbow, and ankles (haemarthroses), are common.
- Median age for the diagnosis is 1y if the disease is severe, but in >9% of cases, the mean age for diagnosis is 15y.
- Despite the inherited nature of the disease, a positive family history is not recorded in 30% of cases.

Clotting studies

- Both forms of haemophilia cause a prolonged APTT and a normal PT.
- The two can only be distinguished by measuring levels of each factor.

Prognosis

- Long-term complications include haemarthropathy (repeated bleeding episodes in the joints).
- Replacement of the missing factor is the key therapeutic intervention.
- Factor concentrates are pooled from multiple donors and carry a much higher risk of transmission of infection.
- Although stringent donor screening and viral inactivation of concentrates reduce this risk, there is a move towards the use of synthetic factors.
- Trials with gene therapy are under way using adenovirus vectors containing the genes for factors VIII and IX.

- Monoclonal antibodies, such as Emicizumab, have been licensed for the treatment of haemophilia. Emicizumab promotes thrombin formation by mimicking FVIIIa activity, regardless the presence of FVIII inhibitors.

Thrombophilia

Definition
- An inherited predisposition to venous thrombosis.
- Thrombophilia is a multigenetic and heterogeneous disease.

Presentation
- Deep vein thrombosis or pulmonary embolus, which may be recurrent.
- Venous thrombosis at unusual sites (e.g. axillary or cerebral veins) may also occur.
- It is associated with pregnancy complications and recurrent miscarriage.

Activated protein C resistance
- The most common form of thrombophilia, affecting 5–10% of people, most commonly Caucasian individuals.
- Due to a single point mutation in the factor V gene (known as factor V Leiden mutation), due to replacement of Arg506 with a Gln.
- Factor V Leiden protein has normal procoagulant activity but is not inhibited in the normal way by activated protein C, resulting in a hypercoagulative state and a tendency to thrombosis.

Prothrombin G20210A mutation
- Affects ~1–5% of people.
- Caused by a single nucleotide change of guanine for adenine at position 20210 of the *PT* gene (called F2).
- Associated with elevated PT levels and an increased risk of venous thrombosis, possibly due to increased rates of thrombin generation, excess growth of fibrin clots, and possibly increased activation of platelets.
- May increase the risk of pregnancy loss.
- Heterozygous and homozygous women with a history of venous thrombosis should avoid use of contraceptive treatment containing oestrogens and HRT.

Protein C and S deficiency
- Protein C deficiency can be found in 1 in 200–500 persons in the general population, but the majority of cases are asymptomatic. Severe homozygous protein C deficiency affects 1 in 500 000 to 1 in 750 000 live births.
- Heterozygous protein C deficiency is an inherited (autosomal dominant) disease. The gene is located in the long arm of chromosome 2.
- More than 200 mutations have been described. The deficiency in protein can be classified as: type I (quantitative) and type II (less frequent and characterized by decreased functional activity of the protein).
- Protein C and S are natural anticoagulants which inactivate clotting factors and regulated normal coagulation.
- Defects in these proteins therefore predispose to thrombosis.

Ancillary tests in the diagnosis of haematological malignancies

Immunohistochemistry

- Immunohistochemistry uses antibodies to detect antigens or specific protein markers in cells or tissues.
- Immunostaining can be performed either directly (primary antibody is labelled) or indirectly (the primary antibody is visualized using a labelled secondary antibody to the species of the primary).
- Steps: 1) Application of a primary antibody (monoclonal or polyclonal) that binds directly to the target antigen; 2) Application of a secondary antibody that binds to the primary antibody, usually to amplify the staining intensity; 3) Detection system: the visualization of the antigen-antibody interaction can be achieved by either conjugation to a fluorescent marker or enzyme followed by colorimetric detection (using chromogens). See Fig. 15.1.

Clonality

- Clonality is used to identify clonal proliferations in lymphoproliferative disorders.
- Rearrangements of the antigen receptor genes (either IgH/IgK/IgL in B-cells or T-cell receptor in T cells) occur during B- and T-cell development. Gene rearrangements generate specific and unique products for each cell that can be detected by polymerase chain reaction (PCR) and differential fluorescence detection on a capillary electrophoresis is used to visualize the products. See Fig. 15.2.

Flow cytometry

- Technique that provides rapid multi-parametric analysis of single cells in a solution and therefore can only be performed in blood samples, bone marrow aspirates, and other tissue fluids. Similar to

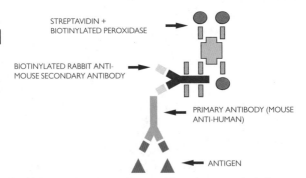

STREPTAVIDIN + BIOTINYLATED PEROXIDASE

BIOTINYLATED RABBIT ANTI-MOUSE SECONDARY ANTIBODY

PRIMARY ANTIBODY (MOUSE ANTI-HUMAN)

ANTIGEN

Fig. 15.1 Immunohistochemistry. There are different detection methods, the avidin/biotin complex (ABC) is the most extended. The primary antibody is detected with a biotic-labelled antibody that interacts with an avidin/biotin complex containing many labels (see Plate 47).

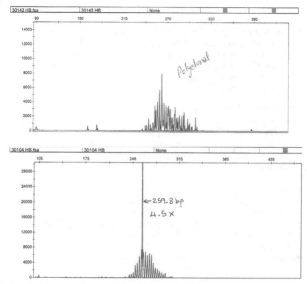

Fig. 15.2 Clonality. Top panel shows an example of a polyclonal result with a variety of different peaks. Bottom panel shows an example of a mononclonal result with a strong peak (arrowed) on a polyclonal background (see Plate 48).

immunohistochemistry with regards to detection of molecules in intact cells but, in distinction to immunohistochemistry, tissue architecture assessment is not possible by flow cytometry.
- Flow cytometry use antibodies (usually 6–8) which are labelled with different fluorescent dyes that emits light of a given colour when excited by a laser. The cells pass through a series of lasers to excite the dyes and detectors measure the emissions from the different dyes on each cell.
- Flow cytometry is very effective in identifying malignant cells in a background of normal cells with high sensitivity.

Fluorescence in-situ hybridization (FISH)
- Technology which allows to locate the position of specific DNA sequences on chromosomes. FISH employs fluorescently labelled DNA or RNA probes to identify regions or genes of interest. The probes hybridize ty complementary base pairing to the nuclei acid sequence of interest and then visualized.
- Steps required: 1) Probe, a labelled DNA or RNA sequence of interest, selection; 2) The labelled probe and the target DNA are denatured; 3) Combining the denatures probe and target allows the annealing of complementary DNA sequences and; 4) And enzymatic or

immunological detection system is used and the signals are evaluated by fluorescence microscopy.

• The most frequent probes used in haematological diagnosis are 'break apart' and 'fusion'. The former is used for translocations, where breaks have occurred at the same time in two chromosomes; and chromosomal deletions and amplifications (parts of the chromosome are lost or there are multiple abnormal copies) are usually detected by fusion probes. See Fig. 15.3.

Sequencing based assays

• Next generation sequencing (NGS) allows the detection of multiple genetic aberrations through large panel-based assays.
• Illumina and Ion Torrent are the two main commercial leaders for NGS. 'Third-generation' sequencing technologies, such as ONT (Oxford Nanopore Technologies) have also been developed, in which PCR is not required for sample preparation.
• NGS can be applied to detect aberrations in.
• The entire genome (whole genome sequencing),
• Protein coding regions (whole exome sequencing) or
• Targeted mutation panels for: a) myeloid malignancies (eg FTL3, NMP1, ASXL1, IDH1/2 in AML); lymphoblastic leukaemia and mature lymphoid neoplasms.
• Detection of complex genomic abnormalities such as translocations and copy number variants (CNVs)

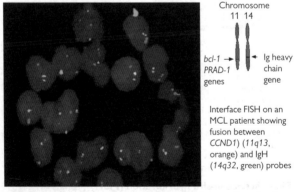

Chromosome 11   14

bcl-1 →   ← Ig heavy
PRAD-1   chain
genes   gene

Interface FISH on an MCL patient showing fusion between *CCND1* (*11q13*, orange) and IgH (*14q32*, green) probes

Fig. 15.3 Fluorescence in situ hybridisation (FISH) result in a case of mantle cell lymphoma (MCL). Tumour cells show abnormal juxtaposition of the orange and green probes due to a t(11;14) chromosomal translocation (see Plate 49).

Acute B-lymphoblastic leukaemia

Definition

- A haematological neoplasm composed of malignant B-lymphoid blasts with bone marrow and blood involvement.
- The WHO classification (2008) includes: acute B-lymphoblastic leukaemia (B-ALL) not otherwise specific and B-ALL with recurrent genetic abnormalities.

Epidemiology

- Incidence 1–4.75/100 000 persons per year.
- Primarily a disease of children (75% of cases occur aged <6y).

Aetiology

- Largely unknown, though there is a suggestion of an inherited component in some cases.

Genetics

- Clonal DJ rearrangement of the *IGH* gene. T-cell receptor gene rearrangement also frequent (up to 70% of cases).
- B-ALL with recurrent genetic abnormalities include: t(9,22) *BCR–ABL1* fusion gene; t(v;11q23) MLL rearranged; B-ALL with hyperploidy, B-ALL with hypoploidy; t(1;19) E2A-PBX1; t(12;21) TEL-AML1.

Pathogenesis

- Mutations in a haematopoietic stem cell leads to the clonal expansion of immature B-lymphoid blasts.
- Rapidly proliferating lymphoid blasts overwhelm the normal bone marrow, spill into the peripheral blood, and infiltrate other organs.

Presentation

- Sudden onset of bone marrow failure with profound anaemia and thrombocytopenia. The leucocyte count may be decreased, normal, or increased.
- Infiltration of other organs is common, causing lymphadenopathy, hepatosplenomegaly, bone pain, headache, vomiting, and cranial nerve palsies.

Microscopy

- See Fig. 15.4.
- By definition >20% of cells in the peripheral blood or bone marrow are lymphoid blasts, relatively monomorphic medium to large cells with a high nuclear-to-cytoplasmic ratio and finely dispersed chromatin.

Immunophenotype

- B-lymphoid blasts usually express CD19, CD79a, CD22, CD10, Pax5, and TdT.
- PAX5 is probably the most sensitive and specific marker for B-cell lineage in bone marrow trephines.
- Myeloperoxidase (MPO) is usually negative.

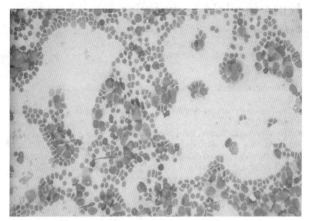

Fig. 15.4 Acute B-lymphoblastic leukaemia. >20% of cells in this preparation are lymphoid blasts characterized by medium to large cells with a high nuclear to cytoplasmic ratio and finely dispersed chromatin (see Plate 50).

T-lymphoblastic leukaemia/lymphoma

Approximately 15% of childhood ALL and 25% of adult ALL are of T-cell lineage (T-lymphoblastic leukaemia/lymphoma).

T-ALL presents with a high leucocyte count and frequently with a mediastinal mass and pleural effusions. Morphologically, blasts are difficult to distinguish from B-lineage blasts and require flow cytometry, immunophenotyping (TdT, CD1a, CD2, CD3, CD4, CD5, CD7, and CD8), and T-cell receptor clonal rearrangement.

T-ALL might be divided in two sub-groups:
1) Early T-precursor ALL (ETP-ALL) with poor prognosis and characterized by FTL3-ITD mutations, DNMT3 mutations, and dysregulation of the RAS pathway
2) Cortical type T-ALL, characterize by TLX1 and / or TAL1 expression.

T-ALL in childhood is more aggressive than B-ALL, with early relapses and CNS involvement.

- Myeloid-associated antigens (CD13 and CD33) are positive in t(9;22) acute lymphoblastic leukaemia (ALL) and CD34+ blasts are common in t(12;21) ALL.

Prognosis
- Modern treatment regimens have excellent success rates, with complete remission achieved in >95% of children. The prognosis in adults is less favourable.
- Central nervous system (CNS) involvement at presentation is associated with aggressive disease and requires specific treatment.
- t(9;22) ALL has the worst prognosis among patients with ALL.

Acute myeloid leukaemias

Definition

- A group of haematological neoplasms composed of malignant myeloid blasts found in the bone marrow and blood.

Classification

- Different classifications have been proposed to classify acute myeloid leukaemia (AML).
- The French–American–British (FAB) scheme is based on morphological findings (M0 to M7).
- The WHO classification relies primarily on cytogenetic findings and includes: AML with recurrent genetic abnormalities; AML with myelodysplasia-related changes; therapy-related myeloid neoplasms; AML NOS; myeloid sarcoma; myeloid proliferations related to Down's syndrome; and blastic plasmacytoid dendritic cell neoplasm.

Epidemiology

- Worldwide incidence is 3.7–4 per 100 000 population per year.
- It shows two peaks in occurrence—in early childhood and later adulthood (mean age at diagnosis is 65y).
- AML represent <2% of all new cancer cases.

Aetiology

- AML may be sporadic or occur as a complication of previous chemotherapy or as a terminal event in a pre-existing myeloproliferative or myelodysplastic disease.

Genetics

- Favourable cytogenetic abnormalities include:

  t(15;17) resulting in *PML-RARA* fusion
  t(8;21), resulting in *RUN1-RUNZ1T1* fusion
  Mutations in *CEBPA*, *GATA2*, or *NMPM1*
  Unfavourable aberrations include:
  t(6;9) resulting in *DEK-NUP214* fusion
  add(5q), del(5q) or -5
  t(9;22) resulting in *BCR-ABL1* fusion
  FLT3-ITD
  Mutations in *DNMT3A*, *TP53*, *RUNX1*, or *ASXL1*
  Chromosomal rearrangements involving the *MLL* gene on chromosome 11 are common in myelomonocytic leukaemias.
  50% of adult AMLs have normal cytogenetics, and gene mutations are frequent in this group; mainly in the *FTL3*, *NPM1* (nucleophosmin member 1), and tumour suppressor *TET2* genes.

Pathogenesis

- Mutations in a haematopoietic stem cell lead to the clonal expansion of immature myeloid blasts.
- Rapidly proliferative myeloid blasts overwhelm the bone marrow and spill into the peripheral blood.
- Infiltration of organs by myeloid blasts can occur in AML, but this is less common than in acute B-lymphoblastic leukaemia.

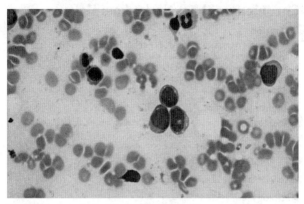

Fig. 15.5 Acute myeloid leukaemia. >20% of cells in this preparation are myeloid blasts characterized by medium to large cells with a high nuclear to cytoplasmic ratio. Some myeloid blasts contain cytoplasmic granules or Auer rods (see Plate 51).

Presentation
- Most cases present with bone marrow failure, leading to anaemia, thrombocytopenia, and neutropenia. There may be leucocytosis.
- Infections, bruising, and haemorrhage are also frequent.
- Organs involved include: lymph nodes, CNS, testes (although this is more frequent in ALL), and skin.

Microscopy
- See Fig. 15.5.
- By definition, >20% of the cells in the peripheral blood or bone marrow are myeloid blasts.
- The blasts are medium- to large-sized cells with a high nuclear-to-cytoplasmic ratio. Some myeloid blasts contain cytoplasmic granules or Auer rods.

Immunophenotype
- Myeloid blasts usually express CD13, CD117, CD33, and CD34.
- They do not express B-lymphoid markers such as CD79a or PAX5, except t(8;21) AML.
- AMLs with *NPM1* mutation express markers of monocytic differentiation such as CD11c, CD68, and CD163.

Prognosis
- Outcome is dependent on the precise type of AML; however, most are aggressive diseases requiring intensive ablative regimes to achieve remission.
- AML associated with previous chemotherapy or a pre-existing myeloid disorder generally has a poor outcome.
- The overall survival as a group is 26% (SEER 2005–2011).

Chronic lymphocytic leukaemia

Definition

- A malignant neoplasm composed of monomorphic small B-cells, involving peripheral blood, bone marrow, spleen, and lymph nodes.
- Small lymphocytic lymphoma (B-CLL/SLL) represent different manifestations of the same disease entity, but with a different anatomical distribution (non-leukaemic).

Epidemiology

- The most common leukaemia in Western countries; incidence of 2–6 cases per 100 000 person per year.
- A disease of older adults, with a peak incidence between 60 and 80 y, although younger individuals might also be affected.
- Men are affected twice as often as women; ratio 1.5–2:1.
- Very rare disease in Eastern countries.

Aetiology

- Unknown.
- Familial predisposition is high; first-degree relatives of CLL patients have a 2–7 times increased risk of developing leukaemia.

Genetics

- Rearrangement of immunoglobulin genes and somatic hypermutation are the most common alterations.
- CLL can be divided in two genetically distinct groups:
  - IGVH-mutated, B-cells have undergone somatic hypermutation of the IGHV locus.
  - IGVH-unmutated, the B-cells have not yet passed through the germinal centre and have an unmutated IGHV locus. This group has a more aggressive course and usually refractory to standard treatment.
  - Expression of the *ZAP-70* gene (tyrosine kinase) is associated with IG unmutated cases.
  - 80% cases have cytogenetic abnormalities, being the most frequent ones 1) del 13q14.3 (50–60% cases) and; 2) trisomy 12 (10–205 of CLL).
  - *TP53* mutations and copy number changes (e.g. as a result of del17p) lead to lack of durable responses to standard chemotherapy. *TP53* mutations are also common in Richter's transformation of CLL.

Pathogenesis

- The neoplastic B-cells gradually fill the bone marrow and then spill into the peripheral blood.
- With progression, lymph nodes become involved, and then the liver and spleen.
- In the final stages of the disease, the neoplastic cells overwhelm the bone marrow and cause bone marrow failure.

Presentation

- Many patients are asymptomatic and diagnosed incidentally when a full blood count reveals a leucocytosis.

- The remainder presents with lymphadenopathy or autoimmune phenomena such as autoimmune haemolytic anaemia or autoimmune thrombocytopenia.
- Splenomegaly, hepatomegaly, and lymphadenopathy are also common.
- The diagnosis requires the presence of lymphadenopathy and/or splenomegaly and lymphocytosis ($>5 \times 10^9$/L monoclonal lymphocytes in the absence of extramedullary disease).

Peripheral blood film

- Excess of mature lymphocytes with clumped chromatin and scanty cytoplasm.
- Proportion of prolymphocytes varies but usually <2%.
- So-called smear cells are characteristic of CLL; these represent neoplastic cells which are smudged during preparation of the film.
- Atypical variants exist and are usually associated with trisomy of chromosome 12.

Histopathology

- Lymph nodes are replaced by small, slightly irregular B-cells with variable numbers of 'lighter areas', the so-called proliferation centres containing larger lymphoid cells (prolymphocytes and paraimmunoblasts).
- Some cases show large cells resembling Reed–Sternberg cells (seen in Hodgkin's disease).
- Involved bone marrow contains collections of monomorphic neoplastic lymphoid cells with round nuclei and coarse chromatin.

Immunophenotype

- Positive for *PAX5*, *CD20*, *CD79a*, *CD5*, and *CD23*.
- CD23 expression is better detected by flow cytometry than immunohistochemistry.
- Negative for cyclin D1.
- LEF1 (lymphoid-enhancer-binding factor 1) is a highly sensitive and specific marker.

Prognosis

- Generally behaves indolently, with many patients surviving for several years after diagnosis, often without treatment.
- However, different risk factors are associated with a worse prognosis: unmutated CLL, expression of ZAP-70, deletions of 11q22-23 and 17p13.
- A small proportion of cases are complicated by the development of diffuse large B-cell lymphoma (DLBCL) (Richter's syndrome) which has a poor prognosis.
- Rare cases (<1%) might develop Hodgkin's disease.

Chronic myelogenous leukaemia

Definition
- A myeloproliferative neoplasm that predominantly involves the granulocyte lineage and is consistently associated with the *BCR–ABL1* fusion gene located on the Philadelphia chromosome.

Epidemiology
- Incidence of 1–2 per 100 000 population per year.
- The peak age of onset is between 50 and 70 y.
- Slight male predominance.

Aetiology
- Unknown.
- An inherited predisposition has not been documented.

Genetics
- By definition, typical cases of chronic myelogenous leukaemia (CML) have the characteristic t(9;22) translocation that results in the Philadelphia chromosome.
- The translocation results in fusion of the *BCR* gene on chromosome 22 to the *ABL1* gene on chromosome 9.
- The *BCR–ABL1* protein (210-kDa protein) has enhanced tyrosine kinase activity, leading to the constitutive activation of signal transduction pathways and deregulated proliferation of myeloid cells.
- Breakpoints on chromosome 2 can be seen outside the major *BCR* region, resulting in different transcripts/shorter fusion proteins (p190), but carrying also an enhanced tyrosine kinase activity.

Presentation
- Most patients are diagnosed during the chronic phase of the disease when a WCC is abnormally raised.
- Symptomatic patients complain of fatigue and night sweats.
- Anaemia and hepatosplenomegaly are often present at diagnosis.
- Several phases are described: chronic phase, accelerated phase, and blastic phase.

Peripheral blood
- Leucocytosis (~100 × 10^9/L) due to the presence of increased numbers of neutrophils in various stages of maturation.
- Basophilia and eosinophilia are common in the chronic phase.
- No dysplasia is present in the chronic phase.

Bone marrow
- Bone marrow trephines are hypercellular due to increased numbers of neutrophils and their precursors.
- Eosinophils might be prominent.
- Megakaryocytes are typically small and hypolobated ('dwarf megakaryocytes').

- Blasts account for <5% of marrow cells in the chronic phase. Immunostaining with CD34 and TdT highlights clusters of blasts (>20%) in the accelerated phase.
- Transformation may be myeloblastic, lymphoblastic, or mixed.
- Reticulin fibrosis in 30% of cases.

Prognosis
- Outcome is much improved since the development of the tyrosine kinase inhibitor imatinib, with 5-year survival rates of 80–90%.
- Quantitative testing of BCR-ABL1 transcripts in peripheral blood and liquid marrow is the base to monitor treatment in CML. A rise in the transcript while a patient is on TKI treatment might indicate development of resistant mutations.
- Disease progression is usually heralded by an increase in circulating blasts to >10% (accelerated phase) and terminates in acute leukaemia when blasts account for >20% of circulating cells.

Rare types of CML
- **Atypical chronic myeloid leukaemia, BCR–ABL1 negative**, now included in the myelodysplastic/myeloproliferative neoplasms (WHO classification 2008), usually with worse prognosis than BCR–ABL-positive cases.
- **Chronic neutrophilic leukaemia**, characterized by peripheral blood neutrophilia and no evidence of myelodysplastic/myeloproliferative neoplasm. In 20% of cases, another neoplasm is present (most frequently multiple myeloma).
- **Chronic eosinophilic leukaemia not otherwise specified**, a multisystemic disease characterized by persistent blood eosinophilia and organ damage by eosinophilic infiltrate (heart, CNS, skin, GI tract, and lungs).
- **Chronic myelomonocytic leukaemia** (myelodysplastic/myeloproliferative neoplasms in the WHO classification 2008), defined by persistent monocytosis, <20% of blasts in the marrow, dysplasia in one or more myeloid lineages and absence of the BCR–ABL fusion gene.
- **Juvenile myelomonocytic leukaemia**, 75% of cases presenting in children <3 years of age. Young infants with Noonan's syndrome and neurofibromatosis type 1 (NF1) are at risk of developing juvenile myelomonocytic leukaemia. Transformation to AML is rare, but if untreated, it is a fatal disorder with children dying from organ failure due to leukaemic infiltration.

Polycythaemia vera

Definition

- A chronic myeloproliferative neoplasm that predominantly involves the erythroid lineage and is almost always associated with a somatic gain-of-function mutation of the *JAK2* gene.

Epidemiology

- Incidence of 1–2.5 cases per 100 000 population per year.
- Affects middle-aged and elderly patients; median age at diagnosis is 60.
- There is a slight male predominance (male:female ratio 1–2:1).

Aetiology

- Unknown in the majority of cases.
- Familial clustering has been reported.
- There are rare cases of primary congenital polycythaemia associated with mutation in genes in the hypoxia pathway (von Hippel–Lindau gene (*VHL*); hypoxia inducible factor (*HIF*) gene).

Genetics

- More than 95% of cases have the *JAK2 V617F* mutation, leading to a deregulated proliferation of all myeloid cells through cytokines and grown factors, including erythropoietin. The erythroid lineage is the most notably increased.
- Philadelphia chromosome or *BCR–ABL1* gene fusion are absent.
- Progression of the disease is associated with the acquisition of cytogenetic abnormalities.

Presentation

- May present incidentally on full blood count or with symptoms related to hyperviscosity (headache, dizziness, visual disturbance, venous or arterial thrombosis).
- Suffusion of the conjunctiva and engorgement of retinal vessels are also present.
- Most patients are plethoric and have hepatosplenomegaly.
- Three phases described: (1) prodromal (mid-erythrocytosis); (2) overt polycythaemic phase; and (3) 'spent' with myelofibrosis, anaemia, and ineffective haematopoiesis.

Full blood count

- ↑ Hb, ↑ red cell count, ↑ haematocrit (HCT), ↑ packed cell volume (PCV).
- Often ↑ WCC and ↑ platelets.
- Subnormal erythropoietin levels.

Bone marrow

- The marrow is hypercellular due to an increase in all myeloid lineages ('panmyelosis'). Haematopoietic tissue makes up to 90% of the intertrabecular space.
- Erythroid precursors and megakaryocytes are most prominent.

- Megakaryocytes form loose clusters and often show significant variation in size and shape.
- There is an increase in reticulin fibre density.

Prognosis

- Median survival is >10y with treatment. Most patients die from thrombosis or haemorrhage.
- Progression to myelofibrosis occurs in ~30% of patients.
- Development of myelodysplasia or AML occurs in 20% of patients, and death from AML occurs in <10% of patients.

Essential thrombocythaemia

Definition
- A chronic myeloproliferative neoplasm that predominantly involves the megakaryocytic lineage.

Epidemiology
- Estimated at 0.6–2.5 per 100 000 people per year.
- Most cases present in adults aged 50–60. A second peak at ~30y of age is also described in women.
- There is no gender predilection.

Aetiology
- Unknown.

Genetics
- No recurring molecular genetic or cytogenetic abnormality is known.
- The presence of a *BCR–ABL1* fusion gene excludes the diagnosis of essential thrombocythaemia (ET).
- A *JAK2 V617F* mutation is found in 50–60% of patients.
- Mutations in the thrombopoietin receptor gene *MPL* detected in 5% of patients.
- Abnormal karyotype in 5–10% of cases.

Presentation
- About half of patients present incidentally when a markedly raised platelet count is found on full blood count.
- The remainder presents with symptoms related to vascular occlusion or haemorrhage (transient ischaemic attacks (TIAs), digital ischaemia and gangrene, major arterial and venous thrombosis).
- Bleeding from the GI tract and less frequently from upper airway or genitourinary tracts.
- Splenomegaly is present in only a minority of patients.

Full blood count
- Sustained elevated platelet count (>450 × 10⁹/L).
- The WCC and red cell count are usually normal, but low Hb levels can be seen with progression to fibrosis.
- Ferritin is usually normal (>20 micrograms/L).

Bone marrow
- The marrow is of normal cellularity but contains increased numbers of large and giant megakaryocytes with abundant cytoplasm and deeply lobated 'stag-horn' nuclei.
- Increase in reticulin fibres is not significant.
- There is no significant erythroid or granulocytic proliferation.
- Absence of increase in myeloblasts.

Prognosis
- Relatively indolent disease with median survival of 10–15y.
- Only a very small proportion of patients progress to bone marrow fibrosis.
- Transformation to AML occurs in <5% of patients and it is usually associated with previous cytotoxic treatment.

Primary myelofibrosis

Definition

- A clonal myeloproliferative neoplasm characterized by predominant proliferation of megakaryocytes and granulocytes in the bone marrow, associated with reactive deposition of fibrous connective tissue and with extramedullary haematopoiesis.

Epidemiology

- Estimated annual incidence of 0.5–1.5 per 100 000 population.
- Occurs mostly in adults aged 60–70, with no gender predilection.

Aetiology

- Unknown in most cases.
- Cases associated with exposure to toxins or ionizing radiation.
- Familial cases are rare, and in a subset of these patients, an autosomal recessive inherited condition might be the cause.
- A previous history of polycythaemia vera (PV) is recorded in 30% of patients.

Genetics

- No specific genetic defect has been identified.
- *JAK2 V617F* mutation detected in 50% of patients.
- 30% of cases have a mutation in CALR.
- Gain-of-function mutation of MPL in 5–8% of cases.
- 12% of cases are triple-negative for any of the aforementioned mutations.
- Abnormal karyotype in 30% of cases, del(20q) and partial trisomy 1q being the most common alterations.
- Absence of Philadelphia chromosome or *BCR–ABL1* fusion gene.

Presentation

- Abdominal discomfort due to massive splenomegaly.
- Symptoms related to hypermetabolism such as night sweats, fever, anorexia, and weight loss.
- Two stages described: prefibrotic/early stage and fibrotic.

Peripheral blood

- ↑ platelets and/or WCC.
- ↓ Hb. Normochromic anaemia.
- Gouty arthritis and renal stones if hyperuricaemia.
- Blood film shows leuckoerythroblastosis with teardrop-shaped RBCs.
- Serum LDH might be increased.

Bone marrow

- Megakaryocytes are markedly abnormal with extensive clustering and marked cytological atypia.
- With progression, there is increasing marrow fibrosis (reticulin grade 2 or 3, on a scale of 0–3) and in 10% of osteosclerosis.
- Increase of myeloblasts not a feature.

- Lymphoid nodules seen in bone marrow trephine biopsies in 20–30% of cases.
- Marked vascular proliferation (tortuous vessels) as fibrosis progresses.
- Extramedullary haematopoiesis can be confirmed in liver biopsies or in splenectomy specimens.

Prognosis

- Survival depends on the extent of marrow fibrosis at diagnosis.
- Patients with marked fibrosis have median survival times of 3–7 y.
- The major causes of death are bone marrow failure, thromboembolic events, portal hypertension, and the development of AML.
- Incidence of AML in primary myelofibrosis (PMF) is 5–30%, some of which might be associated with previous cytotoxic treatment.

Myelodysplastic syndromes

Definition

- A group of clonal haematopoietic neoplasms characterized by dysplasia in one or more of the myeloid cell lineages and associated with ineffective myelopoiesis, cytopenias, and an increased risk of development of AML.

Classification

- The 2008 WHO classification includes: refractory cytopenia with unilineage dysplasia (RCU); refractory anaemia with ring sideroblasts (RARS); refractory cytopenia with multilineage dysplasia (RCMD), 30% of all MDS patients; refractory anaemia with excess of blasts (RAEB), 40% of all patients with MDS; myelodysplastic syndrome with isolated del(5q); myelodysplastic syndrome, unclassified (MDS-U).

Epidemiology

- Estimated annual incidence of 3–5 per 100 000 population.
- Occur mostly in older adults at a median age of 70.
- No significant sex predilection, except del5q (or 5q– syndrome) which is more often seen in women.

Aetiology

- Unknown in most cases.
- Exposure to toxins has been documented.
- Inherited haematological disorders might predispose to MDS (e.g. Fanconi anaemia, Diamond–Blackfan syndrome, dyskeratosis congenita).
- Therapy-related myelodysplastic syndrome (t-MDS) occurs as a late complication of chemo- or radiotherapy treatment and might account for up to 20% of all MDS.

Genetics

- A number of recurring chromosomal aberrations have been described in MDS, in 50% of primary MDS and 90% of secondary MDS:
  - chromosomal deletion or loss (e.g. del5q, 17p loss)
  - chromosomal gains: trisomy 8, trisomy 11
  - chromosome rearrangement: t3q26, t11q23
  - complex karyotypes (>3 abnormalities).
- Cytogenetic and molecular studies are important in proving clonality and determining the prognosis.

Presentation

- Refractory anaemia is the most common presentation.
- Neutropenia and thrombocytopenia are less frequent.
- Symptoms related to bone marrow failure: infective episodes, bleeding abnormalities.

▶ Note that hepatosplenomegaly is uncommon in MDS.

Peripheral blood

- Blood film abnormalities vary, depending on each entity, but cytopenias in one or more myeloid lineages are common.
- Blood films may show macrocytes, abnormal neutrophils with poorly developed nuclear segmentation and hypogranular cytoplasm, and giant platelets.
- Leukoerythroblastic changes are present in patients with RAEB, and thrombocytosis is seen in patients with 5q–.

Bone marrow

- Morphological evidence of myelodysplasia may be seen in one or more myeloid lineages in the bone marrow.
- Dyserythropoiesis is characterized by nuclear budding, internuclear bridging, karyorrhexis, multinuclearity, nuclear hypolobation, megaloblastic changes, ring sideroblasts, and cytoplasmic vacuolization.
- Dysgranulopoiesis is characterized by small size, nuclear hypolobation, irregular hypersegmentation, and cytoplasmic hypogranularity.
- Dysmegakaryocytopoiesis is characterized by small size, nuclear hypolobation, or multinucleation.
- Bone marrow is usually hypercellular and an increase in reticulin fibres is noted (myelofibrosis might be prominent in 10% of cases). Some MDS are hypoplastic (~10%), although *per se* this group has no independent prognostic significance.
- CD34 immunohistochemistry can help to highlight clusters of blasts away from the bone trabeculae and vascular structures, particularly in cases of RAEB.

Prognosis

- Survival depends on a number of factors, including morphological subtype, karyotype, severity of cytopenia, and age.
- A scoring system to predict survival and evolution to AML has been proposed by the International Myelodysplastic Syndrome Working group based on: blasts count in the marrow, number of cytopenias, and karyotype abnormalities.
- Low-risk forms of MDS (RCUD and RARS) tend to have a more prolonged natural history, with a very low incidence of progression into AML.
- High-risk forms (RAEB-2) are more aggressive, with many patients succumbing rapidly to bone marrow failure or AML.

Follicular lymphoma

Definition
- A mature B-cell neoplasm composed of germinal centre cells (centrocytes and centroblasts).

Epidemiology
- Accounts for ~20% of all non-Hodgkin's lymphomas.
- Predominantly affects adults aged 50–60; slight female predominance.
- More common in Western countries.

Aetiology
- Unknown.

Genetics
- 90% of cases have a characteristic t(14;18) translocation which results in fusion of the *BCL2* gene to the *IGH* locus.
- Deregulated production of the anti-apoptotic Bcl-2 protein results in clonal proliferation. However, overexpression of BCL2 is insufficient to induce lymphomagenesis.
- Other chromosomal alterations: random losses of 1p36 and 6q; gains in chromosomes 7 and 18.
- Recurrent mutations in some genes (*MLL2, EZH2*) are detected.
- The microenvironment is essential through expression of CXCR4 and CXCR5 by lymphoma cells, the role of T-regulatory cells and M2 polarized macrophages.

Presentation
- Widespread lymphadenopathy and splenomegaly.
- Patients are otherwise relatively asymptomatic.
- The bone marrow is frequently involved.
- Some variants are recognized: paediatric follicular lymphoma; primary intestinal follicular lymphoma; testicular follicular lymphoma.

Histopathology
- See Fig. 15.6.
- Nodal architecture is replaced by back-to-back neoplastic follicles, but areas of diffuse proliferation of neoplastic cells are also observed.
- Neoplastic follicles lack mantle zones and are composed of randomly distributed neoplastic centroblasts and/or centrocytes.
- Tangible body macrophages are usually absent.
- Interfollicular spread of neoplastic cells is usually present.
- Bone marrow involvement is characterized by paratrabecular aggregates of neoplastic centrocytes and centroblasts.

Immunophenotype
- B-cell markers PAX5, CD20, and CD79a are positive.
- Bcl-2, Bcl-6, and CD10 are also positive in the follicle centres, and CD20/CD10 cells are also detected in the interfollicular areas.
- CD5, CD23, and cyclin D1 are negative.

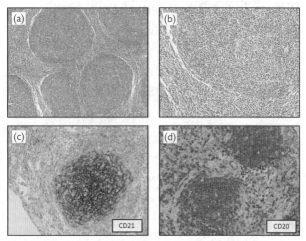

Fig. 15.6 Follicular lymphoma. (a, b) Lymphoma characterized by a nodular pattern. The nodules are well defined and lack mantle areas (haematoxylin and eosin). (c) Follicular pattern highlighted with CD21 (staining follicular dendritic cells). (d) The cells in the follicle centres are CD20-positive (B-cell marker) (see Plate 52).

- CD21/CD23 stain follicular dendritic cells and highlight the follicular growth pattern.
- The proliferation index (assessed with Ki67/MIB1) is usually 20–30%.

Prognosis
- Related to the extent of disease and tumour grade.
- 25–35% progress into a high-grade lymphoma, usually DLBCL, associated with a rapid clinical decline and death.
- Transformation usually associated with acquisition of additional chromosomal abnormalities (e.g. MYC translocations).

Diffuse large B-cell lymphoma

Definition

- A mature B-cell neoplasm composed of large B-lymphoid cells with a diffuse growth pattern.
- Clinically and biologically heterogeneous disease, including a wide range of subtypes and related entities.
- The 2017 WHO classification includes new sub-entities/provisional entities based on genomic aberrations with clinical and therapeutic implications (see box).

Epidemiology

- Accounts for 30–40% of all non-Hodgkin's lymphomas.
- Predominantly affects elderly adults aged >60.
- Slight predominance in males.
- The majority are *de novo*, but some cases represent transformation from pre-existing low-grade lymphomas (e.g. follicular lymphoma, Richter's transformation of small lymphocytic lymphoma/leukaemia).

Aetiology

- Remains unknown in many cases.
- Immunodeficiency/immunosuppression is a risk factor where the lymphoma is driven by Epstein–Barr virus (EBV), HHV-8, or both.

Genetics

- Chromosomal translocations in BCL6 (35–40% cases), Bcl-2 (10–15%), and c-MYC (5–10%) and somatic hypermutations in germinal centre genes (e.g. BCL6, c-MYC, PAX5) are well known.
- Alterations in genes and proteins involved in cell cycle control, cell survival, and apoptosis.
- Activation of the nuclear factor kappa B (NF-κB) pathway, including mutations in CD79A/B, CARD11, and MYD88.
- Different micro-RNA signatures (miR221, miR22, mir93, miR331, and miR491) have been linked with more aggressive disease.
- MYC rearrangements occur in 5–10% of DLBCL.

Presentation

- Rapidly growing mass which may be nodal (60%) or extranodal (40%).
- The most common extranodal site is the GI tract, but virtually any site may be affected.
- Up to one-third of the cases have extranodal involvement at the time of presentation.
- Bone marrow involvement occurs in ~20–33% of patients.

Histopathology

- Involved tissues are replaced by diffuse sheets of large atypical lymphoid cells which are usually more than twice the size of a normal lymphocyte.
- The involved lymph nodes show effacement of the normal architecture, partial or total, with frequent extension of the neoplastic cells into the surrounded perinodal tissue.

- Three variants (immunoblastic, centroblastic, anaplastic), based on the predominant type of neoplastic cell.
- Apoptotic debris are usually seen and there may be confluent areas of tumour necrosis.

Immunophenotype
- Positive with at least one pan B-cell marker (CD20, CD19, CD22, CD79a, Pax5).
- Cyclin D1 usually negative but can be positive in 2% cases.
- Other frequent expressed markers are CD10, Bcl6, MUM1/IRFA4, GCTE1, and FOXP1.
- High proliferation index (usually 40–90% of cells).
- MYC protein expression (>40% cells) is associated with inferior overall survival, particularly when BCL2 protein is co-expressed.

Prognosis
- DLBCL as a group is an aggressive disease but potentially curable with chemotherapy.
- Survival is much improved since the introduction of the anti-CD20 inhibitor rituximab, with long-term survival rates of around 60–75%.
- Bone marrow involvement is generally associated with poor prognosis.
- Non-anti-CD20 antibodies targeting tumour cells and stroma have shown promising results (e.g. proteasome inhibitors, immunomodulatory drugs, anti-CD22).

High-grade B-cell lymphoma
- HGBL is a new entity in the 2017 WHO classification, no longer classified as DLBCL or BL.
- It includes two subgroups:
  1. High-grade B-cell lymphoma with MYC and Bcl2 and/or BCL6 rearrangements, often called 'double' or 'triple-hit' lymphomas
  2. HGBL NOS, characterized features resembling DLBCL or BL or blastoid morphology and lack the genetic alterations described earlier.
- These lymphomas usually present in elderly patients with advanced disease, often with CNS and/or bone marrow involvement, and do not tend to respond to standard chemotherapy (CHOP or R-CHOP)
- Immunophenotypically these lymphomas express CD19, CD20, CD79a and PAX5. There is variable expression of CD10, BCL6, MUM1 and BCL2. The proliferation fraction with Ki67 is 90–95%
- Response rates to R-CHOP and duration of response is low compared with DLBCL.
Insert Inline Figure 1 here

Burkitt's lymphoma

Definition
- An aggressive B-cell tumour of germinal centre cell origin.

Variants
- Three variants have been described: **endemic** (equatorial Africa); **sporadic** (children and young adults); and **immunodeficiency-associated**-Burkitt's lymphoma (BL) in association with HIV infection.

Epidemiology
- BL accounts for 0.3–1.3% of all non-Hodgkin's lymphomas.
- BL is the most frequent childhood malignancy in equatorial Africa in patients between 3 and 7y.

Aetiology
- EBV might a play a role in the aetiology of the disease.
- In endemic areas, there is an epidemiological link with malaria.
- Immunosuppression (HIV, post-transplant) appears to increase the risk.

Genetics
- Translocation and deregulation of the c-*myc* gene (on chromosome 8) is present in the majority of cases.
- The translocation partner is usually *IGH* (14q21) and less commonly *IGK* and *IGL*. The molecular consequence of the different types of translocations is deregulated expression of the *MYC* oncogene, which plays an essential role in cell cycle control.
- Gains in 12q, 20q, 22q, and Xq and losses of 13q have also been described.
- Amplifications in 1q and gains in 7q are associated with a poor clinical outcome.

Presentation
- Bulky disease, rapid and aggressive clinical course with frequent bone marrow and CNS involvement.
- Extranodal involvement is common, jaws/facial bones (endemic variant) and ileocaecal junction (sporadic) being the most frequent sites.
- Nodal involvement is more frequent in adults.

Histopathology
- See Fig. 15.7.
- Diffuse monomorphic infiltrate of small to medium lymphoid cells with rounded nuclei, small nucleoli, and small to moderate amount of basophilic cytoplasm.
- Mitotic figures are frequent, and almost all cases show apoptotic debris.
- Classical 'starry sky pattern', secondary to debris concentrated in the cytoplasm of macrophages admixed with sheets of neoplastic cells.

Immunophenotype
- Prototype CD20+, CD10+, Bcl6+, Bcl2–, IgM+, and TdT– with a proliferation ratio with Ki-67 of nearly 100%.

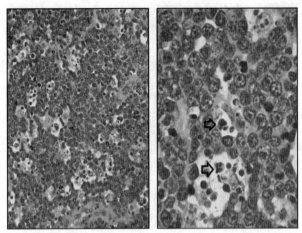

Fig. 15.7 Burkitt's lymphoma. Lymphoma characterized by monomorphic medium-sized lymphoid cells with a 'starry sky' pattern. Detail of tingible body macrophages containing apoptotic tumour cells (arrows) (see Plate 53).

- VpreB3, a protein in the pre-B-cell receptor, is highly expressed in all cases of BL.
- EBER (EBV-encoded small RNAs detected by *in-situ* hybridization) is present in 90% of African BL, but only in 30% of cases in Western areas.

Prognosis

- Overall cure rate for sporadic BL in Western countries is ~90% in the absence of adverse prognostic factors.
- If CNS involvement is present at presentation, the reported 5-year event-free survival is 84%. Older patients have poorer outcomes than young patients on most therapies.
- Treatment consists of initial cytoreduction with cyclophosphamide, prednisolone, and vincristine, followed by intensive chemotherapy in varying combinations.

Burkitt-like lymphoma with 11q aberration

- BL 11q shares the same pathological features and gene expression profile of BL but lacks the MYC rearrangement and harbours an 11q-arm aberration. This is a provisional entity in the revised WHO classification (2017)
- In comparison with BL, BLL-11q seems to have more complex karyotypes, a certain degree of cytological pleomorphism, sporadically a follicular pattern and a high incidence of nodal presentation
- BL 11q usually occurs in younger patients and present with localized lymphadenopathy. The clinical outcome is similar to BL.

Extranodal marginal zone lymphoma of mucosa-associated lymphoid tissue (MALT lymphoma)

Definition

- An extranodal mature B-cell neoplasm composed predominantly of small neoplastic marginal zone (centrocyte-like) cells.

Epidemiology

- Accounts for 7–8% of all non-Hodgkin's B-cell lymphomas.
- Gastric MALT lymphomas account for 50% of all gastric lymphomas.
- Predominantly arises in adults at a mean age of 60.
- Variation in different geographic areas.

Sites of involvement

- The GI tract accounts for 50% of all cases, with the stomach being the most common location.
- Other sites include the lung, salivary gland, skin, thyroid, and breast.
- Involvement of the small intestine is usually in the form of 'immunoproliferative small intestinal disease' (IPSID).

Aetiology

- Gastric cases are typically associated with *Helicobacter pylori*.
- Other implicated organisms include *Campylobacter jejuni* (jejunum) and *Borrelia burgdorferi* (skin).
- Autoimmune diseases are also associated, for example, Hashimoto's thyroiditis (thyroid) and Sjögren's syndrome (salivary gland).

Genetics

- t(11;18) involving the *AP12–MALT12* fusion gene is present in the majority of MALT lymphomas not responsive to *H. pylori* eradication therapy.
- Other well-known chromosomal abnormalities include t(1;14) (p22;q32)/*BCL10–IGH* and t(14;18) (q32;q21)/*IGH–MALT1*.
- These translocations involve genes which play an important role in the activation of the NF-κB pathway.

Pathogenesis

- Most cases are preceded by a chronic inflammatory disorder that causes the accumulation of extranodal lymphoid tissue.
- Prolonged stimulation of lymphoid proliferation eventually leads to transformation into a neoplastic process.
- In the stomach, growth of neoplastic B-cells is stimulated by tumour-infiltrating *H. pylori*-specific T cells through the interaction between B- and T cells involving CD40 and CD40L co-stimulatory molecules.
- *A20* mutation and deletion are commonly seen in MALT lymphoma of the ocular adnexa, salivary glands, and thyroid.

Presentation

- Symptoms relating to a mass at the involved site.

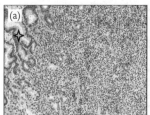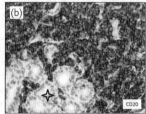

Fig. 15.8 Extranodal marginal zone lymphoma involving the stomach. (a) Gastric mucosa (asterisk indicates gastric glands) infiltrated by a lymphoma composed of small centrocyte-like lymphocytes (haematoxylin and eosin). (b) The lymphoma cells are CD20 diffuse-positive (see Plate 54).

- Patients usually present with low-stage disease.
- Multiple extranodal sites might be affected in the same patient.
- Bone marrow involvement is seen more frequently in extra-gastric MALT lymphomas.
- Advanced disease at diagnosis appears to be more common in MALT lymphomas that arise outside of the GI tract.

Histopathology

- See Fig. 15.8.
- Involved tissues contain a heterogeneous population of small neoplastic B-cells which surround and may overrun background reactive lymphoid follicles.
- The cells include marginal zone cells, cells resembling monocytoid cells, small lymphocytes, and scattered immunoblasts and centroblast-like cells.
- In epithelial-lined tissues, the neoplastic lymphoid cells typically infiltrate and destroy the epithelium, creating so-called lymphoepithelial lesions.

Immunophenotype

- B-cell markers, including CD20, CD79a, and Pax5, are positive.
- CD5, CD10, CD23, and cyclin D1 are all negative.
- Marginal zone markers (CD21 and CD35) are usually positive.
- Neoplastic cells express IgM but lack IgD expression.
- IRTA-1 and MNDA, recently added markers, are positive.

Prognosis

- Tends to show indolent behaviour with prolonged disease-free remissions following treatment.
- Usually favourable outcome; overall survival at 5 y >85%.
- Histologic transformation to large-cell lymphoma in ~10% of cases.
- *H. pylori* eradication therapy is recommended to all localized (stages I–II) gastric lymphomas, independently of histological grade.

Mantle cell lymphoma

Definition

- A mature B-cell neoplasm composed of monomorphic, small to medium-sized lymphoid cells with irregular nuclear contours and a CCND1 translocation.

Epidemiology

- Accounts for 3–10% of all non-Hodgkin's B-cell lymphomas.
- Predominantly arises in adults at a mean age of 60.
- Slight male predominance.

Aetiology

- Unknown in the majority of cases.
- Familial aggregation is recognized, and candidate genes in these familial cases include germline mutations in the ataxia-telangiectasia mutated (*ATM*) and *CHK2* genes.

Genetics

- Virtually all cases show a t(11;14) translocation involving the *CCND1* (cyclin D1) and *IGH* genes.
- Deregulated expression of cyclin D1 results in uncontrolled proliferation of the lymphoid cells.
- Cases with lack of t(11;14) and lack of cyclin D1 expression do exist.
- Many other chromosomal alterations are described.
- Oncogenic mutations in genes targeting the DNA damage response pathway are described.
- *TP53* mutations are present in cases with a high proliferation index.

Presentation

- Most patients present with lymph node involvement and stage III or IV disease.
- The liver, spleen, marrow, or peripheral blood may also be involved.
- Extranodal sites may also be affected, particularly the GI tract.

Histopathology

- Involved tissues are replaced by sheets of monomorphic, small to medium-sized lymphoid cells with irregular nuclear contours.
- Vaguely nodular growth pattern often seen.
- Hyalinized small blood vessels and scattered epithelioid histiocytes are often present.
- Some morphological variants are recognized, some associated with a more aggressive behaviour (e.g. blastoid and pleomorphic variants).

Immunophenotype

- B-cell markers are positive as well as surface IgM/IgD.
- CD5 and cyclin D1 are positive.
- CD23 and CD10 are usually negative.
- SOX11, a neural transcription factor, is expressed in the majority of mantle cell lymphomas, including cyclin 1-negative cases.

In-situ mantle cell neoplasm

- Previously known as 'in-situ mantle cell lymphoma' is also included in the 2017 WHO classification.
- In-situ MC neoplasm is characterized by the presence of cyclin-D1 positive cells restricted to the mantle area of otherwise hyperplastic-appearing lymphoid tissue. The cells harbour CCND1 rearrangements. Compared with classical MCL the expression of CD5 might be low and SOX11(-) cases have been also described.
- This entity usually has an indolent course with stable disease even without any treatment. However, rare cases might progress to overt mantle cell lymphoma.

Classical Hodgkin's lymphoma

Definition

- A lymphoid neoplasm composed of crippled neoplastic B-cells, known as Hodgkin/Reed–Sternberg (HRS) cells, within a rich, non-neoplastic inflammatory background.

Epidemiology

- Bimodal age distribution, with a peak at 15–35y and a smaller peak in adults (>55 years old).
- Classical Hodgkin's lymphoma (cHL) accounts for 20% of all malignant lymphomas.
- Men are more commonly affected than women (ratio 1.5:1), with the exception of the nodular sclerosis variant which has an equal gender incidence.
- Lower incidence in developing countries, with the exception of EBV+ cHL in younger patients.

Aetiology

- Unknown, though EBV infection has been implicated in some types.
- Immunosuppression (e.g. HIV infection) might contribute to the development of EBV+ cHL.
- Familial clustering has been described.

Genetics

- HRS cells are of B-cell lineage and derive from germinal centre B-cells.
- NF-κB pathway is frequently activated, contributing to evasion of apoptosis, survival, and proliferation of neoplastic cells.

Presentation

- Most patients present with localized lymphadenopathy, most frequently cervical, axillary, and inguinal nodes.
- Fever, night sweats, weight loss are common (so-called B symptoms) in 40% of cases.
- Nodular sclerosis subtype typically presents with mediastinal involvement (bulky mass in >50% of cases).
- Bone marrow involvement is infrequent (3–5%) in immunocompetent patients.

Histopathology

- See Fig. 15.9.
- Lymph nodes are replaced by small numbers of neoplastic HRS cells (usually 0.1–2%) within a rich inflammatory background.
- The textbook diagnostic Reed–Sternberg cell is a very large cell with two or more large nuclei, a thick nuclear membrane, and prominent eosinophilic nucleoli.
- Four histological subtypes are recognized, depending on the number and nature of the HRS cells and the reactive background: nodular sclerosis (50–80% cases), mixed cellularity (20–30%), lymphocyte-rich (5%), and lymphocyte-depleted (very rare).

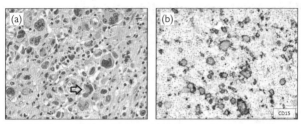

Fig. 15.9 Classical Hodgkin's lymphoma. (a) Mononuclear Hodgkin cells and large atypical Reed–Sternberg cells (arrow), multinucleated with prominent nucleoli. (b) The cells are positive with CD15 (membrane staining) (see Plate 55).

Immunophenotype

- HRS cells are CD30+ and CD15+ with a typical membranous and Golgi staining pattern.
- MUM-1 is strongly positive and there is reduced/weak expression of PAX5. CD45 (pan-leucocyte marker) is negative and a subset of cases express CD20.
- EBV (either latent membrane protein-1 or EBER *in-situ*) positive, depending on age, geographic factors, and subtype (frequently positive in mixed cellularity type and less frequent in nodular sclerosis).

Prognosis

- Modern treatment regimes cure cHL in >85% of cases.
- Histological subtype has limited value to predict prognosis.

Nodular lymphocyte-predominant Hodgkin's lymphoma

A distinct subtype of Hodgkin's lymphoma, known as **nodular lymphocyte-predominant Hodgkin's lymphoma (NLPHL)**, is also recognized.

NLPHL accounts for 5% of all Hodgkin's lymphomas and typically arises in young to middle-aged adults aged 30–50. Localized peripheral lymphadenopathy is the most frequent clinical presentation.

The abnormal B-cells, known as lymphocyte-predominant (LP) or 'popcorn' cells, are immunophenotypically distinct from classical HRS cells; they usually lack CD30 and CD15 and strongly express B-cell markers (CD20, CD79a, Oct2, BOB1) and EMA. Large numbers of follicular T-helper cells (CD57+, PD1+) are noted, forming rosettes around the LP cells.

The disease behaves indolently; it is rarely fatal, but frequent relapses are common. In early stages, radiotherapy is the standard treatment, and in other stages the therapeutic regime is similar to cHL.

Lymphoplasmacytic lymphoma

Definition

- A neoplasm of small B-lymphocytes, plasma cells, and plasmacytoid lymphocytes involving the bone marrow and sometimes the spleen and lymph nodes.
- Cases with lymphoplasmacytic lymphoma (LPL) in the bone marrow and IgM monoclonal gammopathy are referred to as Waldenström macroglobulinaemia.

Epidemiology

- Median age 63–68 y, male predominance.
- Incidence of 3 per 10^6 people per year.
- More frequent in Caucasians, compared with other ethnic groups.

Aetiology

- Family predisposition.
- Chronic hepatitis C, in addition to type II cryoglobulinaemia, drives proliferation of LPL.
- Some patients with Sjögren's syndrome might be at higher risk for LPL.

Genetics

- The most common alteration is a mutation in the *MYD88* gene (90% patients).
- Mutations in *DXCR4* are also frequent.
- Trisomy of chromosomes 4, 3, and 18.

Presentation

- Symptoms related to 'hyperviscosity' such as mucosal bleeding, visual disturbances due to retinopathy, and neurological disorders.
- Precipitation of cryoglobulins results in purpura, arthralgia, and cutaneous vasculitis.

Histopathology

- Nodular, interstitial, and/or diffuse infiltrate of small lymphocytes, plasma cells, and lymphoplasmacytoid cells in the bone marrow.
- Paratrabecular aggregates are also frequent.
- In the lymph nodes, the architecture might be partially preserved or replaced by nodules of neoplastic cells.
- Intranuclear inclusions (Dutcher bodies) are often seen.
- Mast cell hyperplasia is common.

Immunophenotype

- Positive with pan-B-cell markers CD20, CD19, CD20, CD22, and CD79a.
- Usually CD5-negative.
- Negative also with CD10, CD23.
- Plasma cells are highlighted with CD138 and are monotypic with light chains.
- Expression of surface immunoglobulins, mainly IgM and sometimes IgG.

Prognosis

- Indolent disease; median survival 5–10 y.
- Main causes of death are transformation to high-grade lymphoma and infection.
- Standard treatment in symptomatic patients include rituximab (anti-CD20 antibody), cyclophosphamide, and dexamethasone.

Plasma cell myeloma

Definition

- A disseminated bone marrow-based plasma cell neoplasm associated with a serum and/or urine paraprotein (usually M-protein).

Epidemiology

- Incidence 3–5 per 100 000 population.
- Occurs in older adults, with a mean age at diagnosis of 70 y.
- There is a male predominance (1.5:1) and it is more frequent in Afro-Caribbean ethnic groups.
- Cases can occur *de novo*, but the majority are preceded by monoclonal gammopathy of undetermined significance (MGUS).

Aetiology

- Unknown in most cases.
- Chronic antigenic stimulation (chronic bacterial diseases and inflammatory conditions) might play a role in some cases of multiple myeloma.

Genetics

- Frequent translocations involving the heavy chain locus on chromosome 14q32 (see Table 15.1). The most frequent partner is cyclin D1 (11q13). The t(4;14) translocations is associated with adverse prognosis.
- Trisomies of odd-numbered chromosomes (3, 5, 7, 9, 11, 15, 19, and 2).
- Activating mutations of *RAS* (*K*- and *NRAS*).
- MYC overexpression secondary chromosomal gain or translocation is a frequent secondary event, seen in up to 50% of myeloma cases.
- Activation of the NF-κB pathway by mutations in upstream genes.
- Epigenetic changes are also important, mainly DNA methylation, histone modifications, and non-coding RNAs.

Pathogenesis

- The neoplastic plasma cells secrete cytokines which activate osteoclasts, causing lytic bone lesions.
- Circulating paraprotein depresses normal immunoglobulin production, increasing the risk of infections.
- Free light chains passing through the kidney contribute to renal failure.

Table 15.1 Common IgH translocations in myeloma

Translocation (frequency)	Fusion partner
t(11;14) 15–20%	CCND1
t(4;14) 15%	MMSET and FGFR3
t(4;16) 5%	MAF
t(6;14) 1–2%	CCND3
t(14;20) 1%	MAFB

- The interaction between myeloma cells and bone marrow stromal cells increases myeloma cell growth and it is a target for new treatments.

Presentation

- Bone pain, pathological fractures, and recurrent infections.
- Anaemia, increased erythrocyte sedimentation rate (ESR), hypercalcaemia, and renal impairment are common.
- Clinical variants include: asymptomatic (smouldering) plasma cell myeloma; non-secretory myeloma and plasma cell leukaemia (>2 × 10^9/L clonal plasma cells in the peripheral blood).

Histopathology

- Definite diagnosis requires bone marrow biopsy and/or bone marrow aspirate.
- The bone marrow contains an excess of monoclonal plasma cells present in clusters, nodules, or sheets (Figs. 15.10 and 15.11).
- Plasma cells might contain globular inclusions: Russell bodies (cytoplasmic) and less frequently Dutcher bodies (nuclear inclusions).
- Prominent osteoclastic activity can also be seen in bone marrow biopsies.
- Clonality can be proven immunohistochemically by demonstrating kappa or lambda light chain restriction, and tumour burden can be assessed by *CD138* immunostaining.

Immunophenotype

- Positive with *CD138*, *CD38*, *VS38c*, and *CD79a*.
- *CD56* is aberrantly expressed.

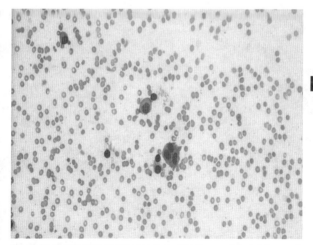

Fig. 15.10 Multiple myeloma bone marrow aspirate. Groups of atypical plasma cells are present (see Plate 56).

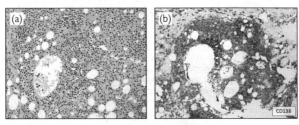

Fig. 15.11 Multiple myeloma bone marrow trephine biopsy. (a) Sheets of plasma cells infiltrate the bone marrow. The plasma cells have a round eccentric nucleus and abundant basophilic cytoplasm (haematoxylin and eosin staining). (b) The plasma cells are diffusely and strongly positive with CD138 (plasma cell marker) (see Plate 57).

- Some cases are cyclin D1-positive and this correlates with the presence of t(11;14).
- Less frequently, plasma cells can express *CD117*, *CD20*, and rarely *CD10*.

Prognosis

- Myeloma remains an incurable disease.
- Typical survival is 3–4 y from diagnosis.
- Prognostic factors include: renal function, β_2 microglobulin levels, cytogenetics abnormalities, and high degree of bone marrow involvement.

Primary amyloidosis

Definition
- A plasma cell neoplasm, or rarely a lymphoplasmacytic disorder, associated with secretion of abnormal immunoglobulin light chains and the deposition of AL amyloid in multiple tissues.

Epidemiology
- Rare disease.
- Median age at diagnosis 65 y, with clear male predominance.

Aetiology
- Up to 20% of patients have an underlying plasma cell myeloma and even a higher proportion will have criteria for MGUS.

Genetics
- Genetic abnormalities similar to those described in MGUS and plasma cell myeloma.
- t(11;14) present in >40% of cases of primary amyloidosis.

Pathogenesis
- AL amyloid is composed of immunoglobulin light chains (intact or fragments) secreted by monoclonal plasma cells which deposit in various tissues in a β-pleated sheet structure.
- Accumulated amyloid includes intact light chain and fragments of the variable NH2-terminus region.
- Rarely, immunoglobulin heavy chains are involved in the pathogenesis.

Presentation
- Clinical features related to the deposition of amyloid in multiple organs.
- Common sites of involvement include the skin, kidney, heart, liver, bowel, and peripheral nerves.
- Typical features include purpura, peripheral neuropathy, cardiac failure, nephrotic syndrome, bone pain, and malabsorption.
- Haemorrhage is a common complication, usually as consequence of blood vessel fragility from amyloid deposition.

Histopathology
- Amyloid can be demonstrated in many tissues as a pink amorphous substance. Congo red stains amyloid red under standard light microscopy and 'apple green' under polarized light.
- Amyloid is usually present in thickened blood vessel walls, and in the bone marrow it is seen in the interstitium.
- Bone marrow biopsies typically show a mild increase in plasma cells which may appear normal or atypical. The plasma cells are monotypic for either kappa or lambda light chains.

Immunophenotype
- Staining for amyloid P component.
- Anti-amyloid fibril antibodies against AL kappa and lambda and amyloid AA component might be useful.

Prognosis
- Poor prognosis with a median survival of only 2 y from diagnosis or shorter for patient with coexisting plasma cell myeloma.
- Treatment options include reduction in the production of the amyloid-forming protein and supporting the function of damaged organs.
- Most frequent cause of death is amyloid-associated cardiac failure.

Mature T-cell non-Hodgkin's lymphomas

Definition
- A group of lymphoid neoplasms derived from natural killer (NK) or T cells.

Classification
- The WHO classification includes >20 entities, accounting for 12–15% of all the malignant lymphomas.
- Peripheral T-cell lymphoma not otherwise specified (PTCL-NOS) and angioimmunoblastic T-cell lymphoma (AITL) are the most common types.
- Other types include enteropathy-associated T-cell lymphoma (EATL), adult T-cell lymphoma (ATLL), anaplastic large-cell lymphoma (ALCL), and extranodal NK nasal-type lymphoma.

Epidemiology
- Some geographic variation, depending on the type (EATL in the UK, ATLL in Japan, extranodal NK nasal-type in the Far East).
- The mature T-cell and NK-cell neoplasms usually affect adults, and most of the entities described are more commonly reported in males than in females. However, some types (e.g. *ALCL*) are commonly seen in children/young adults.

Aetiology
- EBV might play a role particularly in some entities (e.g. EBV+ T-cell lymphoproliferative diseases of childhood).
- Chronic immunosuppression (e.g. post-transplant) contributes to the development of some types (e.g. hepatosplenic T-cell lymphoma).

Genetics
- Monoclonal or oligoclonal rearrangement of the T-cell receptor.
- *RHO-A* mutations are common in AITL.
- *ALK* gene translocation, most commonly t(2;5)(p23;q35)(NPM-ALK), in ALCL–ALK+.
- Complex karyotype with recurrent chromosomal gains (7q, 9q, 17q) and losses (4q, 5q, 6q, 9p) in PTCL-NOS.

Presentation
- Might be nodal (PTCL-NOS, AITL, ALCL), extranodal (nasal-type, EATL, hepatosplenic), cutaneous only, or disseminated (AITL, aggressive NK-cell leukaemia).
- The majority are clinically aggressive.
- Compared to aggressive B-cell lymphomas, patients tend to present with more advanced disease, a poorer performance status, and an increased incidence of B-symptoms.

Histopathology
- Varies, depending on the entity, but effacement of the nodal architecture is common in cases with nodal involvement.

- AITL shows prominent vascularization by arborizing venules and expansion of CD21+ follicular dendritic cell networks. An oligoclonal r monoclonal B-cell population due to the expansion of B-cells infected with EBV can be seen in some cases.
- ALCL are characterized by 'hallmark cells' with a horseshoe-shaped nucleus, infiltrating sinusoids, and diffuse sheets surrounding residual follicles.
- PTCL-NOS is defined by medium-sized or large pleomorphic cells with irregular nuclei, in a diffuse pattern most frequently. Reed–Sternberg-like cells can be seen.

Immunophenotype

- Lack of at least one T-cell marker (CD5 and CD7 the most frequently lost). CD4 and CD8 might be positive or negative.
- CD30 is frequently expressed in ALCL and in a proportion of cutaneous T-cell lymphomas and PTCL-NOS.
- Cytotoxic markers (TIA-1, granzyme B, perforin) are positive in ALCL.
- Follicular T-helper cell markers (CD10, PD1, CXCL13, and ICOS) are expressed in AITL and in some cases of PTCL-NOS.
- ALK (subcellular localization) varies according to the type of translocation in ALCL. EMA is usually positive.
- NK-cell markers: CD56, CD57, CD16.
- AITL and some entities (e.g. EBV+ lymphoproliferative chronic disease of childhood) are EBV-positive (especially by EBER *in-situ* hybridization).

Prognosis

- The 5-year overall survival with standard chemotherapy varies between 25 and 45%.
- A clinical score (peripheral T-cell index PIT) has been proposed to allow prognostic stratification.
- Morphology usually does not correlate with outcome.
- Monoclonal antibodies (e.g. anti-CD30) might improve prognosis in some cases (e.g. ALCL).

Immunodeficiency-associated lymphoproliferative disorders (IA-LPDs)

Definition and classification

- Heterogenous group of diseases with variable pathological features and different clinical outcomes
- The WHO recognizes four types:
  1) LPDs associated with primary immune disorders (ie common variable immunodeficiency, Wiskott-Aldrich syndrome, ataxia; telangiectasia syndrome);
  2) Post-transplant lymphoproliferative disorders;
  3) LPDs associated with HIV infection;
  4) LPDs arising in patients treated with immunosuppressive drugs (methotrexate, anti-TNF antagonists, thiopurines) for autoimmune diseases or other conditions, other than in the post-transplant setting.

HIV-related lymphoma

- Although antiretroviral therapies have reduced the risk of developing lymphomas, Kaposi sarcomas, and AIDS in HIV patient, the risk of lymphoma is higher compared to the HIV-negative population.
- Approximately 95% of HIV-associated lymphomas are the same NHL and HL occurring in non-HIV patients, being DLBCL and BL the most frequent types.
- DLBCL in HIV patient usually have a non-germinal centre phenotype (non-GCB) characterize by MUM1+, CD138+, CD10(-) and BCL6(-) cells.
- In HIV population the incidence of primary CNS lymphomas, primary effusion lymphomas, and plasmablastic lymphomas of the oral cavity is higher than in non-HIV population.

Post-transplant lymphoproliferative diseases (PTLD)

- Heterogenous group of reactive and malignant lymphoproliferative lesions.
- Most PTLDs are associated with EBV infection. In post-transplant patients, immunosuppression reduces T-cell immunity (mainly CD8+ cells), resulting in proliferation of EBV infected cells, overexpression of LMP1 and LMP2 proteins, and escape from apoptosis.
- 20–40% of PTLDs are EBV negative, being the proportion higher in T-cell PTLDs.
- The incidence depends on the transplant organ: bone marrow and kidney represent the lower risk, whereas intestine is associated with the higher risk.
- The clinical presentation varies greatly. Frequently occur in the first year after transplant but late onset (more than 10 years) has been described in 15–25% of cases.
- The WHO recognizes the following types:
  - Non-destructive PTLDs, characterized by architectural preservation of the involved tissue and absence of features diagnostics of malignant lymphoma. Subtypes in this group are: Plasmacytoid hyperplasia, infectious mononucleosis, and florid follicular hyperplasia.

- Polymorphic PTLD are characterize by effacement of the lymph nodes or extranodal tissues by a proliferation of immunoblasts, plasma cells, and medium-sized lymphoid cells. Usually P-PTLDs demonstrate clonal rearrangement of Immunoglobulin genes.
- Monomorphic PTLDs show similar microscopic and genetic features to their non-PTLD counterparts (i.e. B- and T-cell neoplasms). Most B-monomorphic PTLDs show a non-germinal centre phenotype. Clonal immunoglobulin gene rearrangement is present in almost all cases and contain EBV genomes.
- Classical Hodgkin lymphoma PTLD is the less frequent type but fulfil the diagnostic criteria for cHL. Often these are EBV+ and have a 'mixed cellularity' morphology.

Methotrexate-associated LPD

- MTX-associated LPD is a classical example of iatrogenic IA-LPD.
- The relative risk of LPD in patients treated with MTX is 2.5 higher than in general population.
- DLBCL is the most common subtype (50%) and EBV positivity is found in 60% of cases.
- The clinical findings are the same as those see in immunocompetent patients and extranodal involvement occurs in up to 50% of patients.
- Lymphomas in patients treated with anti-TNF alpha agents (ie infliximab, adalimumab) have also been described, with some studies suggesting an increased risk of hepatosplenic T-cell lymphoma, although a true association is yet to be found.

CAR-T immunotherapy

Concepts

- Chimeric antigen receptor (CAR) T cells are T cells that have been genetically modified in the laboratory to express and antigen receptor in the surface, able to recognize a specific surface antigen in the patient's malignant tumour cells.
- CARs are composed of an antigen-recognizing receptor coupled to signalling molecules that lead to activation of T cells.
- B- and T-cell maturation manifests by cell surface expression of cluster of differentiation (CD) antigens. CD antigens are expressed, variably or constantly, throughout lymphocyte maturation. The pattern of expression of these CDs, define the cell of origin in multiple B- and T-cell derived malignancies.
- After ex-vivo proliferation the CAR-T cells are transferred back to the patient with the aim that will selectively recognize the target antigen, and therefore the tumour cells, and kill them more efficiently.
- Two main toxicities associated with CAR-T immunotherapy are cytokine-release syndrome (CRS) and neurotoxicity.

Steps in CAR-T cell therapy

- See Fig. 15.12.
- Leukopheresis of peripheral blood with the aim to collect autologous T cells.

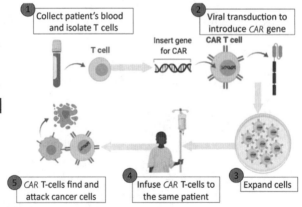

1. Collect patient's blood and isolate T cells

T cell

Insert gene for CAR

2. Viral transduction to introduce *CAR* gene

CAR T cell

5. *CAR* T-cells find and attack cancer cells

4. Infuse *CAR* T-cells to the same patient

3. Expand cells

Fig. 15.12 CAR T immunotherapy (see Plate 58).

- CAR-T engineering: washing of the apheresis product, T-cell selection, T-cell activation, gene transfer, T-cell expansion, and cryopreservation.
- After ex-vivo proliferation the CAR-T cells are transferred back to the patient with the aim that will selectively recognize the target antigen, and therefore the tumour cells, and kill them more efficiently.
- During CAR-T cells production (2–4 weeks) patients usually receive bridging therapy to prevent further progression of the underlying malignancy.

CAR-T-cell therapy in haematological malignancies

Disease	Antigen targeted
Acute lymphoblastic lymphoma/leukaemia (ALL)	CD19, CD22, CD20, CD123
Large B-cell lymphoma, diffuse large B-cell lymphoma, transformed follicular lymphoma, mantle cell lymphoma	CD19, CD20
Chronic Lymphocytic leukaemia / small lymphocytic lymphoma (CLL/SLL)	CD19
Hodgkin lymphoma	CD30, CD19
Multiple myeloma	CD138, BCMA
Myeloid malignancies	CD123, CD33

CAR-T cells in B-cell malignancies

- CD19 is almost uniformly expressed in B-cell development, usually not present in haematopoietic stems cells or plasma cells. CD19 has become an important therapeutic target in B-cell neoplasms.
- CD19 targeted CAR-T-cell therapies are approved for 1) Reaped or refractory large B-cell lymphoma in patients who have received at least two previous lines of treatment.
- Overall response rates vary between 50–80%, but up to 50% of patients will relapse of have progressive disease after treatment.
- Dual CAR-T-cells, targeting both CD19 and CD20 or CD19 and CD22 have been developed.

CAR-T cell therapy in multiple myeloma

- CD19 is rarely expressed in plasma cells.
- The main target in myeloma is the B-cell maturation antigen (BCMA), which binds B-cell activating factor and APRIL (proliferation-inducing ligand).
- Responses rates vary between 50–90% and duration of response range from 4 to 16 months.

Further reading

Hoffbrand AV et al. *Color Atlas of Clinical Haematology*, 4th edition. Mosby Elsevier 2010.

Kumar V et al. *Robins & Cotran Pathologic Basis of Disease*, 10th edition. Elsevier 2020.

Sweerdlow SH et al. *WHO Classification of Tumours of Haematopoietic and Lymphoid Tissues*. Revised 4th Edition. IARC: Lyon, 2017.

Wardford-A and Presnau N (editors). *Fundamentals of Biomedical Science*. Oxford: Oxford University Press, 2019.

Skin pathology

Eczema/dermatitis

Definition

- A group of inflammatory skin diseases characterized clinically by an erythematous papulovesicular rash and histologically by the presence of intraepidermal oedema (spongiosis).

Atopic dermatitis

- Chronic dermatitis occurring in people with atopy.
- Very common disorder with incidences as high as 15%.
- Typically occurs in infants and children.
- Clinically causes an itchy, erythematous papulovesicular rash involving the face and extensor surfaces of the arms and legs.
- Biopsies from acute lesions show epidermal spongiosis and dermal inflammation.
- Biopsies from later lesions show epidermal thickening and hyperkeratosis with mild spongiosis.

Irritant contact dermatitis

- Inflammatory skin disease caused by direct toxic effect of an irritant.
- A common cause of occupational skin disease.
- Clinically causes erythema with vesiculation.
- Biopsies show epidermal spongiosis and dermal inflammation.

Allergic contact dermatitis

- Inflammatory skin disease caused by a delayed-type hypersensitivity reaction to an allergen to which the patient has been sensitized.
- Common occupational skin disease (well described in hairdressers).
- Clinically causes itchy papules and vesicles 12–48h after exposure.
- Common culprits include nickel, cosmetics, and foodstuffs.
- Biopsies show epidermal spongiosis with vesicle formation and an inflammatory infiltrate which usually includes eosinophils.

Nummular dermatitis

- Inflammatory skin disease of unknown cause.
- Clinically shows tiny papules and vesicles that coalesce into coin-shaped patches.
- Biopsies show epidermal spongiosis and inflammation in early lesions. Older lesions show epidermal hyperplasia.

Seborrhoeic dermatitis

- Common inflammatory skin disease affecting 1–3% of people.
- Some evidence suggests it may be the result of an abnormal immune response to *Malassezia* organisms, but this is controversial.
- Clinically causes erythematous, scaly papules, and plaques, sometimes with a greasy appearance, on the scalp, ears, eyebrows, and nasolabial area.
- Biopsies show variable epidermal spongiosis and hyperplasia with parakeratosis centred on hair follicles.

Psoriasis

Definition

- A chronic relapsing skin disorder associated with abnormal hyperproliferation of the epidermis.

Epidemiology

- Common, affecting ~2% of people.
- Mean age of onset 25 y.

Aetiology

- Current evidence suggests that psoriasis is the result of an abnormal immune reaction to an external trigger in a genetically susceptible individual.
- Factors known to trigger or exacerbate the condition include stress, infections, climate, alcohol, smoking, and trauma.
- Genome-wide linkage analysis studies have identified at least nine chromosomal loci associated with psoriasis; most of these appear to be genes encoding human leukocyte antigen (HLA) proteins, cytokines, or cytokine receptors.

Pathogenesis

- Activated plasmacytoid dendritic cells in the skin migrate to draining lymph nodes where they induce the differentiation of naïve T-cells into type 1 and type 17 helper and cytotoxic T-cells.
- Effector T cells circulate to the skin where they elaborate cytokines, including IL-17, IL-22, IFN-γ, and TNF-α, which stimulate the hyperproliferation of epidermal keratinocytes.

Presentation

- Well-demarcated erythematous plaques with adherent silvery scale.
- Sites of predilection are the elbows, knees, and scalp.
- Nail involvement is common with pitting and onycholysis.
- Guttate psoriasis is a clinical variant, characterized by small, 1–5 mm in size, erythematous papules. Many of these cases are preceded by streptococcal infection.
- Severe psoriasis may cause erythroderma (erythrodermic psoriasis).

Histopathology

- Typical lesions show psoriasiform epidermal hyperplasia with thinning of the suprapapillary plates. Plaques of parakeratosis are present, with a diminution of the granular layer beneath the parakeratosis.
- Collections of neutrophils are seen in the stratum corneum (Munro microabscesses) and may also be found within the stratum spinosum.
- The dermis contains dilated capillaries and an inflammatory infiltrate.

Prognosis

- Usually runs a chronic course.
- May have a significant impact on quality of life.

Lichen planus

Definition
- An inflammatory skin disease associated with itchy purple papules clinically and a lichenoid reaction pattern histologically.

Epidemiology
- Affects ~1% of the population.
- Usually arises in middle-aged adults, with a slight female predominance.

Aetiology
- Unknown.

Pathogenesis
- Thought to represent a delayed-type hypersensitivity reaction to an unidentified epidermal antigen.

Presentation
- The skin lesions are small, flat-topped, violaceous papules which are usually intensely itchy.
- Fine white lines (Wickham's striae) usually cross the surface.
- The lesions usually occur on the flexor aspect of the wrists, the extensor aspects of the hands, and the forearms.
- Oral involvement is common, as is genital involvement, particularly in men.

Histopathology
- See Fig. 16.1
- A heavy, band-like inflammatory infiltrate containing lymphocytes and macrophages is present beneath the epidermis.
- The basal layer of the epidermis shows vacuolar damage with cytoid body formation and melanin spillage.
- The epidermis shows irregular acanthosis, hyperkeratosis, and wedge-shaped hypergranulosis.

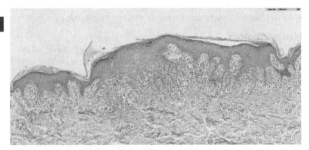

Fig. 16.1 Lichen planus. Histology shows a lichenoid tissue reaction pattern characterized by an irregularly acanthotic squamatised epidermis and an obscuring band of lymphocytic inflammation at the dermo-epidermal junction (see Plate 59).

Prognosis
- In most cases, the disease resolves spontaneously over a variable period of time from weeks to a year.

Erythema multiforme

Definition

- An inflammatory skin disorder associated with distinctive targetoid lesions clinically and an interface reaction pattern histologically.

Epidemiology

- Relatively common.
- Mainly affects young people, including children.

Aetiology

- Most cases are linked to current or previous infections with herpes simplex virus (HSV), which may not always be clinically apparent.
- Other infective agents have also been implicated (e.g. *Mycoplasma*).
- Drugs are also a recognized cause.

Pathogenesis

- Thought to represent a delayed-type hypersensitivity reaction to HSV antigens transported to the skin in circulating lymphocytes.

Presentation

- Discrete, round erythematous patches, 1–2 cm in size, with central discolouration which may blister ('target' lesions).
- Most cases involve the extremities.
- Mild oral involvement is common.

Histopathology

- Biopsies show an interface dermatitis characterized by a superficial lymphohistiocytic inflammatory infiltrate with prominent basal cell vacuolar degeneration and keratinocyte apoptosis.
- Cases with marked basal cell damage may result in subepidermal clefting and blistering.

Prognosis

- Most cases are self-limiting, but recurrent episodes are common.

Granuloma annulare

Definition
- An inflammatory skin disease classically associated with annular lesions clinically and necrobiotic granulomatous inflammation histologically.

Epidemiology
- Common.

Aetiology
- Unknown in the majority of cases.
- *Borrelia* infection has been linked in a small number of cases.

Pathogenesis
- Current evidence suggests it represents a cutaneous reaction pattern to as yet undefined antigens.

Presentation
- Localized lesions of granuloma annulare consist of flesh-coloured or red papules which line up to form an annular lesion of 1–5 cm.
- Acral sites are usually affected, especially the knuckles and fingers.

Histopathology
- See Fig. 16.2.
- The dermis contains a palisading granuloma, characterized by a central area of degenerate (necrobiotic) collagen surrounded by radially arranged histiocytes, lymphocytes, and fibroblasts.
- Mucin is often present within the necrobiotic focus.
- Occasionally, the process forms a more subtle ill-defined lesion in the dermis, rather than a typical well-formed palisaded granuloma (interstitial granuloma annulare).

Prognosis
- About half of cases resolve within 2y of onset, though recurrences are quite common.

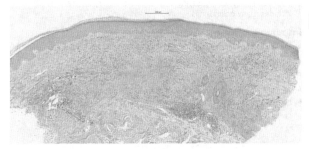

Fig. 16.2 Granuloma annulare. Histology shows a necrobiotic granulomatous inflammation in the dermis characterized by a zone of degenerate collagen surrounded by a palisade of histiocytes and perivascular lymphocytic inflammation (see Plate 60).

Pemphigus vulgaris

Definition
- An immunobullous skin disease due to autoantibodies against epidermal desmosomal proteins.

Epidemiology
- Rare with an incidence of 0.1–1 per 100 000 people per year.
- Usually affects middle-aged adults of 40–60y.

Aetiology
- Production of autoantibodies directed against the epidermal desmosomal cadherin desmoglein-3.

Pathogenesis
- The autoantibody binds to the extracellular domain of desmoglein-3, leading to desmosomal damage and acantholysis.
- The traditional view was that complement fixation led to acantholysis; however, some workers have suggested that the acantholysis may be due to cytoskeletal collapse, independent of the action of complement.

Presentation
- Most cases start with oral erosions and blisters, followed weeks or months later by the development of skin lesions.
- The skin lesions are fragile blisters developing on normal or erythematous skin. The blisters easily rupture, leaving a painful area of erosion.
- The skin lesions typically occur on the face, scalp, axillae, and groins.

Histopathology
- Biopsies show a blister cavity within the epidermis containing acantholytic keratinocytes.
- Typically, the level of the split is suprabasal, such that the floor of the blister is lined by a single layer of intact basal keratinocytes.
- The acantholysis may also involve the epidermis of adnexal structures.
- There is usually an underlying dermal inflammatory infiltrate which includes many eosinophils.

Immunofluorescence
- Direct immunofluorescence on perilesional skin reveals a deposition of IgG and C3 in the intercellular region of the epidermis.

Prognosis
- Mortality rates are low with appropriate immunosuppressive regimes.
- Most complications are therapy-related.

Bullous pemphigoid

Definition
- An immunobullous skin disease due to autoantibodies against epidermal hemidesmosomal proteins.

Epidemiology
- Most common immunobullous skin disorder, but still a rare disease with an annual incidence of 7 per million population.
- Most cases arise in elderly adults aged >70.

Aetiology
- Production of autoantibodies directed against epidermal hemidesmosomal proteins.
- The two key antigens are known as BPAg1 and BPAg2.

Pathogenesis
- Binding of the antibody leads to fixation of complement and an influx of inflammatory cells, including eosinophils.
- Direct cytotoxic action leads to the disruption of the hemidesmosomes anchoring the epidermis to the dermis and the resultant separation of the entire epidermis from the dermis.

Presentation
- The typical skin lesions are large, tense, intact blisters which develop on normal or erythematous skin.
- Sites of predilection include the lower trunk, inner thighs, forearms, axillae, and groins.

Histopathology
- See Fig. 16.3(a)
- Biopsies show a subepidermal blister containing numerous eosinophils.
- The underlying dermis is oedematous and also contains an inflammatory infiltrate rich in eosinophils.

Immunofluorescence
- See Fig. 16.3(b)
- Direct immunofluorescence on perilesional skin reveals linear deposition of IgG and C3 along the basement membrane zone.

Prognosis
- Mortality rates are low with appropriate immunosuppressive regimes.
- Most complications are therapy-related.

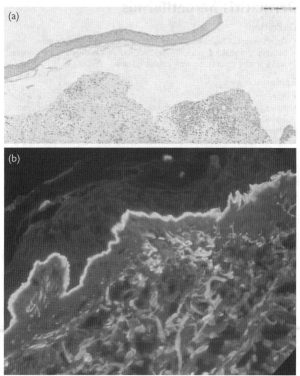

Fig. 16.3 Bullous pemphigoid. (a) Histology of blistered skin shows a subepidermal blister with inflammation in dermis rich in eosinophils. (b) Direct immunofluorescence performed on perilesional skin shows linear deposition of C3 along the basement membrane zone (see Plate 61).

Dermatitis herpetiformis

Definition
- An immunobullous skin disorder characterized by intensely itchy papules and vesicles, granular deposition of IgA in the papillary dermis, and a strong association with coeliac disease.

Epidemiology
- Rare.
- Any age may be affected, but the peak incidence is young adults aged 20–40 y.
- Males are affected twice as often as females.
- The condition is particularly common in Northern Europe and Ireland.
- Up to 90% of people have evidence of coeliac disease, though this may be subclinical.

Aetiology
- IgA transglutaminase antibodies formed in the gut appear to be the key mediator.

Pathogenesis
- IgA transglutaminase antibodies react with transglutaminase enzymes in the skin.
- Fixation of complement stimulates chemotaxis of neutrophils into the papillary dermis.
- Enzymes released from neutrophils lead to blister formation.

Presentation
- The rash is composed of groups of papules and vesicles which are intensely itchy.
- Sites of predilection are the shoulders, back, buttocks, elbows, and knees.

Histopathology
- Biopsies from early lesions show collections of neutrophils within the papillary dermis (papillary dermal microabscesses).
- Biopsies from established lesions show a subepidermal blister rich in neutrophils.

Immunofluorescence
- Direct immunofluorescence of perilesional skin reveals granular deposition of IgA in the papillary dermis.

Prognosis
- The disease is usually chronic and lifelong but shows a dramatic response to the drug dapsone.

Erythema nodosum

Definition

- A syndrome characterized clinically by an acute painful erythematous nodular skin eruption and histologically by a septal panniculitis.

Epidemiology

- Typically affects young adults, with a marked predilection for women.

Aetiology

- Numerous aetiologies have been described.
- Most common associations are sarcoidosis (➔ Sarcoidosis, p. 622), infections, inflammatory bowel disease (➔ Crohn's disease, p. 132 and ➔ Ulcerative colitis, p. 134), and drugs.

Pathogenesis

- Unknown, but probably represents a form of hypersensitivity reaction to infection, drug, or an underlying systemic disease.

Presentation

- Sudden onset of red, warm, tender skin nodules.
- Classically involves the shins, but other sites may be affected.
- Systemic symptoms, such as fever and malaise, may also be present.

Histopathology

- Biopsies show a septal panniculitis characterized by an inflammatory infiltrate centred on the septa of subcutaneous fat.
- The inflammatory infiltrate is composed predominantly of lymphocytes and macrophages.
- Collections of histiocytes surrounded by cleft like spaces are well described (Mieschner's radial granuloma).

Prognosis

- The condition is usually self-limiting over a period of weeks, with the skin nodules eventually fading and discolouring rather like a bruise.

Pyoderma gangrenosum

Definition
- An inflammatory skin disease characterized by the development of one or more large necrotic ulcers with ragged undermined violaceous borders.

Epidemiology
- Uncommon.
- Typically affects middle-aged adults.

Aetiology
- Unknown, though more than half of all cases are associated with a systemic disease (particularly inflammatory bowel disease and arthritis).

Pathogenesis
- Unknown, though many immune abnormalities have been described.
- Whether it represents a form of vasculitis is controversial.

Presentation
- The lesion begins as an erythematous pustule or nodule, typically on the lower extremity.
- Often there is a history of preceding minor trauma (pathergy).
- There is then rapid evolution into a necrotic ulcer with undermined red-purple edges.

Histopathology
- Histology is variable and non-specific.
- There is epidermal ulceration with extensive underlying dermal inflammation and abscess formation.

Prognosis
- Recurrence is common and more than half of patients require long-term therapy to control the disease.

Acne vulgaris

Definition

- A cutaneous disorder of pilosebaceous units leading to comedones ± inflammatory papules and pustules.

Epidemiology

- Extremely common disorder affecting ~85% of adolescents and ~15% of the general population.
- Worldwide distribution with equal sex incidence, though males tend to have more severe disease.

Aetiology

- Most cases are related to increased androgen production during adolescence.
- Endocrine conditions resulting in increased androgen production can also cause acne (e.g. polycystic ovarian syndrome).
- Drugs (e.g. contraceptives, steroids) can exacerbate acne.

Pathogenesis

- Increased sebum production and hyperkeratosis cause blockage to hair follicles and formations of comedones.
- Overgrowth of the bacterium *Propionibacterium acnes* causes secondary inflammation with eventual rupture of the follicle with scarring.

Presentation

- Non-inflammatory acne is characterized by the presence of comedones only, which may be open or closed.
- Inflammatory acne causes superimposed papules and pustules which may be complicated by scarring in more severe cases.

Histopathology

- Comedones show a dilated hair follicle plugged with keratin.
- Inflammatory acne shows an acute inflammatory reaction around the involved hair follicle. More severe cases may shows abscess formation and scarring.

Prognosis

- Most cases can be controlled with treatment and the condition generally improves as the patient passes through adolescence.
- Severe cases can lead to permanent scarring.

Rosacea

Definition
- A chronic skin condition characterized by facial flushing ± persistent erythema, papules, and pustules.

Epidemiology
- Common disease affecting ~3% of the population.
- 2–3 times more common in women.

Aetiology
- Exact cause unknown, but possibilities include vascular abnormalities or a reaction to Demodex mites.
- Numerous triggering factors may exacerbate the condition, including sunlight, stress, exercise, hot/cold weather, alcohol, caffeine, and certain foods.

Pathogenesis
- Triggering factors lead to a vascular reaction with dilation and flushing.
- Some patients develop also an inflammatory reaction leading to papules and pustules.

Presentation
- Erythematous subtype: flushing and persistent facial erythema.
- Papulopustular subtype: persistent facial erythema with papules ± pustules.
- Phymatous subtype: thickened nodular skin on the nose, chin, forehead, cheeks, or ears.
- Granulomatous subtype: hard, brown-yellow or red papules or nodules.

Histopathology
- Erythematous subtype: dermal oedema, telangiectasia, and mild inflammation.
- Papulopustular subtype: acute inflammation around hair follicles. Demodex mites are often present.
- Phymatous subtype: marked follicular dilation and plugging.
- Granulomatous subtype: perifollicular non-caseating granulomas.

Prognosis
- Usually persistent with a relapsing and remitting course.
- Can have significant psychological effects.

Urticaria

Definition
- Vascular reaction of skin characterized by wheals and severe itching.
- Acute urticaria lasts <6 weeks, chronic urticaria lasts >6 weeks.
- **Angio-oedema** is a deeper form of urticaria with subcutaneous swellings particularly affecting the lips, eyelids, and genitals.

Epidemiology
- Very common disease affecting ~20% of the population.

Aetiology
- Most cases are idiopathic but common triggers include drugs and foods (especially shellfish and peanuts).

Pathogenesis
- Mast cells are the primary mediators.
- Histamine and heparin released from activated mast cells causes increased vascular permeability with extravasation of fluid and protein as well as recruitment of leukocytes.

Presentation
- Red or white oedematous plaques that are very itchy (wheals).

Histopathology
- Findings may be mild and subtle.
- Perivascular and interstitial dermal inflammatory infiltrate of eosinophils, neutrophils, and lymphocytes. Neutrophils are often seen in the lumina of dermal vessels.
- Dermal oedema

Prognosis
- Good outcome, usually controllable with antihistamines.

Skin infections

Acute folliculitis

- Infection of hair follicles, usually due to *Staphylococcus aureus*.
- Presents with small, red, tender pustules.
- Deep extension of the acute inflammation may lead to a furuncle with more surrounding erythema and pain.

Impetigo

- Highly infectious superficial bacterial skin infection.
- Very common, particularly in children.
- Caused by either *S. aureus* or *Staphylococcus pyogenes*.
- Presents with vesicles covered by golden yellow crust, typically around the mouth and nose.

Staphylococcal scalded skin syndrome

- A superficial blistering skin disease caused by strains of *S. aureus* producing an epidermolytic toxin.
- Seen almost exclusively in neonates and young children.
- The rash is initially erythematous and then blisters with an appearance likened to a scald.
- Healing occurs within 2–3 weeks without scarring.

Cellulitis

- Deep skin infection caused by *S. pyogenes*.
- Mostly occurs on the legs as an erythematous rash with oedema.
- ▶ Clinically may closely mimic deep venous thrombosis.

Necrotizing fasciitis

- Rapidly progressive necrotizing infection of subcutaneous tissues.
- *S. aureus* and group A β-haemolytic streptococci (dubbed 'flesh-eating bacteria') are the most commonly cultured organisms, but infection is often polymicrobial.
- Fournier's gangrene is a variant on the scrotum.
- Rapid surgical debridement is essential to avoid systemic sepsis.

Cutaneous tuberculosis

- Most caused by haematogenous spread from tuberculous infection elsewhere in the body.
- Lesions occur mostly on the face (particularly around the nose) as red papules and plaques with a gelatinous consistency.
- Biopsies show granulomatous inflammation ± necrosis.

Non-tuberculous mycobacterial infections

- Non-tuberculous environmental mycobacteria may cause infection if inoculated into the skin (e.g. *Mycobacterium marinum*, associated with underwater injuries), *Mycobacterium fortuitum/chelonae*, and *Mycobacterium kansasii*.
- Biopsies typically show areas of suppurative granulomatous inflammation within which small numbers of acid-fast bacilli may be found.

Viral warts

- Very common skin lesions caused by human papillomavirus (HPV) infection.
- May occur anywhere on the skin in people of any age.
- Clinically appear as keratotic papules.
- Immunosuppressed individuals may have them in large numbers.
- Biopsies show marked papillomatosis with hyperkeratosis and tiers of parakeratosis. The keratinocytes show typical viral cytopathic effects with vacuolation and large keratohyaline granules.

Herpes simplex

- Caused by HSV types 1 and 2.
- Infections involve the oral and/or genital areas.
- Infection is lifelong due to viral latency within sensory ganglia.
- Recurrent episodes may be precipitated by many factors and is characterized by the onset of groups of vesicles on an erythematous base.
- Biopsies show ballooning degeneration of keratinocytes with acantholysis. Keratinocyte nuclei contain characteristic pale intranuclear inclusions.

Varicella-zoster

- Varicella-zoster virus (VZV) is highly contagious and most individuals are infected in childhood, leading to chickenpox.
- Infection is lifelong due to viral latency within sensory ganglia.
- Reactivation of the virus in adulthood leads to herpes zoster (shingles), presenting as a band-like vesicular eruption along the distribution of a sensory nerve.

Molluscum contagiosum

- Caused by molluscipoxvirus infection.
- Results in the eruption of groups of small umbilicated papules on the face, limbs, and trunk of young children or the genital region of young adults.
- Biopsies show a highly distinctive lobular epidermal proliferation in which the keratinocytes contain large basophilic cytoplasmic inclusions.

Dermatophytoses
- Common superficial fungal infections caused by 'ringworm' fungi.
- Cause slowly enlarging scaly erythematous annular lesions on the body (tinea corporis), head (tinea capitis), or foot (tinea pedis).

Tinea (pityriasis) versicolor
- Superficial fungal infection caused by the yeast *Malassezia globosa*.
- Presents with multiple areas of hypo- or hyperpigmentation with fine scale in young adults.
- Biopsies show budding yeasts and hyphae within the stratum corneum ('spaghetti and meatballs').

Benign epidermal tumours

Fibroepithelial polyp

- Very common lesion which typically occur as multiple small pedunculated papules around the neck, axillae, and groin.
- Most are removed for cosmetic reasons or because they catch on clothing.
- Histologically, composed of a core of fibrovascular tissue covered by normal or hyperplastic epidermis.

Epidermoid cyst

- Common cutaneous cyst typically arising on the face, neck, upper trunk, vulva, or scrotum.
- Histologically, the cyst is filled with laminated keratin and lined by squamous epithelium with a granular layer.

Pilar (tricholemmal) cyst

- Common cutaneous cyst which almost always occur on the scalp.
- Histologically, the cyst is lined by pale squamous epithelial cells showing abrupt keratinization without formation of a granular layer.

Seborrhoeic keratosis

- Very common lesion seen in middle-aged and elderly adults.
- Appear as brown-black greasy warty lesion which are often multiple.
- May occur anywhere on the body, apart from the palms and soles.
- Histologically composed of a proliferation of basaloid keratinocytes showing variable squamous differentiation, often with hyperkeratosis and horn cyst formation.

Lichenoid keratosis

- Common lesions seen mostly in adults.
- Appear as red scaly lesions.
- Histologically show lichenoid pattern inflammation associated with acanthosis and hyperkeratosis of the epidermis.
- Most are thought to represent regressing benign epidermal lesions or lentigos.

Clear cell acanthoma

- Uncommon lesion seen mostly in middle-aged women.
- Generally found on the lower legs.
- Appear as a solitary pink or red papule or plaque.
- Histologically show acanthosis of the epidermis with keratinocytes having pale or clear cytoplasm. The lesion characteristically is sharply demarcated from the adjacent normal epidermis.

Benign melanocytic tumours

Lentigo simplex

- Very common melanocytic lesion presenting as brown to black well-circumscribed macules which may occur anywhere on the body.
- Simple lentigos may be found at any skin site and may represent a precursor to a junctional naevus.
- Solar lentigos tend to be found on sun-exposed skin of middle-aged and elderly people.
- Those found on mucosal sites such as genitals or lips are often termed melanotic macules.
- Histology shows a slight increase in single melanocytes associated with elongation and hyperpigmentation of epidermal rete ridges.

Melanocytic naevi

- Extremely common melanocytic lesions which are virtually universal in white individuals and may be found anywhere on the body.
- The melanocytic proliferation may be restricted to the epidermis (junctional naevus), dermis (intradermal naevus) or be in both the epidermis and dermis (compound naevus).
- Histologically, junctional naevi show nests of small uniform melanocytes located at the tips of the rete ridges. Intradermal naevi show nests of small melanocytes in the dermis which tend to shrink in size with increasing depth in the dermis ('maturation with depth'). Compound naevi have both junctional and intradermal components.
- Genetically most show activating mutations in *BRAF*.

Common blue naevus

- Relatively common dermal melanocytic naevus which appears as a dark blue papule across a wide age range.
- May occur anywhere on the body, but more commonly on the hands, feet, buttocks, scalp, and face.
- Histologically composed of heavily pigmented spindled and dendritic dermal melanocytes.
- Genetically show mutations of *GNAQ* or *GNA11*.

Spitz naevus

- Uncommon benign melanocytic lesion typically presenting in children or young adults as a pink or red/brown papule or nodule.
- Usually seen on the head, neck, and extremities.
- Histologically, Spitz naevi are usually compound melanocytic lesions composed of large epithelioid and/or spindled cells containing abundant eosinophilic cytoplasm and a conspicuous nucleolus.
- Spitz naevi are of particular importance histologically because the large size of the melanocytes can lead to misdiagnosis as melanoma.
- Genetically show fusions of tyrosine kinase genes such as *NTRK1*, *NTRK3*, *ROS1*, *ALK*, *BRAF*.

Dysplastic naevus

- Very common clinically atypical melanocytic lesion typically presenting as a large (>5 mm) pigmented lesion with irregular margins and variable pigmentation.
- Histologically, the junctional component shows architectural disarray and cytological atypia in some of the melanocytes ('random cytological atypia').
- Lesions may be graded as mild, moderate, or severe, depending on the degree of atypia.
- Mild or moderately dysplastic naevi ae considered low risk lesions and can be excised with narrow margins.
- Severely dysplastic naevi show more histological overlap with in situ melanoma and so are generally excised with a wider (5 mm) margin.
- The biology of dysplastic naevi is somewhat controversial. Whilst the presence of multiple dysplastic naevi is associated with an increased risk of developing melanoma in that individual, current evidence indicates that the risk of a dysplastic naevus transforming into a melanoma appears to be low.

Benign cutaneous soft tissue tumours

Dermatofibroma

- Common benign fibrous tumour of the skin.
- Presents as a reddish-brown papule on the trunk or lower legs.
- Histologically shows an ill-defined dermal lesion composed of short interlacing spindle cells within variable amounts of collagen, foamy macrophages, blood vessels, and inflammatory cells.

Lobular capillary haemangioma

- Benign vascular tumour, also widely known as pyogenic granuloma.
- Present as red papules or nodules which often ulcerate and bleed.
- Occurs mostly on the head and neck or extremities.
- Histologically shows a polypoid dermal lesion composed of lobules of small capillaries.

Neurofibroma

- Common benign cutaneous nerve sheath tumour.
- Most cases are sporadic, but note that multiple neurofibromas and café-au-lait spots are associated with neurofibromatosis type 1.
- Presents as a soft, flesh-coloured papule or nodule at any skin site.
- Histologically shows a dermal tumour containing Schwann cells with wavy nuclei and fibroblasts in a fibrillar background.

Fibrous papule

- Common benign cutaneous fibrous tumour of the skin.
- Presents as a flesh-coloured papule on the nose or face.
- Histologically composed of stellate fibroblasts, collagen, and dilated thin-walled vessels.

Benign skin adnexal tumours

Pilomatrixoma

- Common benign skin tumour showing hair matrix differentiation.
- Presents as a firm papule or nodule in a child or young adult.
- Often occur on the cheek.
- Histologically composed of nodules of basaloid cells showing transformation into anucleate eosinophilic cells ('ghost cells') in the centre of the nodules. Calcification is very common.

Trichoepithelioma

- Benign skin adnexal tumour showing hair germ differentiation.
- Presents as a flesh-coloured papule, usually on the face.
- Histologically composed of organoid nests of basaloid epithelium showing primitive hair follicle formation.

Sebaceous hyperplasia

- Benign hyperplastic skin lesion.
- Presents as a papule on the face in an adult, often mimicking basal cell carcinoma.
- Histologically composed of clusters of enlarged sebaceous glands in the dermis.

Sebaceous adenoma

- Histologically composed of lobules of cells with peripheral basaloid cells with mature sebocytes centrally.
- Multiple sebaceous tumours may be associated with the Muir–Torre syndrome, an inherited syndrome caused by germline mutations in mismatch repair genes.

Cylindroma

- Benign skin adnexal tumour showing sweat gland differentiation.
- Presents as a solitary pink or red lesion, usually on the head or neck.
- Histologically composed of islands of basaloid cells showing ductal differentiation. The tumour islands characteristically fit together like pieces of a jigsaw puzzle.

Poroma

- Benign skin adnexal tumour showing sweat gland differentiation.
- Presents as a solitary lesion with a wide distribution.
- Histologically composed of broad trabeculae of small epithelial cells growing down from the epidermis.

Syringoma

- Benign skin adnexal tumour showing sweat gland differentiation.
- Present as multiple small papules around the eyelids.
- Histologically composed of clusters of small ducts in the dermis with 'tadpole' shapes.

Basal cell carcinoma

Definition
- A group of malignant epidermal tumours composed of basaloid cells.

Epidemiology
- Very common tumours, accounting for 70% of all skin malignancies.
- Seen predominantly in fair-skinned adults with sun damage.

Aetiology
- Cumulative ultraviolet (UV) radiation exposure is the key risk factor.

Carcinogenesis
- Almost all show mutations in genes encoding proteins involved in the sonic hedgehog pathway, most commonly PTCH1.
- A smaller proportion display mutations in SMOOTHENED which encodes the protein normally inhibited by the PATCHED1 protein.

Presentation
- Most appear as pearly papules or nodules on sun-exposed skin. Ulceration may occur.
- Superficial variants present as persistent scaly/erythematous lesions.

Histopathology
- See Fig. 16.4.
- Tumour is composed of groups of basaloid epithelial cells with scanty cytoplasm. Cells at the edge of the groups typically line up in a palisade (peripheral palisading).
- Tumour stroma is typically loose and mucinous.
- Artefactual retraction spaces between tumour cells and stroma are often seen and can be a useful diagnostic feature.
- A number of morphological subtypes are recognized, including nodular, superficial, infiltrative, morphoeic, and micronodular.

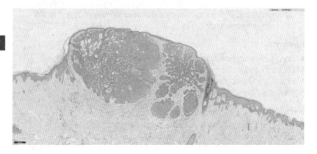

Fig. 16.4 Basal cell carcinoma, nodular subtype. Histology shows well circumscribed nests of basaloid epithelial cells with peripheral palisading and mucinous stroma (see Plate 62).

Prognosis
- Show locally invasive behaviour, but metastasis is extremely rare.
- Complete excision is usually curative.
- Recurrences are more common at high-risk sites (head and neck) and with certain morphological subtypes (infiltrative, morphoeic, micronodular).

Squamous cell carcinoma

Definition
- A malignant epidermal tumour showing squamous differentiation.

Epidemiology
- Common tumours accounting for ~15% of all skin malignancies.
- Most arise on sun-exposed skin of elderly fair-skinned adults.

Aetiology
- Most are related to cumulative UV radiation exposure.
- Immunosuppression increases the risk. Transplant recipients are particularly prone to developing multiple tumours.

Carcinogenesis
- Most arise from **actinic keratoses** which are dysplastic epidermal lesions arising on sun-damaged skin.
- UV radiation, particularly UVB, induces DNA damage in growth-controlling genes such as *KRAS* and *CDK4*.

Presentation
- Skin plaques or nodules, often with a keratinous surface crust.
- Ulceration may be present.

Histopathology
- Nests, sheets, and cords of atypical squamous epithelial cells are seen arising from the epidermis and infiltrating into the underlying dermis.
- Tumours are graded into well, moderately, or poorly differentiated, depending on the extent of keratinization and cytological atypia (higher grades being associated with less keratinization and more atypia).

Prognosis
- Most are only locally infiltrative at the time of diagnosis and cured by surgical excision.
- Risk factors for recurrence or metastasis include depth of invasion, poor differentiation, perineural invasion, narrow excision margins, and immunosuppression.

Merkel cell carcinoma

Definition
- Primary neuroendocrine carcinoma of the skin.

Epidemiology
- Rare tumour with annual incidence of <0.5 per 100 000.
- Mostly seen in older adults with a male predilection.

Aetiology
- 90% are associated with Merkel cell polyomavirus (MCV) infection.
- Chronic high UV exposure and immunosuppression are also associated.

Presentation
- Slowly growing tumour nodule on a sun-exposed site (head and neck 50%; extremities 40%).

Histopathology
- Basaloid 'small round blue cell tumour' centred on the dermis, often with subcutaneous and epidermal extension.
- Cells have scant cytoplasm with 'salt and pepper' chromatin pattern.
- Mitotic activity is abundant.
- Lymphovascular invasion is common.

Immunohistochemistry
- Tumour is positive for cytokeratin Cam5.2 and more specifically cytokeratin 20 which often stains in a paranuclear dot-like distribution.
- Neuroendocrine markers are positive (CD56, chromogranin, synaptophysin) as well as neurofilament.

Prognosis
- Highly aggressive tumour with local recurrence in 40%, regional lymph node metastasis in 55% and distant metastasis in 35%.
- Favourable prognostic features include tumour size <2 cm, location on the limbs, localized disease, younger age, and female sex.

Malignant melanoma

Definition
- A malignant melanocytic tumour arising in the skin.

Terminology
- The vast majority grow initially within the epidermis only (**melanoma in situ**).
- Once a melanoma invades into the dermis (**invasive melanoma**) it acquires metastatic potential.

Epidemiology
- Less common than basal or squamous cell carcinomas of the skin but increasing in frequency and much more often fatal.
- Seen predominantly in fair-skinned individuals with sun exposure.

Aetiology
- UV radiation exposure is the major risk factor.
- An element of genetic susceptibility may also be relevant.

Genetics
- *BRAF* mutations are very common (70%) in melanomas arising in non-chronically sun-damaged skin.
- *KIT* mutations are seen in about 30% of melanomas arising in chronically sun-damaged skin.

Presentation
- Most melanomas present as pigmented skin lesions demonstrating **A**symmetry, irregular **B**orders, uneven **C**olour, and **D**iameter >6 mm (the 'ABCD' acronym).

Histopathology
- **Superficial spreading melanoma** shows a proliferation of atypical melanocytes as single cells and nests within the epidermis with abundant upward spread within the epidermis (pagetoid spread). With invasion, atypical melanocytes are also present in the dermis.
- **Lentigo maligna melanoma** shows a proliferation of single atypical melanocytes in the basal epidermis with extension along adnexal structures. With invasion, atypical melanocytes are also present in the dermis.
- **Nodular melanoma** is composed predominantly of an invasive dermal nodule with only a small overlying epidermal component.
- **Acral lentiginous melanoma** occurs mostly on the foot and shows a proliferation of single and nested atypical melanocytes in the basal epidermis. With invasion, atypical melanocytes are also present in the dermis.
- For all invasive melanomas an important histological measurement is the **Breslow thickness** which is measured from the deepest invasive melanoma cell to the top of overlying granular layer of the epidermis (Fig. 16.5).

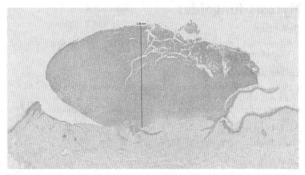

Fig. 16.5 Melanoma Breslow thickness (see Plate 63).

Prognosis

- Invasive melanomas have capacity for extensive metastatic spread to lymph nodes and visceral sites such as lungs, liver, and brain.
- Survival is related to the stage of the disease at diagnosis.
- Key determinants of stage are the Breslow thickness (the thicker the Breslow the higher the stage and the worse the prognosis) and the presence of ulceration.

Mycosis fungoides

Definition

- A low-grade T-cell lymphoma of variably epidermotropic skin-homing T-lymphocytes.

Epidemiology

- Most common form of primary cutaneous lymphoma, but overall an uncommon disease, affecting 0.3 per 100 000 people annually.
- Usually a disease of adulthood but occasionally affects children.

Aetiology

- Unknown.

Genetics

- Disease progression is associated with chromosomal aberrations, particularly involving chromosomes 8 and 17.

Presentation

- Sequential appearance of patches, plaques, and tumours on non-sun-exposed skin (particularly around the buttocks and trunk).
- Patches are multiple large (>10 mm), flat, erythematous, scaly lesions.
- Plaques are elevated lesions arising either within patches or *de novo*.
- Nodules are large exophytic tumour masses.
- Sometimes the disease presents with erythroderma.
- Bone marrow, lymph nodes, and visceral organs may be involved in advanced disease.

Histopathology

- Patch stage shows a mild upper dermal T-cell infiltrate associated with variable epidermotropism. Early disease is often difficult to diagnose as the features overlap with a number of inflammatory conditions.
- Plaque stage shows a more prominent and band-like infiltrate of T-cells with more epidermotropism. Collections of neoplastic lymphocytes within the epidermis may be seen (Pautrier microabscesses). Nuclear atypia of the lymphocytes is more appreciable.
- Tumour stage shows a more diffuse dermal infiltrate which may extend into subcutaneous fat. Epidermotropism may be lost.

Immunophenotype

- Most cases show a T-helper cell phenotype, i.e. CD3+ CD4+ CD8–.

Prognosis

- Risk of progression and death correlates with the stage of disease at presentation.
- 10 year survival rates are high (85-95%) in patch and plaque stage disease, dropping to 40% in tumour stage, and to 20% if there is nodal involvement.

Dermatofibrosarcoma protuberans

Definition
- A superficially located low-grade fibroblastic sarcoma.

Acronym
- DFSP.

Epidemiology
- Rare tumour.
- Most commonly arises in young adults.

Aetiology
- Unknown.

Genetics
- Translocation t(17;22) juxtaposes the *COL1A1* and *PDGFB* genes, resulting in overexpression of PDGFB and autocrine stimulation of tumour cell growth.

Presentation
- Slowly growing plaque with nodules.
- Trunk and proximal extremities most common sites.

Histopathology
- Tumour filling the dermis and extending into subcutaneous fat with a characteristic 'honeycomb pattern'.
- Storiform grown pattern.
- Tumour cells are uniform and spindled with only mild cytological atypia and low mitotic activity.

Immunohistochemistry
- CD34 diffusely positive.
- S100, cytokeratin, desmin negative.

Prognosis
- Locally aggressive growth, often with repeated local recurrences.
- Metastatic behaviour is extremely rare (<0.5%).

Fibrosarcomatous DFSP
A small proportion of DFSPs progress to fibrosarcomatous DFSP (FS-DFSP), in which there is transition into areas where the cells become arranged in cellular 'herringbone' fascicles with more atypia and higher mitotic activity. CD34 expression may be lost in the fibrosarcomatous areas and there is increased p53 expression. FS-DFSP shows a higher risk (10–15%) of metastatic spread.

Atypical fibroxanthoma

Definition

- Low-grade mesenchymal neoplasm of the dermis showing no specific line of differentiation.

Acronym

- AFX.

Epidemiology

- Common tumour seen mostly on chronically sun-damaged skin of elderly individuals.

Aetiology

- Related to UV exposure.
- Immunosuppression may increase the risk.

Presentation

- Rapidly growing exophytic skin tumour, often ulcerated.

Histopathology

- Dermal-based proliferation of highly atypical spindled and/or polygonal cells.
- Abundant mitotic activity.
- Often ulcerated on the surface.

Immunohistochemistry

- This is essential to exclude other malignant tumours that can appear similar.
- Negative for all major lineage markers i.e. keratins, melanocytic, muscle, vascular.
- Usually positive for CD10 though this is not specific for AFX.

Prognosis

- Low rate of local recurrence (<10%).
- Metastatic behaviour is extremely rare.

Pleomorphic dermal sarcoma

This tumour shows identical morphological and immunohistochemical findings as atypical fibroxanthoma but in addition also shows any one of the following: subcutaneous extension or deeper; necrosis; vascular invasion. This tumour is associated with a higher risk of local recurrence (30%) and metastasis (10-20%).

Bone, joint, and soft tissue pathology

Osteoporosis

Definition
- A metabolic bone disease characterized by a generalized reduction in bone density (osteopenia), increased bone fragility and predisposition to fracture.

Epidemiology
- Very common.
- Typically presents in post-menopausal women, though people of all ages may have clinically silent disease.

Aetiology
- Primary: either post-menopausal or age-related (>70 years).
- Secondary: a wide variety of causes, including numerous endocrine diseases (Cushing's syndrome, hyperparathyroidism, hyperthyroidism, hypogonadism), certain chronic diseases (including coeliac disease, inflammatory bowel disease, thalassaemia major), drugs (particularly glucocorticoids), alcohol and poor nutrition.

Pathogenesis
- Bone density in later life is determined by the peak bone density attained in early adulthood and the subsequent rate of bone loss.
- Peak bone density is largely genetically determined but is modified by factors such as nutrition, physical activity and health early in life.
- Bone loss occurs in both women and men with increasing age due to decreasing bone turnover, decreasing physical activity, reduced sex hormones and reduced calcium absorption from the gut.
- In women, post-menopausal oestrogen deficiency markedly accelerates bone loss.
- Glucocorticoids decrease osteoblastic activity and lifespan, reduce calcium absorption from the gut and increase renal calcium loss. Sex hormone production is also suppressed which increases bone turnover and loss.
- There is no biochemical change in osteomalacia, hence the mineral to osteoid ratio is normal.

Presentation
- Most cases are clinically silent until fragility fractures occur.
- Classic sites of fracture include vertebrae (can be spontaneous and leads to loss of height and kyphosis), distal radius (Colles' fracture) and neck of femur following a fall.

Histopathology
See Fig. 17.1.
- Cancellous bone is thinned with disconnectivity of bony trabeculae.
- Cortical bone is thinned with enlargement of Haversian canals.

Prognosis
- Absorptiometry (DEXA) scans can reliably quantify bone density enabling risk of fracture to be estimated.

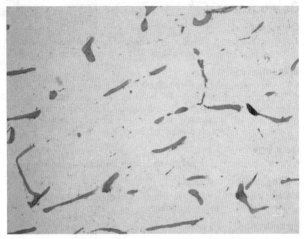

Fig. 17.1 Osteoporosis characterized by thin, disconnected trabeculae of lamellar bone within fatty marrow (see Plate 64).

- Neck of femur fractures require hospital admission and surgical fixation: elderly patients with coexisting medical problems have a significantly increased risk of mortality in the year following a neck of femur fracture.

Osteopetrosis

Definition
- A group of hereditary diseases characterized by dense bones ('marble bone disease') due to failure of osteoclasts to resorb bone adequately.

Epidemiology
- The estimated prevalence is 1 in 100 000–500 000.
- Two major groups presenting in early childhood: autosomal recessive (more severe, affecting children) and autosomal dominant (more frequent); there is also a less common intermediate autosomal dominant osteopetrosis presenting later in life.

Aetiology
- At least ten mutated genes have been implicated in its development.

Pathogenesis
- Mutations interfere either with osteoclast formation or osteoclast function, resulting in dense, brittle bone.

Presentation
- Individuals may be asymptomatic or experience severe symptoms, including visual impairment, stunted growth, and bone marrow failure.
- The most common clinical manifestation is increased fragility of bone, leading to fractures.
- Radiographs show an abnormally high bone density.

Histopathology
See Fig. 17.2.
- If the genetic alteration results in osteoclast formation, very few osteoclasts are present.
- If the genetic alteration results in osteoclast function, abundant and very large osteoclasts are present, but there is little evidence of osteoclast resorption (Howship's lacunae).
- Foci of intra-trabecular hyaline cartilage representing persistent primary spongiosa.

Prognosis
- If severe, there is a high postnatal mortality.
- The only known cure for the infantile malignant form is allogeneic haematopoietic stem cell transplant.

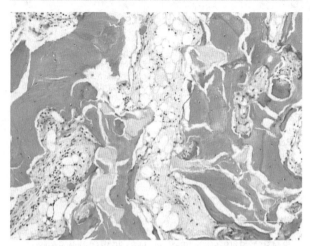

Fig. 17.2 Osteopetrosis is characterized by a distorted bony architecture, with thick trabecular and compact bone largely obliterating the bone marrow space (see Plate 65).

Osteomalacia and rickets

Definition

- Osteomalacia: a metabolic bone disease characterized by softening of bone due inadequate mineralization the mature skeleton.
- Rickets represents the same disease in infants, where there is also inadequate mineralization of the epiphyseal cartilage in the growing skeleton of children.

Epidemiology

- Very common, although true incidence likely underestimated. Reports suggest histological evidence of osteomalacia is present in approximately 25% of European adults.
- Increased risk is largely attributable to low UV-light exposure (e.g. care home residents, wearers of full-body clothing).
- Osteomalacia is becoming more common due to greater public awareness of the link between UV-exposure and skin cancer.

Aetiology

- Almost all cases are due to calcium deficiency which occurs secondary to decreased production (most common cause), decreased absorption, or altered metabolism of vitamin D.
- Decreased vitamin D production is seen in populations with low exposure to UV-light.
- Defective absorption of vitamin D (a fat soluble vitamin) by the small intestine, as seen in Crohn's disease, cystic fibrosis, coeliac disease, and patients with a history of gastrointestinal surgery, can also result in osteomalacia, as can severe nutritional deficiency.
- Altered vitamin D metabolism can be seen in chronic liver disease, chronic kidney disease, and nephrotic syndrome.
- Vitamin D resistance can result in hypophosphataemic rickets, characterized by low serum phosphate levels and resistance to treatment with UV radiation and vitamin D, mainly caused by genetic defects involving renal absorption of phosphate.
- Tumour-induced osteomalacia: mesenchymal tumours secreting fibroblast growth factor (FGF)-23.

Pathogenesis

- Inadequate mineralization of bone matrix (osteoid) due to lack of calcium and, much less commonly, phosphate.
- Bones become abnormally soft and prone to deformity and fracture.
- In children, the soft bone formed at the epiphyseal plate results in skeletal deformity (bowing of the legs) and short stature.

Presentation

- Osteomalacia is often asymptomatic until fracture occurs, although some patients will experience diffuse bone pain and muscle weakness.
- Children with Rickets may present with stunted growth, bowed legs, bone pain, and increased head circumference.
- Radiographs may show an osteoporotic-type pattern with evidence of demineralization: multiple stress factors commonly seen.

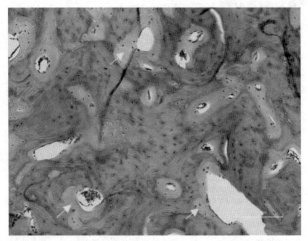

Fig. 17.3 Osteomalacia, as seen in compact bone, showing mature viable bone covered by a thick layer of unmineralized matrix (osteoid)—pale pink (arrows). Similar features are seen in rickets (see Plate 66).

Histopathology

See Fig. 17.3.
- Bony trabeculae are covered by an excessively thick layer of unmineralized osteoid.
- Bone biopsies must not be decalcified if mineralization is to be assessed.

Prognosis

- Vitamin D supplementation usually results in rapid mineralization of bone and resolution of symptoms, though some deformity may remain.
- Failure to respond requires exclusion of vitamin D-resistant rickets.

Paget's disease

Definition

- A localized bone remodelling disease characterized by excessive, chaotic, bone turnover.
- Disease can arise in a single bone (monostotic) or multiple bones (polyostotic): common sites include the skull, pelvis, femur, and vertebrae.
- Originally described by Sir James Paget, an English surgeon and pathologist, in 1877.

Epidemiology

- Second commonest metabolic bone disease after osteoporosis.
- Marked geographic variation, being particularly common in the England (where it is thought to have originated) and Scotland, although incidence appears to be reducing.
- Rare in Scandinavia and many African and Asians populations.
- Seen mostly in older adults (>50 years); slightly more frequent in men.
- Presentation in the young is usually associated with germline alterations (familial Paget's disease).

Aetiology

- Genetic and environmental factors have been implicated.
- Genome wide association studies have identified predisposing polymorphisms in a number of genes involved in the RANK-NFkappaB signalling pathway.
- A proportion of familial cases are associated with mutations in the sequestosome 1 (SQSTM1) gene, transmitted in an autosomal dominant pattern.
- Potential environmental factors include mechanical loading, dietary calcium, and exposure to toxins.
- 'Inclusions' identified on electron microscopy in Pagetic osteoclasts has implicated, a paramyxoviral aetiology, although this is controversial and unproven.

Pathogenesis

- The disease passes through a number of stages, all of which may be seen simultaneously within the same bone or in different bones.
- Initially, there is intense osteoclastic bone resorption.
- Osteoblastic activity then becomes exaggerated with laying down of grossly thickened, poorly organized weak bone which is prone to deformity and pathological fracture.

Presentation

- The vast majority of patients are asymptomatic, the diagnosis being made incidentally on radiology.
- Symptomatic disease usually presents with bony pain and deformity.
- Biochemical studies reveal raised serum alkaline phosphatase with normal calcium levels.
- Radiographic features depend on the phase of the disease.

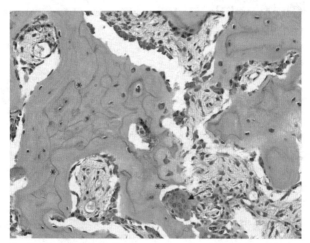

Fig. 17.4 Paget's disease. Diffuse remodelled cancellous bone with prominent cement lines* and deep Howship's lacunae** which, in areas, are associated with osteoclasts, containing very large numbers of nuclei (arrow) (see Plate 67).

Histopathology

See Fig. 17.4.
- Bony trabeculae are thickened with a 'mosaic' pattern of cement lines indicating repetitive phases of bone resorption and formation.
- Striking numbers of osteoclasts with more nuclei than normal.
- Cortical Haversian canals are replaced by irregular trabeculae.
- The bone marrow becomes densely fibrotic.

Prognosis

- Most patients do not suffer from any significant problems.
- Potential complications include pathological fractures and deafness due to compression of cranial nerve VIII by enlarging skull bones.

! Secondary osteosarcoma is the most significant complication of Paget's disease. Although it only occurs in <1% of cases, it has a very poor prognosis. Osteosarcoma should be considered in any patient known to have Paget's disease if their bony pain rapidly worsens.

Osteomyelitis

Definition

- Infection in a bone.

Epidemiology

- May develop at any age.
- At risk groups include smokers, patients with various chronic diseases that impair circulation (including diabetes and sickle-cell disease), immunosuppressed patients (e.g. patients receiving systemic cancer therapies) and intravenous drug users.Aetiology
- Haematogenous spread from a distant infection focus (e.g. pneumonia).
- Penetrating trauma (e.g. open fracture).
- Iatrogenic (e.g. following joint replacement or root canal treatment).
- Direct spread from an adjacent infection (e.g. a foot ulcer in a diabetic patient).
- The vast majority of chronic infections result from unresolved acute osteomyelitis.

Pathogenesis

- Infective agent can be bacterial (including mycobacterial) or fungal: *Staphylococcus aureus*
- Is the commonest isolated organism; anaerobes and Gram-negative bacteria, including Pseudomonas aeruginosa, are also common.
- Sickle-cell disease increases susceptibility to *Salmonella* osteomyelitis.
- Infection leads to an influx of acute inflammatory cells into the bone; subsequent destruction of bone leads to necrotic bone known as sequestrum.
- Failure to eradicate infection may lead to chronic osteomyelitis with areas of infected necrotic bone surrounded by areas of new bone formation (involucrum).Presentation
- Fever and pain in the affected bone, sometimes with overlying warmth and redness of skin.
- Children may present with failure to weight-bear: preferential involvement of proximal/distal portions of long bones in a paediatric population.
- Cultures may be negative in chronic infections due to low levels of causative organisms.

Histopathology

- Infiltration of bone by neutrophil-rich inflammatory infiltrate with bone necrosis and reactive bone formation.
- Granulomatous component often seen in mycobacterial osteomyelitis.
- Plasma cell and xanthogranulomatous variants exist.

Prognosis
- Aggressive treatment with intravenous antibiotics and surgical debridement of any necrotic bone required if cure is to be achieved.
- Development of osteomyelitis following joint replacement may lead to failure of the prosthesis (periprosthetic reactions; ➲ Periprosthetic reactions, p. 531).
- Chronic sinus formation may occur carrying a risk of associated squamous carcinoma (Marjolin's ulcer).
- AA amyloidosis may occur as with other chronic infections.

Osteoarthritis

Definition

- A group of diseases characterized by joint degeneration.

Epidemiology

- The most common joint disease.
- About 2 million people in the UK have symptomatic disease.
- Predominantly a disease of the elderly.

Aetiology

- Primary osteoarthritis: most common, with no clear cause.
- Secondary osteoarthritis: brought about by conditions causing damage to joints (e.g. rheumatoid arthritis (RA), gout, trauma).

Pathogenesis

- Insult to joint tissue (not always understood) initiating a cycle of cellular events, including low-grade chronic inflammation of the synovium, release of metalloproteinases and degradation of articular cartilage matrix (fibrillation, erosion and cracking, and exposure eventually of bone (eburnation)).

Presentation

- Joint pain, tenderness, swelling (seen in small joints), stiffness.
- Symptoms typically worsen during the day with activity.
- Principally affects the hip, knee, spine, and small joints of the hands.

Histopathology

See Fig. 17.5.

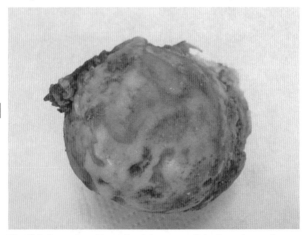

Fig. 17.5 Osteoarthritis. Femoral head shows an eroded and irregular articular surface (see Plate 68).

- Articular cartilage is thinned and lost.
- Subchondral bone is exposed and thickened.
- Subchondral cysts may be present.
- Osteophytes can occur at the periphery of the joint.

Prognosis

- The condition tends to progress with time and requires analgesics.
- Severe disease usually requires joint replacement.

Rheumatoid arthritis

Definition
- A multisystem autoimmune disease in which the brunt of disease activity falls upon synovial joints.

Epidemiology
- Common, affecting about 1% of people.
- Particularly affects young and middle-aged women.

Aetiology
- The initial trigger remains unknown.
- Once inflammation begins, it appears to become self-perpetuating.

Pathogenesis
- Infiltration of synovium by CD4+ T-cells, B-cells, plasma cells, and macrophages.

Presentation
- Symmetrical, swollen, painful, stiff, small joints of hands and feet.
- Symptoms are typically worse in the morning.

Serology
- ~70% of patients are positive for rheumatoid factor (RhF), an autoantibody which binds the Fc portion of IgG. RhF is often positive in other autoimmune diseases and some apparently healthy individuals.
- Newer antibodies, known as anti-citrullinated protein antibodies, have a much greater specificity, though they are not widely available.

Extra-articular manifestations
- Cardiac disease: ischaemic heart disease, pericarditis.
- Vascular disease: accelerated atherosclerosis, vasculitis.
- Haematological disease: anaemia, splenomegaly.
- Pulmonary disease: pulmonary fibrosis, pleuritis.
- Skin: rheumatoid nodules, erythema nodosum, pyoderma gangrenosum.
- Neurological: peripheral neuropathy, stroke.
- Deposition of serum amyloid A as β-pleated sheets in multiple organs (AA amyloidosis).

Histopathology
- Marked synovial hyperplasia with a heavy inflammatory infiltrate of lymphocytes, with germinal centre formation, and plasma cells, along with pannus formation over the articular cartilage (fibroblastic granulation tissue).

Prognosis
- The disease shows variable behaviour, but there have been considerable recent advances in the successful treatment of this disease (anti-TNF-α).

Spondyloarthropathies

Definition

- A group of inflammatory joint diseases characterized by arthritis affecting the spinal column and peripheral joints and enthesitis (inflammation at the insertion site of tendons and ligaments to bone).

Epidemiology

- Common diseases, affecting nearly 1% of people.
- Usually in young adults aged 20–40; slight male predominance.

Genetics

- Strong genetic association with possession of HLA-B27 allele.

Pathogenesis

- Traditional theories proposed that an unidentified 'arthritogenic peptide' is presented by HLA-B27 to CD8+ cytotoxic T-cells, leading to joint inflammation.
- Studies show that misfolded HLA-B27 causes endoplasmic reticulum stress and production of IL-23 via the T-helper 17 axis.

Ankylosing spondylitis

- Affects 0.5% of people, usually in young adults aged 20–40.
- Lower back pain due to sacroiliitis is the typical presentation.
- Extra-articular manifestations include iritis, pulmonary fibrosis, and aortitis.

Reactive arthritis

- Occurs within 1 month of an infection elsewhere in the body.
- Usually related to a genitourinary infection with *Chlamydia* or a gastrointestinal (GI) infection with *Shigella, Salmonella,* or *Campylobacter.*
- May be due to deposition of bacterial antigens and DNA in joints, but this has not been conclusively proven.
- Typically presents with pain and stiffness in the lower back, knees, ankles, and feet. Enthesitis is also common.

Psoriatic arthropathy

- Seen in about 5% of patients with psoriasis (→ Psoriasis, p. 479).
- Mostly affects the distal interphalangeal joints and may lead to severe deformation.

Enteropathic arthropathy

- Seen in about 10% of patients with inflammatory bowel disease.
- Typically affects sacroiliac and lower limb joints asymmetrically.
- Cause unknown.

Crystal arthropathies

Definition

- A group of joint diseases caused by deposition of crystals in joints.

Pathogenesis

- Crystals are deposited in joints.
- Neutrophils ingest the crystals and degranulate, releasing enzymes that damage the joint.

Gout

- Caused by deposition of monosodium urate crystals in a joint.
- Most cases are related to hyperuricaemia due to impaired excretion of urate by the kidneys.
- Acute gout causes an acute, painful, swollen, red joint. Any joint may be involved, but the first metatarsophalangeal joint is typical.
- Individuals with high urate levels may develop chronic tophaceous gout, in which large deposits of urate (tophi—chalky white material) occur in the skin and around joints (Fig. 17.6).

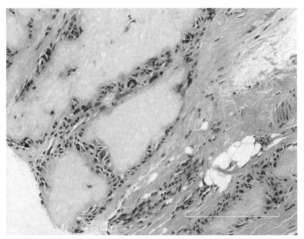

Fig. 17.6 Microscopic features of gout showing amorphous eosinophilic deposits surrounded by epithelioid macrophages and multinucleated giant cells.

Calcium pyrophosphate crystal deposition (CPPD) (pseudogout)

- Caused by deposition of calcium pyrophosphate crystals in a joint.
- Also referred to as chondrocalcinosis.
- Pyrophosphate is a by-product of the hydrolysis of nucleotide triphosphates within chondrocytes of cartilage.
- Shedding of crystals into a joint precipitates an acute arthritis which mimics gout.
- Typically elderly women; usually affects the knee, wrist, and vertebral joints.

Calcific tendinitis

- Caused by deposition of hydroxyapatite crystals in a tendon.
- The most common deposits appear as small granular aggregates within capsular and tendinous tissues without a cellular reaction.
- Macroscopically, deposits have a chalky white appearance; may be bulky or punctate.
- The largest deposits are seen in tumoural calcinosis.

Microscopy

- Joint fluid contains neutrophils and crystals.
- Urate crystals (gout): needle-shaped with negative birefringence.
- CPPD (pseudogout): rhomboid/rod-shaped with positive birefringence (Fig. 17.7).

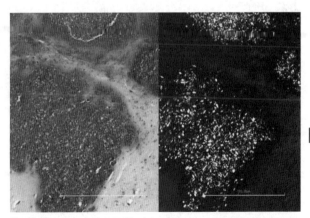

Fig. 17.7 Pseudogout. Rhomboid/rod-shaped crystals under polarized light showing positive birefringence (see Plate 69).

Septic arthritis

Definition
- Infection within a joint.

Epidemiology
- May occur at any age.
- Patients with pre-existing joint disease are at higher risk.

Acquisition of infection
- Infection is usually via haematogenous spread.
- Occasionally may follow penetrating trauma.

Microbiology
- Almost all cases are caused by *Staphylococcus aureus*.

Pathogenesis
- Establishment of infection is favoured by the relative inability of phagocytes to enter the joint space.
- Infection spreads quickly, leading to rapid and irreversible joint destruction if antibiotic treatment is not started early.

Presentation
- An extremely painful, hot, red, swollen joint.

Microscopy
- Joint fluid contains neutrophils but no crystals.

Culture
- Microbiological culture of joint fluid and blood is essential to identify the causative organism and provide antibiotic sensitivities.

Prognosis
- Irreversible joint destruction occurs without treatment.

Periprosthetic reactions

Definition

- Adverse biological reactions (local and systemic) caused by wear debris from prosthetic implants.

Epidemiology

- Mostly seen in total hip arthroplasties or hip resurfacing procedures but can be seen in knee or vertebral disc arthroplasties.
- Affects mainly metal-on-metal (MoM) prosthesis, but also in prosthesis manufactured from other materials (polyethylene, ceramic).

Pathogenesis

- Initiated as a foreign body-type response to wear debris (inflammatory mediators), and the presence of a lymphocytic infiltrate suggests a T-lymphocyte-mediated immune reaction.

Presentation

- Adverse tissue reactions may be systemic or local.
- Local: painful inflammatory synovitis, large joint effusions, osteomyelitis, pseudotumours, and periprosthetic osteolysis with prosthesis loosening.
- Systemic: toxicity due to elevated levels of metal particles and ions.

Histopathology

- Metallosis: stromal deposition of phagocytosed black particulate material, and amorphous intracytoplasmic brown debris (the latter are found in association with MoM prosthesis).
- Necrosis and pseudotumours (granulomatous or destructive cystic lesion, neither infective nor neoplastic).
- Variability in the number, type, and arrangement of inflammatory cells. May show massive synovial surface ulceration and fibrin, synovial hyperplasia, and the presence of thick areas of fibrosis.
- The presence of neutrophil polymorphs suggests an active infection.
- ALVAL score (aseptic lymphocytic vasculitis-associated lesion seen in MoM prosthesis) used for assessment and circulating metal ions.

Prognosis

- Irreversible joint destruction occurs without treatment.

Soft tissue and bone tumours

Primary soft tissue and bone tumours are derived from mesenchymal cells and, therefore, may show various lines of cellular differentiation (e.g. adipocytic, fibroblastic/myofibroblastic, smooth muscle, skeletal muscle, endothelial/vascular, peripheral nerve sheath, osteoblastic, chondroblastic), although in a subset of tumours the line of differentiation/cell of origin remains unknown (e.g. synovial sarcoma).

The overwhelming majority of primary soft tissue and bone tumours are benign. Malignant mesenchymal tumours (sarcomas) are extremely rare and make up <1% of all malignant tumour types in adults (carcinomas and haematological malignancies, by comparison, account of approximately 85% and 15%, respectively). A subset of mesenchymal tumours do not fit neatly into the traditional benign/malignant dichotomy, and may exhibit locally aggressive behaviour but lack metastatic potential or, alternatively, may present a very low risk of metastasis. The World Health Organization categorizes such lesions as 'intermediate' tumours.

The age of the patient along with the anatomical location and size of the tumour are critical considerations when diagnosing tumours of the soft tissues and bone. For example, lipoblastoma occurs exclusively in infants and children whereas well differentiated liposarcoma, on the other hand, almost never occurs in this age group and instead arises in older adults. The vast majority of benign mesenchymal tumours are small and arise in superficial soft tissue (i.e. subcutaneous fat); on the other hand, if a tumour is large and involves the deep soft tissues it is more likely to represent a malignant process. Furthermore, the radiographic appearances of bone tumours in particular forms a critical element of the diagnostic process.

Unlike carcinomas, which typically arise from dysplastic precursor lesions (or 'carcinoma in situ'), xt sarcomas arise 'de novo'. Another notable difference between carcinomas and sarcomas concerns their pattern of spread: while carcinomas typically first metastasize to lymph nodes, it is uncommon for sarcomas to spread via this route; instead, sarcomas usually spread haematogenously and preferentially metastasize to the lungs.

Management of sarcomas without metastatic disease is primarily surgical. Advancements in treatments for metastatic disease have been slow and, overall, approximately 1/3 of patients diagnosed with sarcoma will die from their disease. In recent years molecular genomics has improved our understanding of some sarcoma types and improved diagnostic accuracy; in the future, this will hopefully lead to more effective targeted therapies in at least a proportion of sarcoma subtypes.

Benign soft tissue tumours

Fibroblastic and myofibroblastic tumours

Fibroma of tendon sheath
- **Definition:** Rare benign fibroblastic/myofibroblastic tumour attached to a tendon.
- **Clinical features:** Slow-growing, small nodule arising on a finger tendon. Seen in young and middle-aged adults, with a male preponderance.
- **Gross pathology:** Well-circumscribed, lobular fibrous appearance, firm to palpation.
- **Histopathology:** Well-circumscribed tumour composed of cytologically bland fibroblasts and thin, slit-like blood vessels in a fibrous stroma.
- **Immunohistochemistry:** Positive for smooth muscle actin (SMA).
- **Molecular Genetics:** A translocation t(2;11)(q31;q12) has been reported.
- **Prognosis:** Benign, can occasionally recur.

Fibrous hamartoma of infancy
- **Definition:** Benign soft tissue tumour occurring in newborns and infants.
- **Clinical features:** Rapidly growing, usually solitary; typical sites include trunk and proximal extremities (axilla/groin). Majority occur in first 2 years with a marked male predominance.
- **Histopathology:** Histology shows a triphasic tumour including adipose tissue, bundles of (myo)fibroblastic cells and nodules of primitive mesenchymal cells within a myxoid matrix.
- **Immunohistochemistry:** Myofibroblastic cells are SMA-positive. CD34 expressed by the primitive mesenchymal cells.
- **Molecular genetics:** EGFR exon 20 insertion/duplication mutations are common.
- **Prognosis:** Benign, although occasional cases recur if incompletely excised.

Nodular fasciitis
- **Definition:** A self-limiting, rapidly growing fibroblastic/myofibroblastic tumour. Variants and closely related so-called pseudosarcomatous lesions include intravascular fasciitis, cranial fasciitis, proliferative fasciitis/myositis, ossifying fasciitis, myositis ossificans and fibro-osseous pseudotumour of the digits.
- **Clinical features:** Presents as a rapidly growing lesion, usually over the course of weeks or a few months, in superficial soft tissue. Common sites include upper limb, trunk and head & neck. A history of previous trauma is occasionally reported. Can occur at any age, but often young adults. No gender predilection.
- **Gross pathology:** Almost always <4 cm. Usually arises on the superficial surface of fascia, extending into overlying subcutaneous fat.
- **Histopathology:** See Fig. 17.8. Histological features depend in part on the growth phase, but typically there is a (myo)fibroblastic proliferation with a so-called tissue culture appearance, associated with a myxoid to

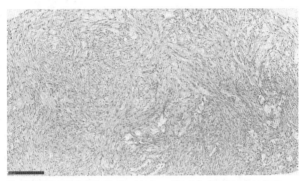

Fig. 17.8 Nodular fasciitis. Myofibroblastic proliferation with a "tissue culture" appearance (see Plate 70).

collagenous stroma, microcystic change, and extravasated erythrocytes. Can be mitotically active, but no atypical mitotic figures are seen.

- **Immunohistochemistry:** SMA positive.
- **Molecular genetics:** Rearrangements of the *USP6* at locus 17p13.2 can be found in >90% of nodular fasciitis cases; the most frequent partner gene is *MYH9*. *USP6* rearrangements are also found in the closely related variants listed above (and also aneurysmal bone cyst).
- **Prognosis:** No malignant potential.

Nuchal-type fibroma

- **Definition:** Benign collagenous lesion; significant histological overlap with Gardner fibroma (a collagenous lesion associated with Familial Adenomatous Polyposis).
- **Clinical** features: Majority of cases occur in the subcutaneous fat of the posterior neck (Gardner fibroma has no such anatomical predilection). Typically adult males. Approximately 50% of patients have diabetes mellitus.
- **Gross pathology:** Small, ill-defined fibrous-appearing lesion.
- **Histopathology:** Ill-defined, paucicellular tumour comprising haphazardly arranged, thick collagen bundles which tend to entrap fat.
- **Immunohistochemistry:** Most cases express CD34.
- **Prognosis:** No malignant potential.

Fibrohistiocytic tumours

Tenosynovial giant cell tumour (TSGCT)

- **Definition:** Benign tumour arising from the synovium of tendon sheaths, joints, and bursa. Classified by site (intra- or extra-articular) and growth pattern (localized and diffuse; diffuse type previously known as pigmented villonodular synovitis, PVNS).
- **Clinical features:** Presents as a painless, slowly growing nodule. Peak age at presentation 20-40 years with a female preponderance.

Localized-type TSGCT is more common and typically occurs in the hands; diffuse-type TSGCT is rarer and arises in the vicinity of larger joints (classically the knee).

- **Gross pathology:** Localized-type is small and well-circumscribed. Diffuse type is larger and a villous appearance may be evidence in intraarticular lesions.
- **Histopathology:** See Fig. 17.9. Both types show a proliferation of round to ovoid mononuclear cells associated with osteoclast-like multinucleated cells and both foamy and haemosiderin-laden macrophages. Localized-type TSGCTs are multinodular and well-circumscribed; diffuse-type TSGCTs have a sheet-like architecture and infiltrative outlines.
- **Molecular genetics:** A proportion of cases demonstrate a *COL6A3–CSF1* fusion, resulting in overproduction of CSF1, a critical growth factor in osteoclast formation.
- **Prognosis:** Localized-type is associated with little morbidity, while diffuse-type TSGCTs are usually locally aggressive with a high recurrence rate.

Lipomatous tumours

Lipoma

- **Definition:** A tumour of mature white fat; commonest mesenchymal neoplasm in humans.
- **Clinical features:** Typically present as a solitary, <5 cm painless subcutaneous mass in adults; can affect virtually any site. Deep soft tissues of the limbs can also be involved (i.e. intramuscular lipoma); these are usually larger than their superficial counterparts.
- **Gross pathology**: Well-circumscribed with a thin capsule and yellow-coloured cut surface.

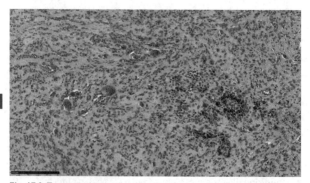

Fig. 17.9 Tenosynovial giant cell tumour. Mononuclear cells in a collagenous background associated with associated with osteoclast-like multinucleated cells and haemosiderin-laden macrophages (see Plate 71).

- **Histopathology:** See Fig. 17.10. Mature adipocytes of uniform size divided into lobules by thin fibrous septa. Secondary changes (e.g. fat necrosis, metaplastic bone formation) frequently seen. Intramuscular lipomas show infiltrative edges with entrapment of skeletal muscle fibres.
- **Prognosis:** Benign. Intramuscular lipomas may recur locally.

Angiolipoma
- **Definition:** Small, subcutaneous adipocytic tumour with capillary-sized vascular component.
- **Clinical features:** Presentation is usually in young adulthood with a male predominance. Lesions typically arise in the extremities, particularly the forearm. Unlike lipomas, angiolipomas are often painful and multiple. A small proportion of cases are familial (autosomal dominant).
- **Gross pathology**: Well-circumscribed, encapsulated tumours with yellow cut surface associated with red-coloured nodules corresponding to aggregates of vessels.
- **Histopathology:** Mature adipocytes with a prominent population of capillary-sized vessels, a proportion of which contain intraluminal microthrombi.
- **Prognosis:** Behaviour is entirely benign.

Spindle cell/pleomorphic lipoma
- **Definition:** Benign adipocytic tumour. Previously separated, spindle cell lipoma and pleomorphic lipoma are now considered to represent two points on a spectrum with shared clinical, morphological, and molecular findings.
- **Clinical features:** Classically presents as a painless subcutaneous mass of the posterior neck/upper back/shoulders ('shawl' distribution) in middle-aged males. Only 10% of cases are in females, where anatomical location is more varied.
- **Gross pathology:** Well-circumscribed tumours; cut surface varies from yellow to white/grey depending on relative proportions of adipocytic and spindle cell components. Some cases are extensively gelatinous, reflecting abundant myxoid stroma.

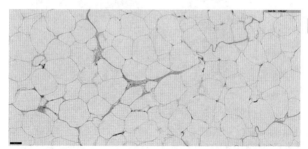

Fig. 17.10 Lipoma. Mature adipocytes with mild variation in size and no atypical stromal cells (see Plate 72).

- **Histopathology:** See Fig. 17.11. Well-circumscribed tumours comprising mature adipocytes and cytologically bland spindle cells set within a fibromyxoid stroma containing thick 'ropy' collagen bundles. The proportion of these individual components is highly variable. In addition, pleomorphic lipomas contain pleomorphic and multinucleated 'floret-like' giant cells.
- **Immunohistochemistry:** CD34 positive. There is loss of nuclear Rb1 expression.
- **Molecular genetics:** Consistent deletions in the long arm of chromosome 13, where the *Rb* gene resides (also seen in mammary-type myofibroblastoma and cellular angiofibroma, tumours which share overlapping morphological features with spindle cell lipoma).
- **Prognosis:** Benign behaviour.

Lipoblastoma/lipoblastomatosis
- **Definition:** Benign tumour of embryonal white fat; can be localized or diffuse (lipoblastomatosis).
- **Clinical features:** Virtually all cases occur in infancy or early childhood. Wide range of sites; extremities and trunk are commonest locations. Localized lipoblastoma usually occurs in superficial soft tissues while lipoblastomatosis typically involves deep soft tissues and may infiltrate around vital structures.
- **Gross pathology**: Variable size with a yellow to white cut surface. Localized lipoblastomas are well-circumscribed while lipoblastomatosis is often infiltrative.
- **Histopathology:** Lobules of adipocytes in various stages of maturation divided by fibrous septa; the more mature areas resemble conventional lipomas with only rare lipoblasts. Myxoid areas containing primitive mesenchymal cells with arborizing vessels are usually seen.
- **Molecular genetics:** *PLAG1* rearrangements (various partners) found in majority of cases.
- **Prognosis:** Benign; recurrences may occur if incompletely excised.

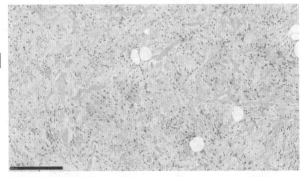

Fig. 17.11 Spindle cell lipoma. Bland spindle cells in a somewhat myxoid background associated with ropey collagen bundles. Occasional mature adipocytes in this example (see Plate 73).

Hibernoma
- **Definition:** Benign adipocytic tumour composed predominantly of brown (fetal) fat.
- **Clinical features:** Longstanding, slow-growing, painless mass in the subcutis of young adults. Metabolically active tumours, hence can be identified incidentally on FDG PET scans. A small proportion are associated with Multiple Endocrine Neoplasia type 1 (MEN1) syndrome.
- **Gross pathology**: Well-circumscribed, wide variation in size. Cut surface has a variable yellow to red/brown appearance, depending on proportions of mature and brown fat.
- **Histopathology:** Mixture of mature fat and brown fat, the latter being characterized by multivacuolated adipocytes with granular, variably eosinophilic cytoplasm and centrally placed nuclei.
- **Molecular genetics:** Rearrangements of the 11q13-21 region seen in most cases.
- **Prognosis:** Benign behaviour.

Peripheral nerve sheath tumours

Neurofibroma
- **Definition:** Commonest peripheral nerve sheath tumour, composed predominantly of Schwann cells. Multiple macroscopic subtypes (see below).
- **Clinical features:** Majority of cases are solitary and sporadic. Cutaneous tumours present as painless dermal masses. Deep soft tissue tumours may induce sensory or motor deficits. Plexiform variant is virtually pathognomonic of neurofibromatosis type 1 (NF1); multiple neurofibromas should also raise the possibility of NF1.
- **Gross pathology:** Macroscopic types include localized cutaneous, diffuse cutaneous, localized intraneural, plexiform intraneural, and diffuse soft tissue tumours. Intraneural forms appear as fusiform masses; the plexiform variant has a so-called bag of worms appearance.
- **Histopathology:** See Fig. 17.12. Relatively low cellularity lesions comprising bland Schwann cells, fibroblast-like cells, and perineural-cells

Fig. 17.12 Neurofibroma. Haphazardly arranged, cytologically-bland spindle cells in a variably collagenous and myxoid stroma (see Plate 74).

haphazardly arranged within a variably collagenous and myxoid stroma.
Scattered mast cells usually seen; occasional axons sometimes present.
Intraneural variants surround by a layer of perineurium. Cytologically
bland lesions although scattered single cells may show degenerative-
type nuclear atypia.
- **Immunohistochemistry:** S100 highlights the Schwann cell
  population; there is also 'finger-print' pattern staining with CD34.
- **Molecular genetics:** Inactivating mutations of one or both copies of
  the *NF1* gene found in both sporadic and NF1-related cases.
- **Prognosis:** Localized cutaneous form is consistently benign. Intraneural
  and plexiform neurofibromas may rarely transform to malignant
  peripheral nerve sheath tumour (MPNST) in the setting of NF1. The
  lifetime risk of MPNST in NF1 patients is approximately 10%.

Schwannoma
- **Definition:** A benign nerve sheath tumour showing Schwann cell
  differentiation.
- **Clinical features:** Slow-growing, painless soft tissue mass affecting
  wide range of ages and sites. Vast majority occur sporadically,
  although multiple schwannomas may be associated with underlying
  neurofibromatosis type 2 (NF2); multiple schwannomas not associated
  with NF2 can also occur (so-called schwannomatosis, which can be
  sporadic or familial).
- **Gross pathology:** Well-circumscribed and encapsulated tumours
  which arise from a nerve. Wide size variation. Cut surface often cystic
  and haemorrhagic in longstanding tumours.
- **Histopathology:** See Fig. 17.13. Encapsulated spindle cell tumour
  comprising cellular areas (Antoni A) alternating with hypocellular
  myxoid areas (Antoni B). Nuclear palisading (Verocay bodies) often
  seen, as are blood vessels with hyalinized walls. Degenerative-type
  atypia may be seen; often accompanied by other degenerative features
  including cystic change, calcification, hyalinization, haemorrhage/
  haemosiderin (so-called ancient schwannoma).
- **Immunohistochemistry:** Strong and diffuse S100 positivity.

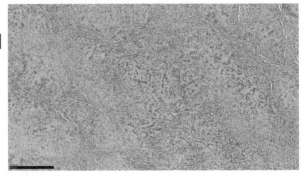

Fig. 17.13 Schwanomma. Nuclear palisading (Verocay bodies) in a schwanomma
(see Plate 75).

- **Molecular genetics:** Approximately 2/3 have inactivation of the *NF2* gene (both sporadic and NF2-related tumours). Familial cases of schwannomatosis harbour a germline *SMARCB1* mutation in approximately 1/3 of cases.
- **Prognosis:** Benign; virtually no potential for malignant transformation.

Perineurioma
- **Definition:** Rare, benign peripheral nerve sheath tumour composed entirely of perineurial cells.
- **Clinical features:** Usually seen in the subcutaneous tissues on the extremities of adults.
- **Gross pathology:** Well-circumscribed and unencapsulated. Wide range of sizes.
- **Histopathology:** Unencapsulated but well-circumscribed spindle cell tumour, typically showing a storiform/whorled architectural pattern with variably collagenous and sometimes myxoid stroma. The spindle cells often have elongated bipolar cytoplasmic processes.
- **Immunohistochemistry:** EMA positive (intensity highly variable); GLUT1 is positive (but not specific) while Claudin-1 is specific but lacks sensitivity.
- **Prognosis:** Conventional form is benign. Malignant perineurioma is extremely rare.

Smooth muscle tumours

(Extra-uterine) leiomyoma
- **Definition:** Benign smooth muscle tumour.
- **Clinical features:** Slow-growing mass in adults. Sites include retroperitoneum/abdomen/pelvis or, rarely, soft tissues of limbs; retroperitoneal/abdominal cases are much more common in females.
- **Gross pathology:** Circumscribed tumour with rubbery, whorled cut surface. Wide variation in size; may become very large.
- **Histopathology:** Paucicellular tumour comprising fascicles of spindle cells with uniform blunt ended ('cigar-shaped') nuclei and eosinophilic cytoplasm, resembling normal smooth muscle cells. Tumours in somatic soft tissue show virtually no mitotic activity; rare mitoses (in the absence of other atypical features) may be seen in retroperitoneal/abdominal/pelvic leiomyomas in females.
- **Immunohistochemistry:** SMA, desmin, and h-caldesmon positive. Retroperitoneal/abdominal cases are oestrogen receptor positive.
- **Prognosis:** Benign with no malignant potential.

Pericytic (perivascular) tumours

Angioleiomyoma
- **Definition:** Benign perivascular smooth muscle tumour.
- **Clinical features:** Small, often painful, and slowly growing tumours arising in subcutaneous fat or dermis; more common in women with a predilection for the lower extremities.
- **Gross pathology:** Well-circumscribed and small (<3 cm).
- **Histopathology:** See Fig. 17.14. Well-circumscribed lesion composed of spindle cells with smooth muscle morphological features (including

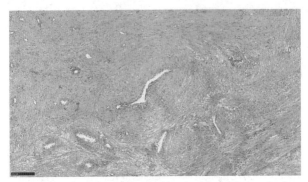

Fig. 17.14 Angioleiomyoma. Spindle cells with eosinophilic cytoplasm asociated with a population of muscularised blood vessels (see Plate 76).

eosinophilic cytoplasm and 'cigar-shaped' nuclei) associated with a population of muscularized blood vessels.
- **Immunohistochemistry:** Smooth muscle markers (SMA, desmin and h-caldesmon) positive.
- **Prognosis:** Benign, no predilection for malignant transformation.

Vascular tumours

Haemangiomas
- **Definition:** Benign neoplasms that usually containing well-formed vessels. Numerous histological subtypes, many of which are now thought to represent vascular malformations.
- **Clinical features:** Can arise in a wide variety of sites including skin, superficial, and deep soft tissues, bone, and viscera. Variable clinical manifestations which are largely site-dependent.
- **Gross pathology:** Often haemorrhagic. Vascular channels may be visible.
- **Histopathology:** Proliferation of vascular structures, the calibre and wall thicknesses of which depends on specific subtype. The vessels are lined by a single layer of cytologically bland endothelial cells. No/very rare mitotic figures.
- **Immunohistochemistry:** Endothelial cells express CD31, CD34, FLI1, and ERG.
- **Prognosis:** Benign, although may recur depending on site and histological subtype.

Arteriovenous malformation
- **Definition:** Vascular anomaly defined by the presence of arteriovenous shunts (i.e. interconnected venous and arterial channels without an intervening capillary bed). Mostly congenital although acquired forms also recognized.
- **Clinical features:** Most occur in the head and neck. Angiography studies required to confirm the presence of high-flow shunting. Severe cases can cause heart failure and/or a consumption coagulopathy

(Kasaback–Merritt syndrome). Congenital cases may not become clinically apparent until childhood or adolescence; acquired forms arise in young adults.
- **Gross Pathology:** Ill-defined lesions containing variably sized vessels.
- **Histopathology:** Proliferation of veins and large arteries in a fibrotic stroma. Capillary-rich areas may be seen. Thrombus formation is common. Shunts difficult to identify histologically.
- **Prognosis:** Benign, although may be difficult to resect hence recurrences are common.

Tumours of uncertain differentiation

Intramuscular myxoma
- **Definition:** Benign, painless, deep-seated tumour characterized by abundant myxoid matrix.
- **Clinical features:** Predominantly affects middle-aged females with a predilection for muscles of the thigh. Most are isolated lesions; some occur as part of Mazabraud syndrome (intramuscular myxoma and fibrous dysplasia).
- **Gross pathology:** Well-circumscribed tumour with a lobulated and gelatinous cut surface. Can reach large sizes.
- **Histopathology:** A sparsely cellular tumour composed of bland stellate to spindle cells embedded in an abundant myxoid stroma. No cytological atypia. Despite appearing well-circumscribed grossly, microscopic examination shows entrapment of skeletal muscle fibres.
- **Molecular genetics:** The majority harbour activating mutations in *GNAS*.
- **Prognosis:** Benign, no propensity for malignant transformation.

Intermediate soft tissue tumours

Fibroblastic and myofibroblastic tumours

Superficial (palmar/plantar) fibromatosis

- **Definition:** Benign fibroblastic/myofibroblastic proliferation typically arising within palmar or plantar aponeuroses. Classified as a 'locally aggressive' tumour by the WHO.
- **Clinical features:** Presents as a small (<3 cm) nodule in middle-aged patients occurring on: volar aspect of hands/digits (palmer fibromatosis/Dupuytren's contracture); plantar aponeuroses (plantar fibromatosis/Ledderhose's disease); dorsal aspect of proximal interphalangeal joints (knuckle/Garrod pads); penile shaft (penile fibromatosis/Peyronie's disease).
- **Gross pathology:** Poorly defined fibrous lesion associated with tendon or aponeurosis.
- **Histopathology:** See Fig. 17.15. Nodules of fibroblastic spindle cells arranged into fascicles and attached to a thickened aponeurosis. Variably collagenous stroma. May be mitotically active and hypercellular during proliferative growth phase (particularly plantar variant).
- **Prognosis:** Significant risk of local recurrence but no potential for malignant transformation.

Deep (desmoid) fibromatosis

- **Definition:** Deep-seated, infiltrative, non-metastasizing (myo) fibroblastic tumour occurring across a wide range of ages. Classified as a 'locally aggressive' tumour by the WHO.
- **Clinical features:** May arise across multiple sites, including abdominal wall (classically young women during or soon after pregnancy, implying a possible hormonal element to tumour growth), extra-abdominal (head & neck, limbs, chest wall, back) and intra-abdominal (mesentery, pelvis, or retroperitoneum). Presenting symptoms may relate to compression of various anatomical structures. Wide range of sizes (up to 20 cm for intraabdominal type).

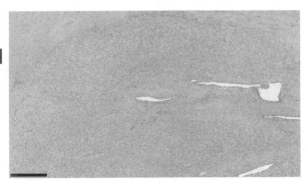

Fig. 17.15 Plantar fibromatosis. Sweeping fascicles in a collagenous background (see Plate 77).

- **Gross pathology:** Poorly circumscribed mass often with a whorled cut surface.
- **Histopathology:** Infiltrative tumour comprising long, sweeping fascicles of bland (myo)fibroblastic cells which entrap native skeletal muscle fibres. Mitotic activity is rare.
- **Immunohistochemistry:** Majority of cases show nuclear expression of beta-catenin (may be focal), reflecting dysregulation of the Wnt signalling pathway.
- **Molecular genetics:** Majority are sporadic and associated with somatic *CTNNB1* mutations; can also occur in Gardner syndrome, a subtype of familial adenomatous polyposis (caused by a germline *APC* gene mutation with an autosomal dominant inheritance pattern).
- **Prognosis:** No metastatic potential but high local recurrence rates. Depending on site, infiltration of vital structures can result in significant morbidity and rare deaths.

Solitary fibrous tumour
- **Definition:** Fibroblastic neoplasm classified within the group of 'rarely metastasizing tumours' by the WHO.
- **Clinical features:** Typically presents as a slow-growing mass in middle aged adults. Historically thought to represent a tumour of the pleura, most cases now recognized to arise at a range of extra-pleural sites including soft tissues and viscera.
- **Gross pathology:** Well-circumscribed tumours (5–10 cm) with tan-coloured cut surface.
- **Histopathology:** Haphazardly arranged fibroblastic cells (so-called patternless pattern) within a fibrous stroma. Dilated, branching, 'haemangiopericytoma-like' blood vessels (a nod to the tumour's previous name) are characteristically seen.
- **Immunohistochemistry:** Strong and diffuse nuclear STAT6 expression. CD34 also positive.
- **Molecular genetics:** Inversion at 12q13 leads to a pathogenic fusion transcript involving *NAB2–STAT6* (reflected in the immunohistochemical expression of STAT6 protein).
- **Prognosis:** Majority are indolent, but rare cases metastasize. Risk stratification models based on patient age, tumour size, mitotic activity and presence/absence of tumour necrosis exist.

Tumours of uncertain differentiation
Angiomatoid fibrous histiocytoma
- **Definition:** Rare soft tissue neoplasm of uncertain histogenesis, classified within the group of 'rarely metastasizing tumours' by the WHO.
- **Clinical features:** Slow-growing painless mass, usually arising in the subcutaneous fat with a predilection for sites rich in lymph nodes (e.g. inguinal region, axilla). Classically occurs in children and young adults; often associated with systemic symptoms (e.g. anaemia, fever).
- **Gross pathology:** Variably sized, well-circumscribed tumour resembling a lymph node or haematoma with a thick pseudocapsule. Cut surface often appears haemorrhagic.

- **Histopathology:** Solid areas of histiocytoid-like cells associated with haemorrhagic/pseudoangiomatoid spaces. There is a surrounding fibrous pseudocapsule rimmed by lymphocytes and plasma cells including germinal centres, simulating a lymph node.
- **Immunohistochemistry:** ~50% cases express EMA and desmin. ALK expression common.
- **Molecular genetics:** Commonest translocation is t(2;22)(q33;q12) resulting in an *EWSR1-CREB1* fusion. A smaller proportion of cases harbour a *EWSR1-ATF1* fusion.
- **Prognosis:** Local recurrence rate between 10–15%. Rare metastases reported.

Malignant soft tissue tumours

Fibroblastic and myofibroblastic tumours

Myxofibrosarcoma

- **Definition:** Malignant fibroblastic tumour with variable amounts of myxoid stroma: one of the most common sarcomas in elderly patients.
- **Clinical features:** Arises in middle-aged to elderly patients, presenting as a slow-growing, painless mass in the extremities, usually superficial to fascia.
- **Gross pathology:** Multinodular with gelatinous cut surface. Deceptively well-circumscribed.
- **Histopathology:** See Fig. 17.16. Variably cellular multinodular tumour with myxoid stroma containing pleomorphic tumour cells and curvilinear blood vessels. Despite often appearing well-circumscribed grossly, microscopic examination frequently reveals an extensively infiltrative growth pattern. Higher grade tumours contain solid areas with marked pleomorphism.
- **Immunohistochemistry/Molecular Genetics:** No characteristic profiles.
- **Prognosis:** High rate of repeated local recurrences, regardless of grade. High-grade tumours metastasize in approximately ¼ of cases (a lower rate than seen in other high-grade sarcomas).

Low-grade fibromyxoid sarcoma

- **Definition:** Rare malignant fibroblastic tumour, first described by Evans in 1987.
- **Clinical features:** Slow-growing mass within the soft tissues of the proximal extremities or trunk in young adults, slight male predilection.
- **Histopathology:** Biphasic collagenous and myxoid stroma, typically abrupt transition between the two. The neoplastic spindle cells have deceptively bland cytology with rare mitotic activity. Collagen rosettes found in a subset of cases. May overlap with sclerosing fibrosarcoma.
- **Immunohistochemistry:** MUC4 positive.

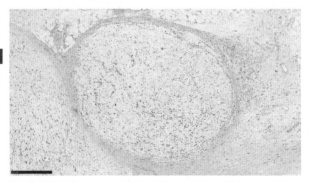

Fig. 17.16 Myxofibrosarcoma. Lobular architecture with myxoid stroma, curvilinear vessels and hyperchromatic tumour cells (see Plate 78).

- **Molecular genetics:** Consistent *FUS–CREB3L2* (or, less commonly, *FUS-CREB3L1*) gene fusions.
- **Prognosis:** Low rates of recurrence and metastases in first 5 years, but a significant proportion of cases recur or metastasize many years later.

Sclerosing epithelioid sarcoma
- **Definition:** Rare malignant fibroblastic tumour with a gene expression prolife overlapping with low-grade fibromyxoid sarcoma.
- **Clinical features:** Most commonly occurs in the soft tissues of the proximal extremities in middle-aged to elderly patients.
- **Histopathology:** Infiltrative tumour composed of (generally) cytologically bland epithelioid cells arranged in cords, set within a densely sclerotic and hyalinized stroma.
- **Immunohistochemistry:** MUC4 expressed in the majority of cases.
- **Molecular genetics:** Gene fusions consistently found, most frequently *EWSR1-CREB3L1*.
- **Prognosis:** More aggressive than related low-grade fibromyxoid sarcoma; metastatic disease occurs in approximately 50% of cases.

Adipocytic tumours
Atypical lipomatous tumour/well differentiated liposarcoma
- **Definition:** Synonymous terms for a group of locally aggressive adipocytic tumours without metastatic potential (unless dedifferentiation occurs—see next); the preferred diagnostic term depends on anatomical site (see below). Commonest liposarcoma subtype.
- **Clinical features:** Occurs in adults, typically middle-aged. Commonest sites include the deep soft tissue of proximal lower limbs and trunk; a significant number of cases arise in the retroperitoneum. Less common sites include spermatic cord, mediastinum and head & neck. Often very large at time of diagnosis (particularly in the retroperitoneum; frequently >20 cm).
- **Gross pathology**: Well-circumscribed and lobulated; yellow-coloured cut surface with variable amounts of white-grey areas.
- **Histopathology:** See Fig. 17.17. Most are 'lipoma-like', being composed of mature adipocytes which vary in size. Cytologically atypical hyperchromatic cells are seen, often within fibrous bands and/or blood vessel walls. Lipoblasts may be seen but are not required for diagnosis. Histological variants exist.
- **Immunohistochemistry:** MDM2 overexpression.
- **Molecular genetics:** Fluorescence in situ amplification (FISH) shows amplification of *MDM2* and/or *CDK4* in almost all cases.
- **Prognosis:** Prognosis is determined by site. Tumours occurring in somatic soft tissue are cured by surgical resection, hence the term 'atypical lipomatous tumour' is applied at these sites. Tumours in the retroperitoneum almost all recur and the majority of patients eventually succumb to the disease (either due to uncontrollable local disease or, in the event of dedifferentiation, metastatic disease).

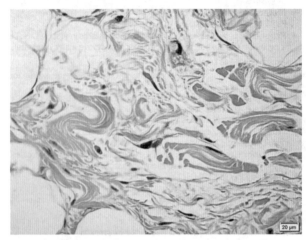

Fig. 17.17 Atypical lipomatous tumour. Mature adipocytes with scattered hyperchromatic spindled stromal cells (see Plate 79).

Dedifferentiated liposarcoma
- **Definition:** Morphological progression from atypical lipomatous tumour/well differentiated liposarcoma to a (usually high-grade) non-lipogenic sarcoma. The majority of cases arise *de novo* although a small proportion occur following recurrence(s) of a well differentiated liposarcoma.
- **Clinical features:** Most frequently occurs in the retroperitoneum of adults as a large, multinodular mass. Spermatic cord and mediastinum are also sites of predilection. Dedifferentiation is a rare event in atypical lipomatous tumours/well differentiated liposarcomas of somatic soft tissue.
- **Gross pathology**: Heterogeneous appearance, including areas with a yellow cut surface (representing the well differentiated adipocytic component) and white-grey areas (representing the non-lipogenic component). Areas of necrosis may also be seen.
- **Histopathology:** A low-grade adipocytic component and a typically high-grade non-lipogenic component which, in most cases, shows features of an undifferentiated pleomorphic sarcoma. The transition between the two components is often abrupt. Various heterologous elements (e.g. rhabdomyosarcomatous differentiation) can be seen in a small proportion of cases.
- **Immunohistochemistry:** MDM2 overexpression.
- **Molecular genetics:** As with well differentiated liposarcomas, dedifferentiated liposarcomas these tumours show amplification of *MDM2* and/or *CDK4*.

- **Prognosis:** Although less aggressive than most pleomorphic sarcomas, almost all patients with retroperitoneal tumours eventually succumb to the disease following (multiple) recurrences; a smaller proportion of cases will metastasize.

Myxoid liposarcoma

- **Definition:** Second commonest form of liposarcoma, accounting for approximately 30% of liposarcomas.
- **Clinical features:** Occur in deep somatic soft tissue, classically thigh. Usually middle-aged adults. Rarely occurs in children/adolescents (commonest liposarcoma in this age group, although still extremely rare). Virtually never occurs in the retroperitoneum (tumours with myxoid liposarcoma histological features in the retroperitoneum are almost always dedifferentiated liposarcomas or metastatic deposits).
- **Gross pathology**: Well-circumscribed tumour with gelatinous appearance.
- **Histopathology:** See Fig. 17.18. Uniform, small oval shaped cells which lack morphological features of adipocytes, set within a myxoid stroma containing a characteristic delicate, arborizing ('chicken-wire') capillary network. Univacuolar lipoblasts are usually seen. More cellular areas comprising round cells with increased mitotic activity found in a minority of cases (high-grade myxoid liposarcoma, previously known as round cell liposarcoma).
- **Molecular genetics:** Pathognomonic *DDIT3* rearrangements (usually *FUS-DDIT3*; rarely *EWSR1-DDIT3*).
- **Prognosis:** ~30–60% metastasize, with an unusual predilection for other soft tissue sites.

Pleomorphic liposarcoma

- **Definition:** Rarest liposarcoma subtype (5% of liposarcomas).
- **Clinical features:** Usually arises in elderly population as a rapidly growing mass of extremities (usually deep soft tissue, although ~25% occur in subcutaneous fat).

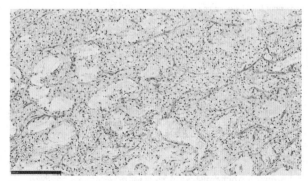

Fig. 17.18 Myxoid liposaroma. Small oval shaped cells set within a myxoid stroma containing a delicate, arbororising capillary network (see Plate 80).

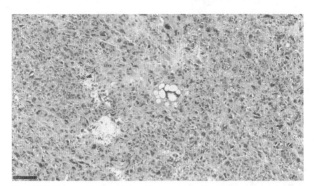

Fig. 17.19 Pleomorphic liposarcoma. Pleomorphic lipoblast amongst a population of pleomorphic cells with eosinophilic cytoplasm (see Plate 81).

- **Gross pathology**: Large, variably circumscribed tumours with yellow to white cut surface.
- **Histopathology:** See Fig. 17.19. Identification of pleomorphic lipoblasts is required for diagnosis (although not pathognomonic as can also be seen in well dedifferentiated and dedifferentiated liposarcomas). Present in variable numbers, hence thorough tumour sampling is critical. Other findings include spindle/pleomorphic cells, often with extreme pleomorphism; some tumours contain abundant epithelioid cells, while others can resemble myxofibrosarcoma.
- **Molecular genetics:** Complex karyotypes, no fusions; absence of *MDM2* amplification facilitates distinction from dedifferentiated liposarcoma.
- **Prognosis:** Very aggressive tumour with a mortality rate ~50%.

Peripheral nerve sheath tumours

Malignant peripheral nerve sheath tumour (MPNST)
- **Definition:** Sarcoma arising from/showing differentiation towards components of a peripheral nerve. 50% of patients have NF1.
- **Clinical features:** Rapidly growing deep-seated tumour arising most commonly in the proximal extremities in association with a major nerve trunk.
- **Gross pathology:** Large tumour with fusiform expansion of associated major nerve branches. A pre-existing plexiform neurofibroma may be seen in patients with NF1.
- **Histopathology:** Alternating hypercellular and hypocellular fascicles of atypical spindle cells with brisk mitotic activity and often extensive necrosis. Occasional tumours show rhabdomyoblastic differentiation (malignant Triton tumour) or osteo/chondro-sarcomatous differentiation. Epithelioid variant accounts for approximately 5% of MPNSTs.
- **Immunohistochemistry:** Totally negative/very focally positive for S100; diffuse staining argues strongly against MPNST (except in the

epithelioid variant, which is diffusely positive). Complete absence of staining with H3K27me3 frequently reported, particularly in high-grade tumours. Loss of INI-1 expression reported in approximately 70% of epithelioid MPNSTs.
- **Molecular genetics:** Complex alterations. Germline *NF1* inactivation in NF1 patients.
- **Prognosis:** Very poor, particularly NF1-associated tumours and malignant Triton tumours.

Smooth muscle tumours

(Extra-uterine) leiomyosarcoma
- **Definition:** Malignant smooth muscle tumour presenting as a range of clinicopathological subtypes determined by anatomical location: retroperitoneal, soft tissue, cutaneous, and gastrointestinal. A subgroup of tumours arise from the walls of large blood vessels, particularly the inferior vena cava.
- **Clinical features:** Incidence increases with age: retroperitoneal tumours and those arising from the inferior vena cava have a strong predilection for females.
- **Gross pathology:** Large, usually well-circumscribed, often whorled/fleshy cut surface.
- **Histopathology:** Cellular tumours comprising fascicles of spindle cells (or, in some high-grade tumours, epithelioid cells) with eosinophilic cytoplasm showing variable degrees of nuclear pleomorphism. Usually numerous mitoses. Necrosis may be seen.
- **Immunohistochemistry:** Positivity for SMA and at least one of desmin and H-caldesmon.
- **Molecular genetics:** Complex karyotypes, not diagnostically relevant.
- **Prognosis:** Overall metastatic rate is high, although very dependent on grade, depth, and anatomic site.

Skeletal muscle tumours

Embryonal rhabdomyosarcoma
- **Definition:** Sarcoma arising from the undifferentiated mesoderm showing morphological and immunophenotypical features of embryonal skeletal muscle. Commonest paediatric sarcoma.
- **Clinical features:** Sarcoma of childhood (3–12 years). Vast majority occur in either the head & neck (including nasopharynx, orbit) or the genitourinary system. Rare in somatic soft tissue.
- **Gross pathology:** Infiltrative tumour. Botryoid variant has a 'grape-like' appearance.
- **Histopathology:** Small, primitive, round to spindle shaped cells; rhabdomyoblasts with cross striations may sometimes be seen. The botryoid variant is characterized by aggregates of tumour cells immediately beneath the epithelial-lined surface (so-called cambium layer).
- **Immunohistochemistry:** Positive for skeletal muscle markers (extent of staining typically less than seen in alveolar rhabdomyosarcoma).
- **Molecular genetics:** Absence of FOXO1 fusions.

- **Prognosis:** Favourable in the absence of metastatic disease. Botyroid subtype has a particularly excellent prognosis.

Alveolar rhabdomyosarcoma
- **Definition:** Primitive round cell sarcoma with skeletal muscle differentiation.
- **Clinical features:** Occurs in adolescents and young adults (generally older population than seen in embryonal rhabdomyosarcoma), usually within the deep soft tissues of the extremities.
- **Gross pathology:** Infiltrative tumour with a soft, grey-coloured cut surface.
- **Histopathology:** Nests of monomorphic small to medium sized tumour cells surrounded by fibrovascular bands; cellular discohesion within the centre of the nests imparts an 'alveolar' appearance. Solid sheets of cells seen in solid variant.
- **Immunohistochemistry:** Diffuse nuclear expression of skeletal muscle markers MyoD1 and myogenin. MUC4 also reported to be frequently positive.
- **Molecular genetics:** ~80% of cases characterized by *PAX3/PAX7-FOXO1* fusions.
- **Prognosis:** Aggressive tumour (much worse prognosis than embryonal rhabdomyosarcoma).

Pleomorphic rhabdomyosarcoma
- **Definition:** High-grade sarcoma of adults showing skeletal muscle differentiation.
- **Clinical features:** Adults, often elderly, present with a rapidly growing mass in deep soft tissues of extremities (usually lower limb).
- **Gross pathology:** Large, well-circumscribed tumours often with areas of necrosis.
- **Histopathology:** Sheets of markedly pleomorphic cells, a proportion of which contain abundant eosinophilic cytoplasm imparting a rhabdoid appearance.
- **Immunohistochemistry:** Positivity (often focal) for myogenin and/or MyoD1.
- **Prognosis:** Highly aggressive tumour with short survival times.

Vascular tumours

Angiosarcoma
- **Definition:** Malignant tumour showing vascular (or lymphovascular) differentiation.
- **Clinical features:** Numerous clinical forms. **Cutaneous angiosarcoma** appears as bruise-like lesions and may be sporadic (head and neck of elderly sun-damaged patients), lympeoedma-associated (e.g. following axillary clearance for breast cancer; Stewart-Treves syndrome) or radiation associated (classically occurring within the skin overlying a previously irradiated breast). **Soft tissue angiosarcoma** is rare and occurs in the deep soft tissues of the extremities or retroperitoneum. **Angiosarcoma of bone** is a rare tumour preferentially arising in long and short tubular bones. **Primary mammary angiosarcoma** is an extremely rare tumour arising in the breast parenchyma of young adult females with no history of breast irradiation.

- **Gross pathology:** Variably defined and often multifocal haemorrhagic tumours.
- **Histopathology:** May be vasoformative, solid, or mixed. Vasoformative tumours are poorly defined and comprise anastomosing vessels with irregular outlines dissecting around native tissue

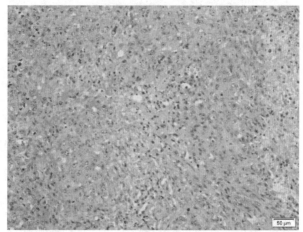

Fig. 17.20 Epithelioid sarcoma, classic-type. Atypical epithelioid cells forming aggregates and surrounding necrotic areas in a granuloma like pattern. This could be mistaken for a carcinoma (see Plate 82).

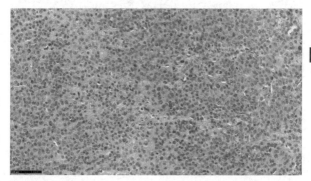

Fig. 17.21 Epithelioid sarcoma, proximal-type. Sheets of pleomorphic epithelioid cells (see Plate 83).

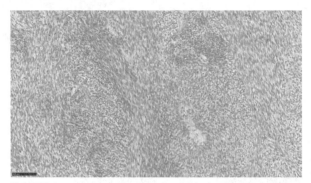

Fig. 17.22 Synovial sarcoma, monophasic-type. Cellular fascicles of monomorphic, blue-appearing spindle cells (see Plate 84).

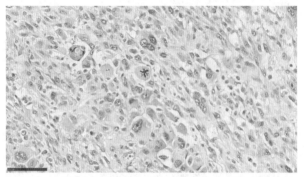

Fig. 17.23 Undifferentiated pleomorphic sarcoma. Sheets of markedly pleomorphic cells with atypical mitotic figures (see Plate 85).

components. The lining endothelial cells are hyperchromatic and may show multi-layering. Solid tumours comprise sheets of pleomorphic spindle cells, often with associated haemorrhage; vasoformative areas may be difficult to identify.

- **Immunohistochemistry:** Positive for ERG, CD31, CD34 and FLI1 (CD34 and FLI less specific). Radiation and lymphedema associated angiosarcomas usually express MYC.
- **Molecular pathology:** *MYC* amplification in radiation and lymphedema associated angiosarcomas can be detected by fluorescence in situ hybridization.

- **Prognosis:** Very aggressive tumour with high rates of recurrence and metastatic disease.

Epithelioid haemangioendothelioma
- **Definition:** Malignant epithelioid vascular tumour.
- **Clinical features:** Commonest sites include soft tissue, bone, liver, and lung. Symptoms are site-dependent. Soft tissue tumours are solitary; bone, liver, and lung lesions frequently multifocal. Patients typically middle-aged, although younger in cases arising in bone.
- **Gross pathology:** A proportion of soft tissue tumours arise in associated with a medium sized vessel, which may be visible macroscopically.
- **Histopathology:** Epithelioid cells arranged into cords set within a myxohyaline stroma; characteristically, tumour cells contain a single intracytoplasmic vacuole, sometimes containing a red blood cell ('blister cells'). Usually no well-formed vessels.
- **Immunohistochemistry:** Positive for ERG, CD31, CD34, and FLI1. Cytokeratins may be positive. CAMTA1 often positive, reflecting the underlying *CAMTA1* gene fusion.
- **Molecular pathology:** *WWTR1-CAMTA1* fusion present in the majority of cases. A small subset of tumours harbour *YAP1-TFE3* fusions.
- **Prognosis:** Less aggressive than angiosarcoma; mortality rate of between 15–20% for tumours arising in soft tissue or bone, higher (approximately 40%) for lung and liver cases.

Tumours of uncertain differentiation (in alphabetical order)

Alveolar soft part sarcoma
- **Definition:** Very rare tumour occurring in children/adolescents/young adults.
- **Clinical features:** Slow-growing tumour with female predominance. Head & neck is the commonest site in children; in adults there is a predilection for deep soft tissues of the thigh.
- **Gross pathology:** Multilobulated tumour with haemorrhage and necrosis.
- **Histopathology:** See Fig. 17.25. Well-formed nests (hence 'alveolar') of monomorphic cells with central nuclei and abundant eosinophilic cytoplasm. Classically the tumour cells appear to be 'falling apart' within the centre of the nests. Nests are surrounded by thin-walled vessels.
- **Immunohistochemistry:** TFE3 nuclear positivity.
- **Molecular genetics:** *ASPSCR1-TFE3* fusion present in most cases.
- **Prognosis:** Slow clinical course but prognosis ultimately poor with late metastases (lung and brain). Prognosis may be better in children with small tumours.

Clear cell sarcoma of soft tissue
- **Definition:** Rare malignant soft tissue tumour showing melanocytic differentiation (formerly known as malignant melanoma of soft parts).
- **Clinical features:** Slow-growing, deep-seated tumours frequently associated with tendons or aponeuroses of distal extremities (particularly the foot and ankle). Mostly occur in adolescents/young adults.

- **Gross pathology:** Usually relatively small tumours with infiltrative outlines.
- **Histopathology:** See Fig. 17.26. Round to spindle cells with clear/eosinophilic cytoplasm and prominent central nucleoli, arranged in lobules separated by fibrous septa. No pleomorphism. Intracellular melanin pigment and scattered 'wreath-like' giant cells may be seen.
- **Immunohistochemistry:** Positive for melanocytic markers (S100, Sox10, HMB45, Melan-A).
- **Molecular genetics:** Characterized by t(12;22)(q13;q12) resulting in an *EWSR1–ATF1* fusion (not specific as also seen in angiomatoid fibrous histiocytomas – but facilitates distinction from melanoma).
- **Prognosis:** Protracted clinical course with recurrences and late metastases—outcome ultimately poor. Unusually for a sarcoma, lymph node metastases are not uncommon.

Desmoplastic small round cell tumour
- **Definition:** Rare, aggressive intraabdominal tumour with characteristic histological, immunophenotypic, and molecular genetic features.
- **Clinical features:** Primarily occurs in children and young adults with a striking male predominance. Presenting symptoms/signs include abdominal pain and ascites relating to usually extensive peritoneal spread.
- **Gross pathology:** Dominant tumour mass associated with multiple smaller deposits coating the peritoneal surface.
- **Histopathology:** Nests of small, round cells with uniform hyperchromatic nuclei, separated by desmoplastic stroma.
- **Immunohistochemistry:** Polyphenotypic differentiation with expression of epithelial, muscle (desmin) and neural (NSE) markers. Antibodies directed against the C-terminus of WT1 often positive.
- **Molecular genetics:** Characterized by t(11;22)(p13;q12) producing an *EWSR1–WT1* fusion.
- **Prognosis:** Very aggressive tumour; overall survival is poor.

Epithelioid sarcoma
- **Definition:** Rare tumour (0.6–1% of all sarcomas) with epithelioid morphology. Two distinct clinicopathological forms of epithelioid sarcoma (ES): classic ES and proximal-type ES.
- **Clinical features:** Classic ES typically seen in male adolescents and young adults, presenting as a slowly growing, painless nodule(s), usually on the volar surfaces of the distal extremities. Proximal-type ES tends to arise in the deep soft tissues of the trunk/pelvis/proximal extremities and affects slightly older patients. Unusually for sarcomas, ES may metastasize to lymph nodes.
- **Gross pathology:** Single or multiple nodules with areas of necrosis and haemorrhage.
- **Histopathology:** See Figs 17.20 and 17.21. Classic ES is formed by a multinodular arrangement of epithelioid and spindle cells, with extensive, central 'pseudogranulomatous' necrosis, round vesicular nuclei, prominent nucleoli, and ample eosinophilic cytoplasm. Proximal-type ES comprises pleomorphic epithelioid cells which often exhibit a rhabdoid appearance; necrosis frequent but not 'pseudogranulomatous' as in classic ES.

- **Immunohistochemistry:** Positive for cytokeratins and EMA; CD34 usually positive. Loss of nuclear INI1/SMARCB1 protein expression seen in almost all cases.
- **Molecular genetics:** Inactivation of the *SMARB1* (*INI1*) tumour suppressor gene.
- **Prognosis:** Classic ES associated with a protracted clinical course including late recurrences and late metastasis. Proximal-type ES has a more aggressive behaviour and higher mortality.

Ewing sarcoma
- See malignant bone tumour section, p. 566.

Synovial sarcoma
- **Definition:** High-grade sarcoma of uncertain differentiation, representing 10–15% of adult soft tissue sarcomas. Monophasic (majority), biphasic, and poorly differentiated forms.
- **Clinical features:** Presents in young adults as a palpable mass in the deep soft tissues (usually in the extremities). May be associated with pain and can be deceptively slow-growing and longstanding.
- **Gross pathology:** Wide variation in size and consistency. Calcifications sometimes seen.
- **Histopathology:** See Fig. 17.22. Monophasic tumours comprising highly cellular fascicles of monotonous spindle cells with minimal cytoplasm. Biphasic forms contain additional epithelial component (i.e. glands/cords/nests). Haemangiopericytoma-like vessels common.
- **Immunohistochemistry:** Variable EMA positivity. BCL2 and CD99 positive (non-specific). Highly sensitive and specific SSX-SS18 fusion specific antibody now available.
- **Molecular genetics:** chromosomal translocation t(X;18), producing fusion genes between *SS18* (*SYT*) and *SSX1*, *SSX2*, or *SSX4*.
- **Prognosis:** Variable, although many behave aggressively with 40% metastatic rate.

Undifferentiated pleomorphic sarcoma
- **Definition:** Heterogeneous group of high-grade pleomorphic sarcomas showing no specific line of differentiation (a diagnosis of exclusion). Previously known as malignant fibrous histiocytoma (MFH). Account for 5–10% of sarcomas in adults older than 40 years.
- **Clinical features:** Large, deep-seated tumours arising in older patients. Most occur in the extremities, particularly the lower limbs.
- **Gross pathology:** Large tumours with grey to cream coloured cut surface. Usually well-circumscribed; often compresses adjacent soft tissue structures.
- **Histopathology:** See Fig. 17.23. Highly pleomorphic spindled and/or epithelioid cells in a collagenous stroma. Various architectural patterns. High mitotic activity, tumour necrosis frequently seen.
- **Immunohistochemistry:** No evidence of a specific line of differentiation.
- **Molecular genetics:** Complex karyotypes.
- **Prognosis:** An overall aggressive sarcoma type with 5 year survival of approximately 50%.

Benign bone tumours

Cartilage-forming tumours

Osteochondroma (exostosis)

- **Definition:** Common tumour comprising a bony projection with a cartilaginous cap.
- **Clinical features:** Majority are solitary and sporadic, typically arising in the metaphyseal region of long bones (e.g. distal femur). 15% of cases occur in the setting of an inherited disorder, primarily the syndrome of multiple osteochondromas (hereditary multiple exostoses) which shows an autosomal dominant pattern of inheritance.
- **Gross pathology:** Tumour on the bone surface showing continuity with the cortex and medulla. May be flat (sessile osteochondroma) or, more commonly, attached to pre-existing bone via a stalk (pedunculated osteochondroma). Overlying cartilaginous cap usually <2 cm in thickness.
- **Histopathology:** See Fig. 17.24. A paucicellular cartilaginous cap, the base of which shows enchondral ossification merging with trabecular bone of the medullary cavity.
- **Molecular genetics:** Hereditary multiple exostosis is associated with germline *EXT1/EXT2* mutations; homozygous deletion of *EXT1* also seen in many sporadic osteochondromas.
- **Prognosis:** Benign; small minority may transform into peripheral chondrosarcoma.

Chondroma

- **Definition:** Benign conventional cartilage-forming tumour of bone. **Enchondromas** arise in the medullary cavity (typically within the small bones of hands and feet) while **periosteal chondromas** arise on the bone surface (often long tubular bones, the proximal humerus being a characteristic site).
- **Clinical features:** Most enchondromas are solitary and usually represent an incidental finding. Multiple lesions can be seen in the

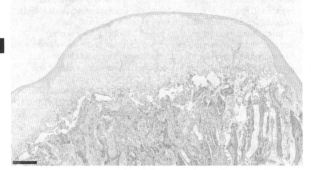

Fig. 17.24 Osteochondroma. Cartilaginous cap showing enchondral ossification merging with trabecular bone (see Plate 86).

setting of enchondromatosis (Ollier's disease and Maffucci syndrome). Periosteal chondromas often present as a painful palpable mass.
- **Gross pathology:** Multilobulated tumours with a glistening cut surface.
- **Histopathology:** Lobules of mature hyaline cartilage; generally paucicellular although enchondromas of hands and feet and periosteal chondromas tend to be more cellular. No mitoses and no permeation of pre-existing bone.
- **Molecular genetics:** *IDH1/IDH2* somatic point mutation detected in ~50% of cases.
- **Prognosis:** Benign. Very rare cases may transform to chondrosarcoma.

Chondroblastoma
- **Definition:** A rare benign, chondrogenic bone tumour with a predilection for the epiphyseal/apophyseal region of long bones.
- **Clinical features:** Majority of cases seen in skeletally immature patients but may present later in life. Pain is a common symptom.
- **Gross pathology:** Well-circumscribed with a sclerotic rim; sometimes haemorrhagic reflecting secondary aneurysmal bone cyst-like changes.
- **Histopathology:** Sheets of round to polygonal cells with grooved nuclei and distinct cytoplasmic borders admixed with islands of eosinophilic chondroid matrix. Classically pericellular 'chicken-wire' calcification is seen and there are also numerous multinucleated osteoclast-like giant cells.
- **Immunohistochemistry:** Variable S100 and DOG1 positivity. Antibodies against (H3F3B)(K36M) are highly sensitive and specific.
- **Molecular genetics:** A p.Lys36Met substitution in gene *H3F3B* (or, less frequently, *H3F3A*) in >90% of cases.
- **Prognosis:** Benign—no malignant potential.

Chondromyxoid fibroma
- **Definition:** Rare, slow-growing, non-conventional benign cartilaginous bone tumour with myxoid and fibroblastic components.
- **Clinical features:** Most cases occur before the age of 40, typically arising in the metaphyses of long bones in the lower extremity. May present with pain.
- **Gross pathology:** Well-circumscribed, lobulated tumour.
- **Histopathology:** Lobules of stellate cells set in a fibro/chondro-myxoid matrix, with greater cellularity at the lobule peripheries.
- **Molecular genetics:** Structural rearrangement of *GRM1* gene.
- **Prognosis:** Benign; occasionally recurs, no malignant potential.

Bone-forming tumours
Osteoid osteoma
- **Definition:** A benign bone-forming neoplasm accounting for ~10% of primary bone tumours.
- **Clinical features:** Most commonly arises in the cortex of a long bone of a child or young adult, especially the femur and tibia. Characteristically painful, especially at night; relieved with non-steroidal anti-inflammatory drugs (NSAIDs). Readily identified on plain radiographs as a small lucent nidus <2 cm in size.
- **Gross pathology:** Small, round, red-coloured, and gritty lesion.

- **Histopathology:** A central nidus comprising anastomosing trabeculae of woven bone rimmed by osteoblasts with a peripheral zone of dense osteosclerosis.
- **Molecular genetics:** *FOS* gene arrangements may be seen.
- **Prognosis:** Low rates of recurrence and no risk of malignant transformation.

Osteoclast giant cell-rich tumours

Non-ossifying fibroma/fibrous cortical defect
- **Definition:** Commonest bone tumour; occult lesions estimated to be present in ~1/3 of children. Non-ossifying fibroma is distinguished from fibrous cortical defect by size (>2 cm) and intramedullary location.
- **Clinical features:** Generally found in the metaphysis of long bones of lower extremities in children/adolescents. Usually an incidental finding.
- **Gross pathology:** Well-defined with sclerotic borders.
- **Histopathology:** Fig. 17.25. Fibroblastic spindle cells arranged into a storiform architecture with admixed osteoclast-type giant cells and both foamy and haemosiderin-laden histiocytes.
- **Prognosis:** Benign.

Aneurysmal bone cyst (ABC)
- **Definition:** A destructive and expansile lesion characterized by cyst-like, blood-filled spaces. Primary ABCs are true neoplasms while secondary ABCs represent a reactive process occurring secondarily in a range of benign and malignant neoplasms.
- **Clinical features:** Most commonly seen in children/adolescents/ young adults. Can arise in any bone although preferentially occur in the metaphyseal region of long bones where they are usually located within the medulla. A significant proportion of cases arise in vertebrae.
- **Gross pathology:** Well-defined lesion; multiloculated with blood-filled spaces.

Fig. 17.25 Non ossifying fibroma. Fibroblastic cells in a storiform arrangement with scattered osteoclast-type giant cells (see Plate 87).

- **Histopathology:** Large blood-filled spaces divided by fibrous septa containing osteoclast-like giant cells and a fibro-osteoid membrane.
- **Molecular genetics:** *USP6* gene arrangement in primary ABCs (not in secondary ABCs).
- **Prognosis:** Benign although may recur following curettage in a proportion of cases.

Vascular tumours

Haemangioma of bone
- Definition: Benign tumour with a predilection for vertebral bodies.
- Miscellaneous benign mesenchymal tumours of bone.

Simple (unicameral) bone cyst
- **Definition:** A common non-neoplastic cystic bone lesion.
- **Clinical features:** Usually incidental finding in childhood, more common in males. Lesions in children tend to arise in the metaphysis of the proximal humerus or proximal femur.
- **Gross pathology:** Large cystic cavity, usually unilocular, containing translucent fluid.
- **Histopathology:** The 'cyst' wall is formed by a thin layer of fibrous tissue +/− osteoid. Fibrin deposition may also be seen and there are often multinucleated giant cells.
- **Prognosis:** Benign. Fracture may occur through simple bone cysts.

Fibrous dysplasia
- **Definition:** Benign intramedullary fibro-osseous tumour; usually solitary (monostotic) although multifocal (polyostotic) lesions in ~25% of cases.
- **Clinical features:** Typically presents in children/adolescents/young adults. Any bone can be affected although predilection for craniofacial bones and femur. Polyostotic form can be associated with McCune-Albright and Mazabraud syndromes.
- **Gross pathology:** Tan/white-coloured with gritty consistency.
- **Histopathology:** Curvilinear trabeculae of woven bone lacking osteoblastic rimming, set within a pauci- to moderately cellular fibrous stroma. Secondary ABC changes may be seen.
- **Molecular genetics:** Activating *GNAS* mutations found in most cases.
- **Prognosis:** Benign, although some cases may cause skeletal deformities. Malignant transformation is a very rare event.

Intermediate bone tumours

Cartilage-forming tumours

Synovial chondromatosis

- **Definition:** A rare cartilaginous tumour comprising multiple nodules involving the joint space or, less commonly, tenosynovium (i.e. extra-articular). Classified as a 'locally aggressive' tumour by the WHO.
- **Clinical features:** Typically presents in young adult males; the knee joint is the commonest site.
- **Gross pathology:** Multiple, variably sized grey-coloured nodules free in the joint space and/or attached to synovium.
- **Histopathology:** See Fig.17.26. Nodules of hyaline-type cartilage containing clusters of chondrocytes.
- **Molecular genetics:** *FN1-ACVR2A* fusions present in most cases.
- **Prognosis:** Recurs in 15–20% of cases. Malignant transformation occurs in about 5–10% of tumours, usually limited those which have undergone multiple recurrences (although can rarely occur *de novo*).

Bone-forming tumours

Osteoblastoma

- **Definition:** A benign bone-forming tumour, histologically similar to osteoid osteoma but >2 cm and lacking the nocturnal pain relieved by NSAIDs as is classical of osteoid osteoma. Classified as a 'locally aggressive' tumour by the WHO.
- **Clinical features:** Most commonly presents in children or young adults but can present later in life. Axial skeleton is a common site; can present with pain, scoliosis. Radiographs may show focal cortical expansion or destruction that can be misdiagnosed as a malignancy.
- **Gross pathology:** Usually well-defined with cortical thinning. Can appear haemorrhagic, particularly in the presence of an associated secondary ABC.

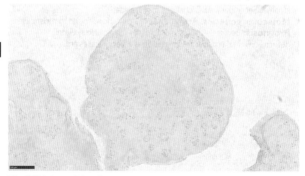

Fig. 17.26 Synovial chondromatosis. Multiple nodules of hyaline cartilage with clustering of chondrocytes (see Plate 88).

- **Histopathology:** Features similar to osteoid osteoma. May be mistaken for osteosarcoma histologically, hence correlation with the radiological appearances is essential.
- **Prognosis:** Virtually no risk of malignant transformation, but can recur.

Osteoclast giant cell-rich tumours

Giant cell tumour of bone

- **Definition:** Classified as a 'locally aggressive, rarely metastasizing' tumour by the WHO. Arises in the epiphysis of long bones.
- **Clinical features:** Only seen in the mature skeleton, typically presents between 20 and 45 years with pain and swelling over the site of the tumour. Distal femur, proximal tibia, and distal radius are commonest sites.
- **Gross pathology:** Usually well-circumscribed with cortical thinning or destruction, sometimes with a soft tissue component. May also erode subchondral bone plate.
- **Histopathology:** Sheets of neoplastic ovoid mononuclear cells of osteoblastic lineage interspersed with non-neoplastic, uniformly distributed, large osteoclast-like giant cells. Brown tumour of hyperparathyroidism can show very similar morphological appearances (serum calcium and phosphate levels should therefore be evaluated).
- **Molecular genetics:** Somatic driver mutations in the *H3F3A* gene (p.G34W/L) in >90% of cases (can be detected by immunohistochemical antibody).
- **Prognosis:** Local recurrence following excision occurs in about 25% of cases. Benign lung metastases/implants rarely occur (believed to represent an embolic event, possibly partly due to surgical manipulation); these tend to be slow-growing (and sometimes regress spontaneously). Bona fide malignant transformation of giant cell tumours can also rarely occur, usually after multiple recurrences.

Malignant bone tumours

Bone metastases

- **Definition:** Deposits of tumour in bone via haematogenous spread from a malignancy at a distant site. The vast majority of malignant tumours found in bone represent metastatic carcinoma, with most originating from the lung, breast, kidney, thyroid, and prostate.
- **Clinical features:** Presents with pain or fracture, or may be identified as part of staging. Usually patients have a history of carcinoma, although bone involvement can sometimes be the presenting complaint. Any bone can be involved although predilection for femur, humerus, and axial skeleton. Bony metastases are one of the common causes of hypercalcaemia.
- **Gross pathology:** Most metastatic deposits are osteolytic (i.e. they destroy bone; e.g. lung, renal), but some metastases are osteoblastic/sclerotic (i.e. they induce bone formation; e.g. prostate). Usually haemorrhagic appearances on gross examination.
- **Histopathology:** Typically retain the morphological features of the primary tumour.
- **Immunohistochemistry:** Cytokeratins positive; precise profile depends on site of origin.
- **Prognosis:** Prognosis determined by primary tumour type.

Cartilage-forming tumours

Conventional chondrosarcoma (CS)

- **Definition:** Malignant cartilage-forming tumour. Can be classified by histological grade, that is, low-grade (atypical cartilaginous tumour/grade 1 CS) vs. high-grade (grade II/III CS); location (i.e. central; intramedullary) vs. peripheral (exostotic) vs. periosteal; and aetiology, that is, primary (arising in normal bone) vs. secondary (arising in an enchondroma or osteochondroma).
- **Clinical features:** Mostly older adults >50 years presenting with pain. Commonest sites include pelvis, femur, proximal humerus, and ribs. Incidence of CS arising in an enchondroma (i.e. secondary central CS) occurs at a higher rate in Ollier's disease and Maffucci syndrome.
- **Gross pathology:** Usually large, lobulated tumours with glistening blue-grey cut surface. A pre-existing osteochondroma may be identifiable in secondary peripheral CS.
- **Histopathology:** See Fig. 17.27. Atypical cartilaginous tumours/grade 1 CS show very similar histological appearances to enchondromas (i.e. lobules of hyaline cartilage of low cellularity with no/minimal cytological atypia and no mitoses); however, there is permeation of pre-existing lamellar bone which is a key diagnostic feature. Grade II/III CS shows higher cellularity and often myxoid areas; the chondrocytes exhibit larger nuclei and there is often mitotic activity (occasional mitoses only in grade II CS, more frequent mitoses in grade III).
- **Molecular pathology:** Mutations in *IDH1* or *IDH2* in most cases.
- **Prognosis:** Low-grade tumours (atypical cartilaginous tumours/grade 1 CS) are locally aggressive carrying a risk of recurrence but essentially no metastatic potential. The term 'atypical cartilaginous tumour' can

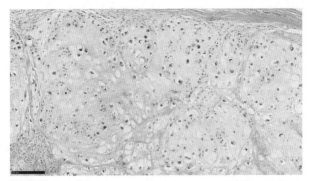

Fig. 17.27 Grade III chondrosarcoma. Cartilaginous tumour displaying markedly atypical chondrocytes (see Plate 89).

be utilized in the appendicular skeleton while 'grade 1 CS' is applied to tumours of the axial skeleton to reflect the increased morbidity and mortality relating to locally aggressive disease at sites such as the pelvis and skull base. Grade II and III CS are high-grade sarcomas with metastatic potential (particularly Grade III CS).

Dedifferentiated CS
- **Definition:** Highly malignant CS comprising a conventional CS component showing abrupt transition to a high-grade non-cartilaginous sarcoma. Dedifferentiation occurs in ~10% of central CSs.
- **Clinical features:** Mostly older adults presenting with pain or fracture. Commonest sites include femur and pelvis.
- **Gross pathology:** Conventional CS component is usual central and appears lobulated with a glistening blue-grey cut surface. The dedifferentiated component is usually tan-coloured.
- **Histopathology:** The conventional low-grade component is formed by hyaline cartilage which abruptly transitions to a high-grade non-cartilaginous sarcoma (usually undifferentiated pleomorphic sarcoma, occasionally osteosarcoma).
- **Molecular pathology:** Mutations in *IDH1* or *IDH2* in most cases.
- **Prognosis:** Very poor with high rates of lung metastases.

Mesenchymal chondrosarcoma
- **Definition:** Rare, high-grade biphasic tumour distinct from conventional chondrosarcomas.
- **Clinical features:** Wide age range; peak in young adults. Most occur in bone (particularly craniofacial and rib) although can also arise in soft tissue and intracranial location.
- **Gross pathology:** Large destructive tumour with partly calcified and partly fleshy cut surface. Conventional CS component is usual central and appears lobulated with a glistening blue-grey cut surface. The dedifferentiated component is usually tan-coloured.

- **Histopathology:** Sheets of primitive small round cells associated with haemangiopericytoma-like vessels and islands of low-grade hyaline cartilage.
- **Immunohistochemistry:** Small round cells may be positive for CD99 and S100.
- **Molecular pathology:** *HEY1-NCOA2* gene fusion is consistently found.
- **Prognosis:** Aggressive tumour; 5-year survival ~60%. May follow a protracted clinical course.

Bone-forming tumours

Malignant bone-forming tumours, known as osteosarcomas, are the most common non-haematological malignant primary bone tumours. Numerous subtypes exist: they can be divided by location (intramedullary vs. surface), grade, or whether they arise in normal bone or diseased bone (primary vs. secondary).

Conventional (intramedullary) osteosarcoma
- **Definition:** A high-grade bone-forming tumour located in the medullary cavity. Most common osteosarcoma subtype.
- **Clinical features:** Most present between 14–18 years although there is a second peak in older adults (many representing 'secondary osteosarcoma', mainly arising in the setting of Paget's disease or previous radiation therapy). Mainly arise in the metaphysis of long bones; most cases occur around the knee. Presentation is with pain +/– a palpable mass.
- **Gross pathology:** Large, ill-defined destructive tumour often with cortical breach and involvement of soft tissue compartment. Most patients receive neo-adjuvant chemotherapy hence therapy-related changes (e.g. fibrosis and necrosis) are expected in the resection specimen.
- **Histopathology:** See Fig. 17.28. Atypical pleomorphic tumour cells associated with lace-like osteoid production; divided into osteoblastic,

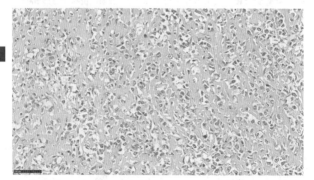

Fig. 17.28 Conventional (osteoblastic) osteosarcoma. Atypical cells associated with abundant osteoid formation (see Plate 90).

chondroblastic or fibroblastic types (many cases show a combination of morphologies).

- **Prognosis:** Highly malignant tumour which shows early and rapid haematogenous dissemination, particularly to the lungs Prognosis largely determined by preoperative chemotherapy response: the 5-year survival for 'good responders' is 60%, whereas non-responders have poor survival rates of <15%.

Low-grade central osteosarcoma

- **Definition:** Rare low-grade osteosarcoma variant arising in medullary cavity.
- **Clinical features:** Older peak age than conventional osteosarcoma (~30 years). Similar anatomical distribution to conventional osteosarcoma.
- **Gross pathology:** Large, relatively well-circumscribed gritty mass in medullary cavity.
- **Histopathology:** Fibroblastic-type spindle cells with only relatively mild atypia set in a collagenous stroma. Variable amounts of osteoid and woven bone which may be arranged into trabeculae. Permeation of pre-existing bone identified.
- **Molecular pathology:** *MDM2* amplification identified in a proportion of cases.
- **Prognosis:** Excellent if completely excised; low metastatic rate.

Parosteal osteosarcoma

- **Definition:** Low-grade surface OS. Commonest surface OS.
- **Clinical features:** Affects young adults in 3rd–4th decades (older than peak conventional OS age group), more common in females. Involves long bones (especially posterior aspect of distal femur).
- **Gross pathology:** Ossified lobulated mass on bone surface.
- **Histopathology:** Trabeculae of woven and lamella bone in a fibrous stroma which contains mild atypical spindle cells; cartilaginous differentiation often seen.
- **Molecular pathology:** *MDM2* amplification in majority of cases.
- **Prognosis:** Excellent if completely excised.

Periosteal osteosarcoma

- **Definition:** Rare, intermediate grade OS arising on the bone surface.
- **Clinical features:** 2nd–3rd decade. Diaphyseal lesion, commonly arising in the anteromedial aspect of the tibia.
- **Gross pathology:** Lobulated tumour attached to cortical surface. Glistening cut surface.
- **Histopathology:** Lobules of cartilage showing moderate to severe cytological atypia associated with osteoid production.
- **Prognosis:** Better prognosis than conventional OS (~90% disease free survival at 5 years).

High-grade surface osteosarcoma

- **Definition:** Very rare high-grade OS subtype.
- **Clinical features:** 3rd–4th decade. Diaphyseal region of femur, tibia, or humerus.
- **Gross pathology:** Well-circumscribed tumour on bone surface.
- **Histopathology:** Identical to conventional OS.
- **Prognosis:** Aggressive tumour with high rate of metastatic disease.

Vascular tumours

Angiosarcoma and epitheliod haemangioendothelioma of bone—see malignant soft tissue tumour section p. 548 & p.551

Notochordal tumours

Chordoma

- **Definition:** Malignant tumours derived from the embryonic notochord. Almost all occur in the axial skeletal, specifically the sacrococcygeal region (50%) and skull base/clivus (35%).
- **Clinical features:** Usually arises in middle-aged to elderly adults with a male predominance. Symptoms include pain and site-related neurological symptoms.
- **Gross pathology:** Lobular tumour with a gelatinous cut surface.
- **Histopathology:** Epithelioid cells forming cords and nests in a myxoid stroma. The cells often have 'bubbly' cytoplasm (physaliphorous cells). Rarely, chordomas can undergo dedifferentiation into an undifferentiated pleomorphic sarcoma. A poorly differentiated variant also exists.
- **Immunohistochemistry:** Pancytokertatin positive, variable S100. Brachyury is a highly specific marker.
- **Prognosis:** Median survival of 7 years.

Undifferentiated small round cell sarcomas

Ewing sarcoma

- **Definition:** Malignant round cell tumour of neuroectodermal origin defined by a gene fusion involving a gene in the FET family (almost always *EWSR1*) and a member of the ETS family of transcription factors. Most cases arise in bone (Ewing sarcoma is the 2nd commonest malignant bone tumour in children after osteosarcoma).
- **Clinical features:** Majority (>80%) of cases occur in childhood and adolescence, arising in the diaphyseal region of long bones, flat bones, or the spine. A small proportion arise outside the skeleton (more commonly in adults). Very rare in people of African ancestry. Pain is the commonest presenting symptom.
- **Gross pathology:** Soft, grey-white coloured cut surface.
- **Histopathology:** See Fig. 17.29. Sheets of monomorphic small round cells with hyperchromatic nuclei and scant cytoplasm. Necrosis is commonly seen.
- **Immunohistochemistry:** Strong and diffuse membranous CD99 staining (highly sensitive but not specific). NKX2.2 is a more specific marker.
- **Molecular genetics:** t(11;22)(q24;q12) resulting in a *EWSR1–FLI* translocation found in >85% of cases. Most of the remaining cases contain a *EWSR1–ERG* fusion. Other rare undifferentiated small round cell sarcomas with alternative molecular signatures, previously falling under the umbrella-term 'Ewing-like sarcomas' have now been defined: these include round cell sarcomas with *EWSR1*-non-*ETS* fusions, *CIC*-rearranged sarcoma (a soft tissue tumour) and sarcomas with *BCOR* alterations.

Fig. 17.29 Ewing Sarcoma. Sheets of monotonous small round cells (see Plate 91).

- **Prognosis:** Ewing sarcoma has a relatively high cure rate for localized disease (>65%), although metastatic tumours carry a much poorer prognosis. Tumours arising at certain sites, such as the pelvis, are also associated with more aggressive disease.

Further reading

BoSTT App. Available at: https://www.rnoh.nhs.uk/our-services/cellular-and-molecular-pathology/bostt-app.

Campbell P, Ebramzadeh E, Nelson S, Takamura K, De Smet K, Amstutz HC. Histological Features of Pseudotumour-like Tissues from Metal-on-metal Hips. *Clin Orthop Relat Res* 2010;468:2321–2327.

Coindre JM. Grading of Soft Tissue Sarcomas: Review and Update. *Arch Pathol Lab Med* 2006;130:1448–1453.

Hornick J L (2013). *Practical Soft Tissue Pathology: A Diagnostic Approach*. Philadelphia, PA: Elsevier/Saunders.

WHO Classification of tumours Editorial Board. Soft tissue and bone tumours. Lyon (France): International Agency for Research on Cancer; 2020.

Neuropathology

Nervous system malformations

Neural tube defects

- Due to defective closure of the neural tube during embryogenesis.
- Both genetic and environmental factors are involved.
- Maternal folate deficiency in early gestation is a risk factor.
- **Anencephaly** is a uniformly fatal malformation of the anterior neural tube leading to absence of the brain and cranial vault.
- **Encephalocele** is a protrusion of malformed brain tissue through a midline skull defect, usually in the occipital region. Large encephaloceles are usually fatal.
- **Spina bifida** is a group of malformations of the spinal cord due to defective closure of the caudal end of the neural tube and lack of fusion of the vertebral arches and skin coverings. There may be associated outpouchings of meninges (**meningocele**) or meninges and spinal cord (**myelomeningocele**). The latter may cause problems such as urinary incontinence, constipation, and variable degrees of motor and sensory impairment of the legs.

Agenesis of the corpus callosum

- Occurs if the glial bridge fails to form between the two cerebral hemispheres or if axons fail to cross it. May be complete or partial.
- Often associated with other malformations (e.g. holoprosencephaly).
- May cause varying degrees of psychomotor retardation.

Congenital aqueduct stenosis

- Developmental anomaly causing narrowing of the cerebral aqueduct.
- Most common cause of congenital hydrocephalus.
- Rarely may be inherited in an X-linked recessive pattern.

Chiari malformations

- Condition in which brain tissue extends into the spinal canal.
- Part of the skull is misshapen and pushes brain tissue downwards.
- Type 1 is milder and occurs as the skull and brain are growing such that it presents in late childhood or early adulthood, usually with headaches.
- Type 2 is present at birth and causes more displacement of the cerebellar vermis together with a myelomeningocele. Diagnosis is usually made prenatally on ultrasound.

Dandy-Walker malformation

- Absent or rudimentary cerebellar vermis leading to filling of the posterior fossa by a large cyst representing a dilated fourth ventricle.
- May be associated with other malformations.

Syringomyelia

- Fluid-filled cavity within the central grey matter of the spinal cord.
- Usually affects the cervical and upper thoracic segments. Extension of the syrinx into the medulla is known as syringobulbia.
- Expansion of the syrinx causes atrophy of the adjacent spinal cord.
- Presents in early adulthood with isolated loss of pain and temperature in the upper limbs due to damage to spinothalamic tracts.

Epilepsy

Definition

- A recurrent tendency to spontaneous episodes of abnormal electrical activity within the brain which manifest as seizures.

Epidemiology

- Common (1–2% of population worldwide affected), 2nd most common neurological disorder after stroke.

Aetiology

- Very often idiopathic with no clear cause found.
- May be associated with underlying structural lesions (trauma, neoplasms, malformations), metabolic conditions (alcohol, electrolyte disorders), infections and rare genetic diseases (e.g. ion channel mutations).

Partial seizures

- Features attributable to a localized part of one hemisphere.
- In simple partial seizures, consciousness is unimpaired (e.g. a focal motor seizure).
- In complex partial seizures, consciousness is impaired (e.g. motionless staring).

Generalized seizures

- No features referable to one hemisphere (no focality); consciousness is always impaired.
- Absence seizures ('petit mal') cause brief (<10 s) pauses (e.g. stopping talking in mid-sentence, and then carrying on where left off).
- Tonic-clonic ('grand mal') cause sudden loss of consciousness with stiffening (tonic) of limbs and then jerking (clonic).
- Myoclonic jerks cause sudden violent movements of the limbs.

Temporal lobe epilepsy

- Typical onset in late childhood and adolescence.
- Usually presents with complex partial seizures (e.g. strange feeling in gut or sense of déjà vu or strange smell followed by automatism).
- Secondary generalized tonic-clonic seizures may also occur.
- In most cases an epileptogenic focus is present in medial temporal structures (e.g. hippocampal sclerosis).

Childhood absence epilepsy

- Idiopathic generalized epilepsy syndrome affecting children aged 4–12.
- Characterized by recurrent absence seizures.
- Some children also develop tonic-clonic type seizures.

Juvenile myoclonic epilepsy

- Idiopathic generalized epilepsy syndrome affecting children and adolescents aged 8–20.
- Most common seizure type is a myoclonic jerk, but tonic-clonic and absence seizures may also occur.

Hippocampal sclerosis

- Loss of pyramidal neurons and gliosis most often in the CA1 region of the hippocampus.
- Frequent feature of temporal lobe epilepsy.
- Most common cause of drug-resistant epilepsy in adults.

Focal cortical dysplasia (FCD)

- Malformation of cortical development which is restricted to a localized area of the cortex.
- Common cause of drug-resistant epilepsy in children.

Sudden unexpected death in epilepsy (SUDEP)

- Affects 1 in very 1000 adults with epilepsy each year (less common in children).
- Whilst rare it represents the most common cause of premature death in adults with epilepsy.
- Main risk factor: Poorly controlled epilepsy / tonic-clonic seizures.
- Often nocturnal and unwitnessed.
- Alternative cause of death has to be excluded at post mortem (e.g. drowning, status epilepticus).
- Exact mechanism unclear but centrally mediated depression of cardiac and respiratory regulation is favoured.

Head injury

Epidemiology

- About 50 000 severe head injuries occur each year in the UK.
- Responsible for some 20% of deaths in young people aged 5–45.
- May cause severe disability in those who survive.

Skull fracture

- Severe head injury may cause skull fracture at the site of impact.
- A marker of serious head injury with increased risk of underlying intracranial injury such as contusions and haematomas.
- Base of skull fractures may cause lower cranial nerve palsies or cerebrospinal fluid (CSF) discharge from the nose or ear or so-called raccoon eyes.

Cerebral contusions

- Bruises on the surface of the brain.
- Occur when the brain suddenly moves within the cranial cavity and is crushed against the skull.
- Typically there is injury at the site of impact (the 'coup' lesion) and at the site diagonally opposite this point (the 'contrecoup' lesion).
- Oozing of blood into the brain parenchyma and associated cerebral oedema are important contributors to raised intracranial pressure.

Extradural haematoma

- Due to haemorrhage between the dura and the skull.
- The bleeding vessel is often the middle meningeal artery which is torn following fracture of the squamous temporal bone.
- Accumulation of extradural blood is slow as the firmly adherent dura is slowly peeled away from the inner surface of the skull.
- Patients may appear well for several hours following head injury ('lucid' interval'), but then quickly deteriorate as the haematoma enlarges and compresses the brain.

Subdural haematoma

- Due to haemorrhage between the dura and the arachnoid.
- Results from tearing of delicate bridging veins that traverse the subdural space to drain into the cerebral venous sinuses.
- Blood from these veins spreads freely through the subdural space, enveloping the entire cerebral hemisphere on the side of the injury.
- Usually occur after severe head trauma (acute subdural haematoma) but can be seen following relatively minor trauma (chronic subdural haematoma) particularly in older people, those taking anticoagulant medication or people who misuse alcohol.

Traumatic axonal injury

- Typically follows sudden acceleration-deceleration injuries.
- The most severe form is known as **diffuse axonal injury**, which causes immediate unconsciousness and almost inevitable death.
- Histologically there is widespread axonal swelling with increased numbers of microglia and eventually degeneration of the involved fibre tracts.

Cerebral infarction

Definition

- Ischaemic necrosis of an area of the brain.

Epidemiology

- Common, accounting for about 80% of strokes.
- Mostly seen in the elderly.

Aetiology

- Most are caused by thromboemboli from either the internal carotid artery or the left side of the heart lodging in a cerebral artery.
- A small proportion are due to *in situ* thrombosis of an atherosclerotic plaque within a cerebral artery.

Pathogenesis

- Sustained occlusion of a cerebral artery leads to ischaemic necrosis of the territory of brain supplied by the affected artery.

Presentation

- Rapid onset of focal CNS signs and symptoms related to the distribution of the affected artery (stroke, cerebrovascular accident).
- The majority involve the territory of the middle cerebral artery of a cerebral hemisphere resulting in varying degrees of contralateral hemiplegia and hemiparesis, homonymous hemianopia, and dysphasia.

! Transient ischaemic attacks (sudden episodes of focal CNS signs which resolve within 24 hours or less) are important warning signs to the risk of future cerebral infarction.

Macroscopy (Fig. 18.1)

- After 24 hours, the infarcted area softens and there is loss of the normal sharp definition between the grey and white matter. Cerebral oedema within and around the infarct often causes midline shift.
- From 48 hours to 10 days the infarct becomes gelatinous and the distinction between the infarct and normal brain becomes clearer.
- From 10 days to 3 weeks the infarct liquefies and undergoes cystic change.
- In some cases, reperfusion leads to bleeding into the infarct visible as punctate haemorrhages ('haemorrhagic infarct').

Histopathology

- Within the first 48 hours, there are ischaemic neuronal changes (shrunken eosinophilic neurones) with influx of neutrophils.
- Mononuclear cells then phagocytose myelin breakdown products and astrocytes proliferate as the infarct organizes over 2–3 weeks.

Prognosis

- One in eight strokes are fatal within the first month and 25% within the first year. The more severe the disability the more likely death will occur.

- Common complications include pneumonia, depression, contractures, constipation, bed sores. Emotional effects may be significant.

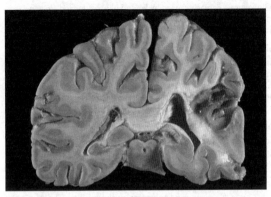

Fig. 18.1 Cerebral infarction (see Plate 92).

Reproduced with permission from Clinical Pathology (Oxford Core Texts), Carton, James, Daly, Richard, and Ramani, Pramila, Oxford University Press (2006).

Hypoxic ischaemic brain damage

Definition

- Global brain damage caused by limited blood flow and oxygen deprivation to the brain.
- It is also referred to as hypoxic ischaemic encephalopathy (HIE).

Epidemiology

- In children neonatal HIE is an important manifestation and related to hypoxic ischaemic damage around the time of birth (before, during, after). The incidence in developed countries is 1.5 per 1000 live births.
- In older children drowning and asphyxiation remain common and in adults the commonest setting is post cardiac arrest.

Aetiology

- It is the combination of hypoxia (reduced oxygen) and ischaemia (reduced energy supply), which causes the damage. The brain is relatively more resistant to hypoxia alone.
- Different brain regions have different susceptibilities to hypoxic ischaemic brain damage. They vary between the developing and the adult brain. This is termed **selective vulnerability**. The developing brain is relatively more resistant to hypoxia. In general, grey matter structures due to their high metabolic requirements are more susceptible (e.g. cerebral cortex, cerebellar cortex, basal ganglia, thalami). In the hippocampus, the CA1 region is well known for its selective vulnerability to hypoxia-ischaemia.

Presentation

- Reduced level of consciousness / coma in the acute stages.
- Persistent vegetative state (absence of higher cerebral functions with brainstem function retained) is a well known late sequela.

Macroscopy

- In the acute setting the brain is oedematous and there may be dusky discolouration of grey matter structures with blurring of the grey white matter borders (best seen along the cortical ribbon).
- In patients with prolonged survival the cortical ribbon may appear thinned with linear discoloration corresponding to cortical laminar necrosis (even within the cortex there are horizontal layers of neurons, which are more metabolically active and are affected first).

Histopathology

- In the first 48 hours there are ischaemic neuronal changes in aereas of susceptibility similar to those described in the early stages of cerebral infarction (see *Cerebral Infarction*).
- In long term survivors cortical laminar necrosis is a feature (necrosis of the more metabolically active layers of the cerebral cortex; Layers 3 and 5).

Intracerebral haemorrhage

Definition
- Spontaneous (non-traumatic) bleed into the substance of the brain.

Epidemiology
- Accounts for about 20% of strokes.
- Mostly occurs in late middle age.

Aetiology
- Hypertension is the commonest cause.
- Rarer causes include cerebral amyloid angiopathy, rupture of an arteriovenous malformation, and coagulation disorders.

Pathogenesis
- Most cases related to hypertension are due to ruptured Charcot-Bouchard microaneurysms.
- A haematoma forms which destroys the brain structure and causes a sudden rise in intracranial pressure.

Presentation
- Sudden onset of focal CNS signs related to the area of the haemorrhage together with symptoms and signs of raised intracranial pressure.
- Large haemorrhages are a common cause of sudden death due to a rapid rise in intracranial pressure and tonsillar herniation.
- Even small haemorrhages within the brainstem may cause sudden death if they disrupt areas vital for cardiorespiratory function.

Macroscopy (Fig. 18.2)
- A haematoma is seen replacing the underlying brain structure with associated mass effect (midline shift, herniation).
- Hypertensive bleeds typically involve deep brain structures (basal ganglia/internal capsule) but also pons or cerebellum.
- Bleeds related to other causes are more likely to be lobar (out in the lobes and less deep).

Histopathology
- Early lesions show blood clot surrounded by brain tissue characterized by hypoxic neuronal changes and oedema.
- Reactive astrocytes then proliferate and the damaged area organizes much like an area of infarction.
- Histological examination of the surrounding tissue may give important clues to the underlying cause of the haemorrhage (e.g hypertensive small vessel disease or cerebral amyloid angiopathy).

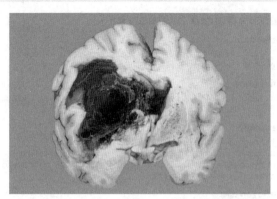

Fig. 18.2 Intracerebral haemorrhage. This is a slice of brain taken at post-mortem from a patient who suddenly collapsed and died. There is a massive intracerebral haematoma which led to a huge rise in intracranial pressure and herniation. The cause in this case was hypertension, and other changes of hypertension at post-mortem included left ventricular hypertrophy and nephrosclerosis of both kidneys (see Plate 93).

Reproduced with permission from *Clinical Pathology* (Oxford Core Texts), Carton, James, Daly, Richard, and Ramani, Pramila, Oxford University Press (2006).

Prognosis

Mortality is high (over 40%) due to effects of raised intracranial pressure.

Subarachnoid haemorrhage

Definition
- Primary subarachnoid haemorrhage is a spontaneous (non-traumatic) bleed into the subarachnoid space.

Epidemiology
- Incidence 8 per 100 000 per year.
- Most occur in adults aged 35–65.

Aetiology
- Most commonly due to rupture of a **berry aneurysm**.
- It has been hypothesized that a congenital defect in the tunica media of the cerebral vessels leads to aneurysm formation later in life due to atherosclerosis and hypertension.

Pathogenesis
- Most berry aneurysms arise at sites of arterial bifurcation at the base of the brain.
- Rupture of the aneurysm usually results in extensive bleeding through the subarachnoid space. The haemorrhage may extend into the brain tissue as well as the ventricular system.

Presentation
- Sudden severe headache often described as like 'being struck on the back of the head'.
- May be precipitated by exertion or straining.
- There may be loss of consciousness or instant death in severe cases.
! Complications, such as re-bleeding from the aneurysm, CSF malabsorption problems, and arterial vasospasm may cause further deterioration.

Macroscopy (Fig. 18.3)
- Blood is present within the subarachnoid space, often with abundant clot around the circle of Willis at the base of the brain.
- After clearing the blood clot, the ruptured berry aneurysm may be found in the circle of Willis.

Histopathology
- The aneurysm sac itself is composed of a thick fibrous intimal layer and an outer adventitial layer. No muscular media is present.

Prognosis
- One-third die instantly from tonsillar herniation caused by a massive rise in intracranial pressure.
- One-third become unconscious with a high risk of mortality or permanent neurological deficit.
- One-third have a good outcome provided there is no re-bleeding.

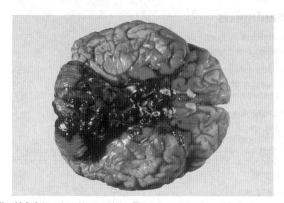

Fig. 18.3 Subarachnoid haemorrhage. This is the undersurface of the brain removed at post-mortem from a patient who suddenly cried out, collapsed, and died. Blood is seen filling the subarachnoid space. When the blood clot was cleared away, a ruptured berry aneurysm was found in the circle of Willis (see Plate 94).

Reproduced with permission from *Clinical Pathology* (Oxford Core Texts), Carton, James, Daly, Richard, and Ramani, Pramila, Oxford University Press (2006).

Meningitis

Definition

- Infection of the meninges.

Epidemiology

- Incidence of viral meningitis about 11 per 100 000 per year.
- Incidence of bacterial meningitis about 3 per 100 000 per year.

Microbiology

- Viruses are the most common cause, usually echoviruses or coxsackieviruses.
- Most cases of bacterial meningitis are caused by *N. meningitidis* or *S. pneumoniae*. *E. coli* and group B streptococci are important causes in neonates.

Pathogenesis

- Bacteria usually reach the meninges via the bloodstream from the nasal cavity, often following a viral upper respiratory tract infection.
- Both the meningococcus and the pneumococcus have capsules which render them resistant to phagocytosis and complement.
- The bacteria enter the subarachnoid space where the blood-brain barrier is weak (e.g. the choroid plexus).
- Once in the CSF, the bacteria multiply rapidly and stimulate an acute inflammatory response within the meninges.

Presentation

- Headache, fever, neck stiffness, photophobia.
- The symptoms are usually more severe in bacterial meningitis.

Microbiology

- Examination of CSF fluid obtained through lumbar puncture shows a predominance of lymphocytes in viral meningitis and many neutrophils in bacterial meningitis.
- Gram staining helps narrow down the likely cause in cases of bacterial meningitis.
- Culture of CSF and/or blood cultures should grow the causative organisms in cases of bacterial meningitis.
- No organism will be cultured in cases of viral meningitis.

Prognosis

- Viral meningitis usually runs a mild course with complete recovery.
- Bacterial meningitis is a much more serious, potentially life-threatening, infection if not treated early with appropriate antibiotics. Survivors of severe cases may be left with permanent neurological sequelae including hearing loss, learning difficulties, paralysis, and epilepsy.

Cerebral infections

Encephalitis

- Infection of the brain parenchyma.
- Viruses are the most common cause, usually herpes simplex virus.
- HSV encephalitis occurs following reactivation of the virus in the trigeminal ganglion, from which the virus can pass into the temporal lobe.
- Simultaneous perioral involvement may be a clue to the diagnosis.
- Presents with confusion, behavioural changes, and altered consciousness. Seizures may occur in severe cases.
- Brain imaging may highlight abnormalities in the temporal lobe.
- PCR on a CSF sample can identify the virus.
- Histologically there is a necrotizing inflammation with typical herpetic intranuclear inclusions within neurons and glial cells.
- ▶▶ Urgent antiviral treatment is essential.

Cerebral abscess

- Foci of infection associated with destruction of brain tissue.
- Usually bacterial infections, often with a mixture of organisms.
- Most arise by direct spread from an infection in a paranasal sinus, the middle ear, or a tooth.
- Can also arise from haematogenous spread, usually from septic emboli originating from infective endocarditis.
- Presents with symptoms of an infected intracranial mass i.e. headache, nausea, vomiting, fever, seizures, and localizing neurological signs.
- CT scanning is usually diagnostic.
- Treatment requires surgical drainage and prolonged antibiotics.
- Considerable risk of mortality (20%) and morbidity (50% of survivors are left with persistent neurological deficits or epilepsy).

Progressive multifocal leukoencephalopathy

- Caused by the JC virus of the polyoma group of papovaviruses.
- Seen almost exclusively in the immunocompromised.
- Infection causes multiple small foci of demyelination within white matter which may coalesce into larger cystic areas. Histologically viral inclusions are found within the enlarged nuclei of oligodendrocytes towards the periphery of demyelinated areas. The inclusions stain with SV40 antibody (which also labels JC virus). A striking feature (particularly in older lesions) is the presence of very large astrocytes with bizarre pleomorphic hyperchromatic nuclei.
- Diagnosis relies on presenting neurological features, characteristic brain MRI findings and presence of JC virus DNA in CSF.
- Progression is usually relentless and mortality may be up to 50% within the first 3 months. Treatment of the cause for the underlying immunosuppression can lead to remission of progressive multifocal leukoencephalopathy (PML). However, reconstitution of the immune system (e.g. in AIDS therapy) can occasionally result in an increased inflammatory response to the virus with exacerbation of disease.

Multiple sclerosis

Definition

- A relapsing and remitting demyelinating disease of the CNS in which episodes of neurological disturbance affect different parts of the CNS at different times.

Epidemiology

- Commonest demyelinating disease of the CNS.
- Peak age of onset age 20–30 years.
- Females slightly more commonly affected.
- Increased risk in family members, highest in monozygotic twins (30%).
- Striking geographical variation with annual incidence rates up to 1 in 500 at highest latitudes and near absence near the equator.

Aetiology

- Precise cause remains unknown but thought to involve a complex interaction of both environmental and genetic factors.
- It has been hypothesized that immune-mediated demyelination is trigged by an unknown pathogen (e.g. infective organism?) acquired during childhood or adolescence in genetically susceptible individuals.
- Candidate genes are involved with regulation of immune responses.
- More recently, sun exposure has been implicated as a factor for the geographical variation with vitamin D deficiency due to low ultraviolet light exposure. Vitamin D, a secosteroid, is known to influence the immune system and the expression of genes relevant to the disease.

Pathogenesis

- Episodes of demyelination lead to attacks of acute neurological deficit, which develop over a period of a few days and remain for a few weeks before symptom recovery.
- In the early stages of the disease, complete or almost complete recovery from an episode of demyelination is typical.
- As the disease progresses, recovery is slower and residual deficit remains as a critical threshold of axons die. Eventually extensive axonal death results in permanent neurological disability characteristic of progressive disease.

Presentation

- Symptoms may be highly variable depending on lesion site in the CNS.
- Blurred vision/loss of colour vision due to optic nerve demyelination.
- Vertigo and incoordination due to cerebellar demyelination.
- Eye movement disorders due to brainstem demyelination.
- Patchy numbness and tingling in a limb with progression to paraplegia, incontinence, and sexual dysfunction due to spinal cord demyelination.
- CSF examination typically shows oligoclonal bands (raised intrathecal immunoglobulin synthesis)

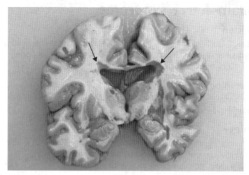

Fig. 18.4 Multiple sclerosis plaques. Brown appearance of multiple sclerosis plaques, seen here in a characteristic location around the lateral ventricles (arrows) (see Plate 95).

Reproduced with permission from *Clinical Pathology* (Oxford Core Texts), Carton, James, Daly, Richard, and Ramani, Pramila, Oxford University Press (2006).

Macroscopy (Fig. 18.4)

- Well circumscribed grey plaques are present most clearly seen within the CNS white matter (grey matter demyelination such as in the cortex does occur but is not readily seen macroscopically).
- Chronic plaques feel hardened / 'sclerosed' on palpation, hence the name 'multiple sclerosis'.
- Sites of predilection include the optic nerves, periventricular white matter, brainstem, and cervical spinal cord.

Histopathology

- Active plaques contain a prominent inflammatory infiltrate with destruction of myelin sheaths. There are sheets of macrophages containing myelin debris and there is perivascular lymphocytic inflammation.
- Established plaques show complete loss of myelin with a reduction in oligodendrocytes. There is relative preservation of axons. However, axonal loss does occur and may vary in extent. There is astrocytosis (reactive astrocytes), which is responsible for the firmness of the plaques. Astrocytosis or glial scarring is the equivalent of fibrous scarring elsewhere in the body.

Prognosis

- Most patients eventually suffer progressive disease where irreversible accumulation of disability is a key feature and complications related to this are common (pneumonia, urinary tract infections, pressure sores etc.). An overall reduction of life expectancy is recognized.
- A small proportion of patients can present with an aggressive form of MS ('Marburg's disease') where life expectancy can be weeks to months in the most severe cases.

Guillain–Barré syndrome

Definition
- Classical Guillain–Barré syndrome (GBS) is an acute demyelinating polyneuropathy which usually follows 1–2 weeks after an upper respiratory tract or gastrointestinal infection.

Epidemiology
- Rare disease.
- Annual incidence 1–2 per 100 000.

Aetiology
- Common triggers are *C. jejuni*, *Mycoplasma*, CMV, HIV, VZV, EBV.
- Other associations include vaccination, surgery, malignancy.
- In many cases no clear cause can be identified.

Pathogenesis
- Theories suggest that the immune response mounted to an antigen on a pathogen cross reacts with components of peripheral nerve, particularly myelin.
- Demyelination leads to an acute polyneuropathy.

Presentation
- Sudden onset of tingling and numbness of fingers and toes.
- Over a period of weeks, the weakness spreads proximally.
- Classical form is acute inflammatory demyelinating polyneuropathy (AIDP). Antibodies to gangliosides, basal lamina components, and several myelin proteins.
- 'Axonal' form increasingly recognized (acute motor axonal neuropathy or AMAN), more aggressive, more common in Japan and China. Immune target is the axon.
- Acute motor sensory axonal neuropathy (AMSAN) has more extensive sensory involvement.
- Miller Fisher syndrome has a triad of ataxia, areflexia, and ophthalmoplegia). Anti-GQ1b ganglioside autoantibodies are common.

! Progressive ventilatory failure is the main danger and ventilatory support may be required. Lumbar puncture typically shows increased CSF protein with a normal cell count (albuminocytological dissociation).

Prognosis
- Plasmapheresis and intravenous immunoglobulins reduce morbidity.
- >85% make a complete or near complete recovery.
- 10% are unable to walk unaided at 1 year.
- Modern mortality rates 1–2.5%.

Myasthenia gravis

Definition

- An autoimmune disease caused by production of autoantibodies directed against various antigens of the neuromuscular junction, typically the nicotinic acetylcholine receptor (nAChR) rarely MuSK (a tyrosine kinase receptor) and very rarely LRPP4 (low density lipoprotein receptor related protein 4).

Epidemiology

- Uncommon disease with annual incidence of 20 per 100 000.
- Mostly seen in women under 50 and men over 50 years old.

Aetiology

- Precisely what leads to production of the autoantibodies is unclear.
- Interestingly up to 75% of patients with nAChR autoantibodies have an abnormality of the thymus, either a neoplasm (thymoma) or hyperplasia. Thymectomy may help in these patients. The autoantibodies may be generated in the abnormal thymus.

Pathogenesis

- The nAChR is the receptor at the motor end plate through which the neurotransmitter acetylcholine acts to stimulate muscular contraction.
- Autoantibodies binding to the nAChR limit depolarization at the end plate and thus impair muscular contraction.
- MuSK is involved with clustering of nAChR, which is important for its normal function.

Presentation

- The key feature is muscular fatiguability.
- Muscle groups affected, in order are: extraocular, bulbar, face, neck, limb girdle, trunk.
- Symptoms can be very subtle and the diagnosis is easily missed or mistaken for other conditions.
- Lambert-Eaton myaesthenic syndrome is typically a paraneoplastic syndrome (most commonly associated with small cell carcinoma of the lung) and patients develop autoantibodies against voltage gated calcium channel on the presynaptic nerve terminal.
- There are also a rising number of very rare genetic mutations described as the cause of congenital myasthenic syndromes which may present later in life and may mimic myasthenia gravis.

Prognosis

- Most patients respond to medical treatment, which typically involves a combination of acetylcholinesterase inhibitors (such as pyridostigmine) and immunomodulatory therapies. Patients tend to have relapsing, but not progressive, symptoms.
- Patients with an aggressive form of thymoma may have a lower life expectancy.

Autoimmune encephalitis

Definition
- Inflammation of the brain parenchyma caused by the body's immune system attacking healthy cells and tissues.

Epidemiology
- Important cause of non-infectious encephalitis.
- Commonly tumour-associated (paraneoplastic manifestation of disease). There are well recognized associations of certain tumours with certain onconeuronal autoantibodies (e.g. NMDA receptor encephalitis and ovarian teratoma in young women).

Aetiology
- Autoimmune-mediated (attack by body's immune system).

Pathogenesis
- Some involve antibodies to intracellular antigens, such as anti-Hu. These have a strong tumour association with poor prognosis due to T-cell responses and irreversible neuronal killing. Antibodies not directly pathogenic but useful tumour markers.
- Some involve antibodies to extracellular antigens, such as the NMDA receptor. Variable tumour association and better prognosis. Antibodies thought to be directly pathogenic with reversible effects and little neuronal death.
- There are forms in which precise antigens are less clearly established.

Presentation
- Subacute presentation with decreased level of consciousness, fluctuation, and changes in cognition. Psychiatric manifestations and abnormal movements may also occur.
- Several distinct syndromes are recognized (e.g. 'stiff-person syndrome' with GAD65, GlyR, and amphiphysin autoantibodies).

Alzheimer's disease

Definition

- A neurodegenerative disease characterized clinically by dementia and histopathologically by neuronal loss in the cerebral cortex in association with numerous amyloid plaques and neurofibrillary tangles.

Epidemiology

- Most common cause of dementia.
- Increasing incidence with age (5% people >65, 20% of people >80).
- Represents an enormous social and financial burden to healthcare.

Aetiology

- Unknown in the vast majority of cases.
- The allele $\varepsilon 4$ of the apolipoprotein E gene (APOE) is a major risk factor for the disease. A single allele increases the risk of developing the disease threefold, two allelles increase it more than tenfold.
- A very small proportion of cases are familial, typically occurring in younger individuals and linked to autosomal dominant genetic mutations in genes such as amyloid precursor protein (APP) on chromosome 21, presenilin 1 (PSEN1) on chromosome 14 and presenilin 2 (PSEN2) on chromosome 1.
- Patients with Down's syndrome (trisomy 21) invariably develop Alzheimer's disease in later life. This is attributed to the presence of three copies of the APP gene on chromosome 21 resulting in increased production of $A\beta$.

Pathogenesis

- Current evidence suggests Alzheimer's disease is a 'proteinopathy' related to abnormal accumulation of $A\beta$ amyloid and the protein *tau*.
- $A\beta$ peptides are derived from APP by the action of secretase enzymes (presenilin forms part of the γ secretase complex).
- Precisely how $A\beta$ amyloid interacts with *tau* and how the accumulations leads to neuronal loss is unclear.
- Progression of tau pathology is more tightly linked to anatomical connections than progression of $A\beta$ pathology. This is probably responsible for the hierarchical distribution of the lesions ('march of the tangles') which forms the basis of the Braak neurofibrillary tangle staging.

Presentation

- Typically it begins with memory loss, particularly day-to-day memory and new learning which correlates to the early involvement of the medial temporal lobe and the hippocampus. Over time there is increasing disability in managing daily activities such as finances and shopping.
- Loss of motor skills then causes difficulty dressing, cooking, cleaning.
- Late in the disease there is agitation, restlessness, wandering, and disinhibition. This may cause considerable upset to family and carers.
- Terminal stages cause reduced speech, immobility, and incontinence.

- It is recognized that the disease has a long preclinical phase and there is an active search for biomarkers which might help with early diagnosis. Positron emission tomography (PET) scanning for amyloid in living persons is now possible and is one of the tests which might help in the appropriate clinical context. A variety of CSF biomarkers are also under evaluation.

Macroscopy (Fig. 18.5)

- Brain weight reduced, often to less than 1000 g.
- Cortical atrophy involving narrowing of gyri and widening of sulci, particularly in the medial temporal lobe and hippocampus.
- Compensatory enlargement of the temporal horns of the lateral ventricles is often seen with significant medial temporal lobe atrophy.

Histopathology

- There are positive and negative signs.
- The key microscopic features are the presence of abundant **neuritic plaques** and **neurofibrillary tangles** in the cerebral cortex (positive signs). The positive signs form the basis of the diagnostic criteria.
- There is associated loss of neurons and synapses, which is more difficult to measure on microscopy (negative signs).

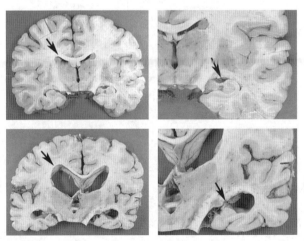

Fig. 18.5 Alzheimer's disease. The top images are from a normal patient aged 70, whilst the bottom images are from a patient with Alzheimer's disease. Note the ventricular dilation (left- hand side) and cortical atrophy in the brain from the patient with Alzheimer's disease, particularly marked in the hippocampus (right- hand side) (see Plate 96).

Reproduced with permission from *Clinical Pathology* (Oxford Core Texts), Carton, James, Daly, Richard, and Ramani, Pramila, Oxford University Press (2006).

- Neuritic plaques are spherical collections of tortuous neuritic processes surrounding a central amyloid core. The key component of the amyloid core is the Aβ protein.
- Neurofibrillary tangles are neuronal cytoplasmic inclusions composed of paired helical filaments, the main constituent of which is *tau* protein.
- Aβ deposits may also be found in the vessels (referred to as cerebral amyloid angiopathy). Varying amounts of vascular amyloid are present in Alzheimer's disease.

Prognosis
- Death occurs ~10 years from diagnosis, often from terminal pneumonia.

Vascular dementia

Definition

- A disease characterized clinically by dementia and histopathologically by injury to the brain parenchyma associated with a wide range of cerebrovascular lesions (e.g. diffuse white matter chronic ischaemic damage, multiple infarcts, strategic infarcts),

Epidemiology

- Common cause of dementia (estimated 4.2% of people >85).
- Cerebrovascular disease often not the sole cause of dementia. It frequently co-exists with other pathologies, particularly Alzheimer's.

Aetiology

- Risk factors similar to those for cerebrovascular disease or stroke.
- Hypertension and age linked to small vessel disease (arteriolosclerosis), the most common pathological substrate for vascular dementia.
- CADASIL (cerebral autosomal dominant arteriopathy with subcortical infarcts and leukoencephalopathy) is a rare genetic cause of small vessel disease due to mutations in the NOTCH3 gene.

Pathogenesis

- Small vessel disease (arteriolosclerosis) may cause chronic ischaemia and diffuse white matter injury (was known as Binswanger's disease).
- Multiple infarcts caused by vascular occlusion due to thrombosis or thromboemboli commonly due to atherosclerosis. Hypoperfusion may contribute.

Presentation

- Impairment of executive function and slowing of mental processing may be prominent, particularly with diffuse subcortical involvement. May be difficult to capture on standard cognitive testing (MMSE).
- May present with stepwise progression (multi-infarct dementia) and focal neurology (depending on infarct location).

Macroscopy

- Atherosclerosis affecting the Circle of Willis at the base of the brain.
- Small infarcts (lacunar infarcts) in the basal ganglia.
- Subtle findings such as loss of white matter bulk.
- Multiple large infarcts are relatively rare.
- Small strategic infarcts (e.g. thalamus) are also rare.

Histopathology

- Atherosclerosis (large vessels), arteriosclerosis (small vessels).
- Parenchymal damage: myelin pallor (diffuse ischaemic damage) with perivascular accentuation and microinfarcts.

Prognosis

Highly variable given the heterogenous nature of the disease.

Dementia with Lewy bodies

Definition

- A neurodegenerative disease characterized clinically by dementia and histopathologically by the presence of Lewy bodies in cortical and subcortical neurones.

Epidemiology

- Common cause of dementia (10–25% in hospital-based series).
- About 5% of people over 85 are affected.
- Slightly more common in men.

Aetiology

- Unknown.

Pathogenesis

- Presumably accumulation of Lewy bodies within neurones leads to damage and cellular loss.

Presentation

- Progressively worsening dementia very similar to Alzheimer's disease.
- Useful distinguishing features from Alzheimer's disease include fluctuating levels of cognition, recurrent visual hallucinations, features of parkinsonism and hypersensitivity to neuroleptics (antipsychotics, major tranquilizers). Autonomic nervous system problems (dysautonomia) and sleep disorders are also described.

Macroscopy

- Cerebral atrophy, particularly in the temporal and parietal lobes. May be similar to Alzheimer's disease but atrophy tends to be milder.
- Loss of pigment from the substantia nigra.

Histopathology

- Intracytoplasmic inclusions known as Lewy bodies are present within neurones of cortical grey matter and subcortical nuclei. Cortical Lewy bodies are best demonstrated by immunohistochemistry for α-synuclein or p62. Immunohistochemistry also labels Lewy neurites (neurites involved by synuclein pathology).
- Lewy bodies are composed of α-synuclein and other proteins such as ubiquitin, p62, and parkin.
- Changes typical of Alzheimer's (amyloid plaques and neurofibrillary tangles) are also often present though areas severely involved in Alzheimer's disease (e.g. the hippocampus) are usually spared.

Prognosis

- Highly variable, but survival following diagnosis is usually 5–7 years.

Parkinson's disease

Definition

- A neurodegenerative hypokinetic movement disorder characterized clinically by parkinsonism and histologically by neuronal loss and Lewy bodies concentrated in the substantia nigra.

Epidemiology

- Commonest hypokinetic movement disorder.
- Occurs mostly in the elderly.
- Higher incidence in men.
- Prevalence of 1% in people aged over 60.

Aetiology

- Unknown in the majority of cases.
- Rare cases are due to inherited mutations in *SNCA* on chromosome 4 which encodes α-synuclein, a component of Lewy bodies. Inherited mutations also found in a number of other genes including LRRK2, PARK2 (encoding parkin) and PINK1.
- Around 10% of cases thought to be familial.

Pathogenesis

- Neurones from the substantia nigra connect to the putamen and globus pallidus where they release dopamine and control movement.
- Lack of dopamine release results in movement disorder.
- It is recognized that other parts of the nervous system are involved resulting in the additional symptoms (see next).
- One hypothesis advocates the caudorostral progression of pathology from the enteric nervous system and olfactory bulb to the lower brainstem and then up to the neocortex along a network of interconnecting neurons (possible even with 'prion-like' propagation).

Presentation

- Onset is typically unilateral (e.g. 'pill rolling' tremor at rest).
- Classic triad of tremor, rigidity, and bradykinesia (parkinsonism).
- Autonomic dysfunction, cognitive neurobehavioural disturbances, and sleep dysfunction are also common. Rapid eye movement (REM) sleep behaviour disorder may precede parkinsonism.
- Dysphagia may be seen with disease progression.
- Patients may develop dementia (overlap with Dementia with Lewy bodies; if clinical onset one year after parkinsonism it is called Parkinson's Disease with Dementia).

! Note that parkinsonism is not specific to Parkinson's disease; it merely reflects dysfunction of the substantia nigra system. Other causes of parkinsonism include drugs, toxins, infections, trauma.

Macroscopy (Fig. 18.6)

- Pallor of the substantia nigra and locus ceruleus.
- Brain weight within normal limits for age.

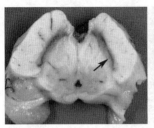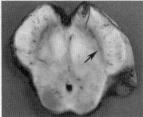

Fig. 18.6 Substantia nigra in Parkinson's disease. Slices through the midbrain of a normal person (left) and a patient with Parkinson's disease (right) showing loss of pigmentation in the substantia nigra in Parkinson's disease (arrows) (see Plate 97).

Reproduced with permission from *Clinical Pathology* (Oxford Core Texts), Carton, James, Daly, Richard, and Ramani, Pramila, Oxford University Press (2006).

Histopathology

- Loss of pigmented neurones from the substantia nigra in the midbrain and locus ceruleus in the pons; dorsal motor nucleus of the vagus nerve in the medulla may also be affected (clinical correlate: parasympathetic nervous system effects).
- Residual neurones contain intracytoplasmic inclusions known as Lewy bodies. Immunohistochemistry for α-synuclein labels Lewy bodies. It also labels Lewy neurites, which show abnormal α-synuclein deposition.
- Other regions may be involved (e.g. cerebral cortex, autonomic nervous system). Alpha-synuclein pathology has been demonstrated in the gut (enteric nervous system) of Parkinson's disease patients. The possibility of diagnosing Parkinson's disease or its early stages based on gut biopsies is an active area of research.

Prognosis

- Treatment with dopaminergic drugs eases symptoms of parkinsonism but does not slow the progression of the disease. Patients on long term treatment with levodopa (commonest medication used for the disease) develop severe dyskinesias (involuntary flailing or jerking body movements) as a side effect.
- Deep brain stimulation of the subthalamic nucleus works by rebalancing aspects of the basal ganglia circuit and is helpful in a small number of selected patients with severe tremor.
- Loss of balance may cause falls and difficulty swallowing may cause aspiration pneumonia.
- The speed of progression varies considerably between individuals.

Huntington's disease

Definition
- An inherited neurodegenerative disorder caused by mutation of the *HTT* gene.

Epidemiology
- Worldwide prevalence 5–10 per 100 000 population but there is considerable geographical variability.
- Most cases present between 35–45 years but can occur at any age.
- Men and women are affected equally.
- Inherited in an autosomal dominant fashion.

Genetics
- HTT contains a sequence of CAG trinucleotide repeats which usually number less than 36.
- Mutant HTT has more than 36 trinucleotide repeats. The higher the number of trinucleotide repeats, the fuller the penetrance and the younger the age of onset.
- Instability of the repeat sequences tends to result in their expansion in each successive generation, a phenomenon known as **anticipation**.

Pathogenesis
- Huntingtin, the protein coded by HTT, interacts with many other proteins and has many biological functions. It is expressed in all cells but is present in highest concentration in the brain and testis.
- Mutated huntingtin is thought to be cytotoxic to certain cell types, most notably neurones in the caudate nucleus and putamen.

Presentation
- Uncontrolled, random, jerky movements (chorea).
- Over time there is motor, neuropsychiatric, and cognitive decline, ultimately terminating in dementia.

Macroscopy
- Striking atrophy of the caudate nucleus and putamen.
- Cortical atrophy may also be present.

Histopathology
- Marked neuronal loss from the caudate nucleus.
- Surviving neurones contain intranuclear dot-like inclusions composed of huntingtin protein aggregates.

Prognosis
- Survival is on average 20 years from onset of symptoms but this is dependent on the length of triplet repeat.
- Death is usually due to pneumonia or cardiac failure (abnormal huntingtin is expressed in cardiac muscle). Suicides are a recognized feature in this patient group.

Motor neurone disease

Definition
- A group of neurodegenerative also known as amyotrophic lateral sclerosis (ALS) diseases characterized by selective loss of motor neurones.

Epidemiology
- Annual incidence 1–5 people per 100 000.
- Men slightly more commonly involved than women.
- Most present between ages 50–70 years old.

Aetiology
- Large proportion of cases are idiopathic with no clear cause.
- ~10% are inherited with a Mendelian pattern.
- Largest group of genetically determined ALS in both sporadic and familial ALS setting is due to an intronic hexanucleotide repeat expansion in *C9ORF72* (European founder mutation).
- A number of other genes have been linked to familial motor neurone disease including *SOD1*, *TDP-43*, and *FUS*.

Pathogenesis
- Little is still known, though research into familial cases has provided interesting insights into the disease.
- *TDP-43* and *FUS* are both RNA/DNA binding proteins with very similar molecular structures.
- Theories suggest that defects in RNA metabolism may be a key event leading to motor neurone degeneration.

Presentation
- Asymmetric weakness, wasting, fasciculation, and spasticity of limb muscles.
- Difficulty swallowing, chewing, speaking, coughing, and breathing.
- Cognitive changes may also occur (overlap with frontotemporal dementia)

Macroscopy
- Anterior roots of the spinal cord appear grey and thinned.

Histopathology
- Selective loss of motor neurones is seen within the motor cortex and anterior horns of the spinal cord.
- The hypoglossal nucleus in the medulla may be selectively affected
- In most sporadic cases, residual motor neurons contain inclusions with TDP-43. Inclusions are also labelled with p62 and ubiquitin.
- Cases linked to C9ORF72 mutations also show TDP-43 pathology. Additional p62 positive inclusions are present, particularly in the hippocampus and the cerebellar granule cell layer.

Prognosis
- The disease is usually progressive and fatal within a few years.
- Death is usually from aspiration pneumonia.

Creutzfeldt–Jacob disease

Definition
- A spongiform encephalopathy caused by accumulation of an abnormal form of prion protein (PrP) which is resistant to proteinase breakdown.

Epidemiology
- Rare, but the most common human prion disease.
- Annual incidence of about 1 per 1,000,000.

Aetiology
- Sporadic cases are thought to be due to chance spontaneous conversion of PrP into the abnormal form.
- Familial cases are due to inherited mutations in the *PRP* gene which predispose the protein to converting into the abnormal form.
- Variant Creutzfeldt–Jacob disease (CJD) is thought to be transmitted through consumption of beef contaminated with abnormal PrP derived from cows with BSE.

Pathogenesis
- Presence of abnormal PrP promotes refolding of normal native PrP proteins into the abnormal form.
- An exponential increase in abnormal PrP results in cell death.

Presentation
- Sporadic CJD typically presents in the middle aged and elderly with an obvious neurological illness that follows a rapidly progressive course.
- Variant CJD is clinically distinct. It affects younger people aged under 30 and initially presents with psychiatric symptoms followed by cerebellar ataxia and dementia.

Histopathology
- Sporadic CJD is associated with vacuolation of grey matter (spongiform change) with neuronal loss and gliosis.
- Variant CJD also shows spongiform change, neuronal loss, and gliosis together with numerous so-called 'florid plaques' composed of deposits of amyloid forms of PrP.
- Florid plaques are the neuropathological hallmark of variant CJD and do not occur in other forms of CJD.

! Given the transmissible nature of prion disease special precautions are taken for patients with suspected CJD if they undergo surgery, particularly brain surgery. Special precautions also apply to suspected CJD autopsy cases.

Prognosis
- No specific treatment currently exists and the disease is usually fatal.

Astrocytoma (including glioblastoma)

Definition

- CNS tumours formed by glial cells showing astrocytic differentiation.
- Include the common diffusely infiltrative astrocytomas (e.g. glioblastoma) as well as the less common low grade circumscribed variants (e.g. pilocytic astrocytoma). Biologically these two groups are distinct. The diffusely infiltrative astrocytomas are subdivided by degree of malignancy into diffuse astrocytoma (WHO grade II), anaplastic astrocytoma (WHO grade III) and glioblastoma (WHO grade IV).
- The diffusely infiltrative astrocytomas are further subdivided into IDH (isocitrate dehydrogenase)-wildtype and IDH-mutant astrocytomas (e.g. glioblastoma, IDH-wildtype, WHO grade IV).

Epidemiology

- Diffusely infiltrating astrocytomas are the most frequent primary CNS tumours (60% primary CNS tumours) and glioblastoma (GBM) is the most common tumour in this subgroup (incidence: 3–4/100 000). 90% of glioblastomas are IDH-wildtype. In comparison, the majority of lower grade diffuse astrocytomas are IDH-mutant.
- On average, grade correlates directly with age of presentation (pilocytic astrocytoma (WHO grade I) in childhood and adolescence, diffuse astrocytoma (WHO grade II) in young adults and GBM (WHO grade IV) in the sixth decade).

Aetiology

- The majority of tumours are sporadic (previous irradiation plays a role in an insignificant fraction of tumours).
- Increased risk of astrocytomas in neurofibromatosis type 1 (mostly pilocytic astrocytomas of the optic pathways).
- Very rare glioblastomas due to inherited tumour syndromes (e.g. TP53 mutations in Li Fraumeni syndrome).

Pathogenesis

- It is suggested that malignant gliomas arise from neural stem or progenitor cells. It is thought that the tumours maintain a primitive population of cells responsible for repopulating tumours as they grow.
- Astrocytomas with IDH mutations (Fig 18.7) are biologically distinct from IDH wild type astrocytomas. IDH mutations are common in grade II and III diffusely infiltrative gliomas (astrocytomas and oligodendrogliomas) and are present in 70–80% of them. 90% of IDH-mutated tumours harbour a hotspot mutation within codon 132 leading to an amino acid substitution from arginine to histidine (R132H). IDH mutations result in the production of an oncometabolite (2-hydroxygutarate) which leads to a hypermethylator phenotype.
- It is believed that IDH mutations occur early on in the development of diffuse gliomas and that further genetic alterations determine whether the tumour shows astrocytic (TP53 and *ATRX* mutations) or oligodendroglial differentiation (1p19q losses).

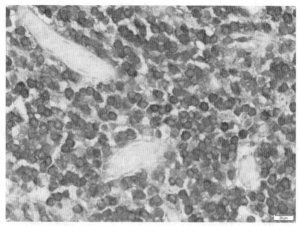

Fig. 18.7 Astrocytoma demonstrating IDH mutation by immunohistochemistry (see Plate 98).

Reproduced with permission *from Clinical Pathology* (Oxford Core Texts), Carton, James, Daly, Richard, and Ramani, Pramila, Oxford University Press (2006).

- IDH mutations are seen in secondary GBMs, which arise from lower grade diffuse astrocytomas. They are typically absent from primary (*de novo*) GBMs, which commonly show *EGFR* amplifications.
- Evolution from grade II astrocytomas into higher grade tumours is characterized by mutations in *CDKN2A* and *RB*.
- Methylation of the promoter of the *MGMT* gene is associated with increased progression free survival of adult GBMs and a better response to temozolamide (standard alkylating chemotherapy agent).
- A tandem duplication or fusion event between the *KIAA1549* and *BRAF* genes is the most common genetic alteration in pilocytic astrocytomas. It results in constitutive activation of the *MAPK/ERK* signalling pathway.
- Fig 18.7 Astrocytoma demonstrating IDH mutation by immunohistochemistry.

Presentation

- Focal neurology is related to tumour location (e.g. weakness, sensory, visual symptoms). GBM typically occurs in the cerebral hemispheres.
- Seizures may be the main or only symptom in low grade tumours.
- As tumours progress increased intracranial pressure symptoms (headaches, vomiting) develop due to mass effect.
- Primary GBMs present with a short history (months, even weeks) and increased intracranial pressure symptoms early on.

Macroscopy

- GBMs are poorly delineated grey-pink tumours with central areas of yellowish necrosis (Fig 18.8).
- Lower grade diffusely infiltrative astrocytomas typically enlarge and distort involved brain structures. They may be firm to the touch.

- Pilocytic astrocytomas are relatively well circumscribed often cystic tumours.

Histopathology

- Diffuse astrocytoma (WHO grade II) shows a mild to moderate increase in glial cellularity compared to normal brain and mild nuclear atypia. There may be microcystic change.
- Anaplastic astrocytoma (WHO grade III) is more cellular with greater nuclear atypia and presence of significant mitotic activity.
- Glioblastoma (WHO grade IV) is a highly aggressive neoplasm composed of atypical astrocytes similar to those seen in anaplastic astrocytoma but with superadded areas of necrosis and / or microvascular proliferation (Fig. 18.9).
- Pilocytic astrocytoma shows a biphasic pattern of compact areas with bipolar astrocytes and loose areas with multipolar astrocytes. Rosenthal fibres are typically seen in the compact areas. Mitoses are rare.
- The concept of integrated diagnosis specifically refers to integrating the histological and molecular data to arrive at an integrated diagnosis. In neuropathology this can be represented using the following 'layered diagnosis' format using the example of an IDH-mutant glioblastoma:
  - *Layered diagnosis*
  - **Integrated diagnosis:** *glioblastoma, IDH-mutant (WHO grade IV)*
  - **Histological diagnosis:** *glioblastoma*
  - **Histological grade:** *WHO grade IV*
  - **Molecular data:** *IDH1 R132H mutation confirmed, no 1p/ 19q-codeletion.*

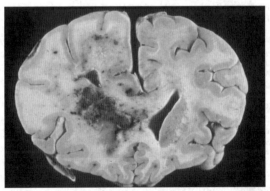

Fig. 18.8 Glioblastoma. This is a section of the brain from a patient who presented with signs of raised intracranial pressure, rapidly deteriorated, and died. There is an ill-defined tumour with areas of haemorrhage. Microscopy revealed this to be a glioblastoma which was much more extensive than was apparent macroscopically (see Plate 99).

Reproduced with permission from *Clinical Pathology* (Oxford Core Texts), Carton, James, Daly, Richard, and Ramani, Pramila, Oxford University Press (2006).

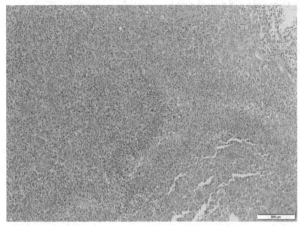

Fig. 18.9 Glioblastoma multiforme histology characterized by atypical astrocytes showing areas of palisading necrosis (see Plate 100).

Prognosis

- Average survival for diffuse astrocytoma (WHO grade II) is about 5 years. For anaplastic astrocytomas (WHO grade III) it is reduced to about 3 years and for GBMs it is less than 1 year. With gold standard treatment (surgery plus chemoradiotherapy) the 2-year survival can reach ~20–25% and 3-year survival ~10%. IDH-mutant diffuse astrocytomas have a better survival when compared to IDH-wildtype astrocytomas of a similar grade.
- Long survival is the rule for pilocytic astrocytoma (95% 5-year survival).

Oligodendroglioma

Definition

- Diffusely infiltrative CNS tumours formed by glial cells showing oligodendroglial differentiation. They are subdivided by degree of malignancy into 'classical' oligodendrogliomas (WHO grade II) and anaplastic oligodendrogliomas (WHO grade III).
- IDH mutations and 1p/19q co-deletions are entity-defining, hence the formal designation of 'oligodendroglioma, IDH-mutant and 1p/19q-codeleted'. There are rare exceptions (paediatric setting).

Epidemiology

- Majority occur in adults (peak incidence: 30–60 years of age).
- 2.5% of all primary brain tumours and 5–6% of all gliomas.

Aetiology

- The tumours are generally sporadic (previous irradiation plays a role in an insignificant fraction of tumours).

Pathogenesis

- Thought to derive from neural stem or progenitor cells similar to diffuse astroglial tumours. IDH mutations are believed to be an early event in tumourigenesis and are shared with low grade diffuse astrocytomas.
- They show co-deletions of chromosomal arms 1p and 19q, CIC, and FUBP1 mutations in addition to IDH mutations.
- Progression to anaplastic histology is associated with the loss of 9p and 10q and mutations in CDKN2A.

Presentation

- Most occur in the cerebral hemisphere. They frequently involve the cortex and hence seizures are the most common presenting symptom. Focal neurological deficits, headaches, and other signs of increased intracranial pressure may also occur.

Macroscopy

- Well circumscribed greyish pink tumours with areas of mucoid change, cystic degeneration, focal haemorrhage, and calcification.

Histopathology

- Oligodendroglioma (WHO grade II) is composed of cells resembling normal oligodendrocytes with round nuclei and fine chromatin surrounded by clear cytoplasm. There is a fine network of branching (chicken-wire) capillaries. Calcification is very commonly seen.
- Anaplastic oligodendroglioma (WHO grade III) is an oligodendroglial neoplasm in which there are areas of higher cellularity, atypia and increased mitotic activity.

Prognosis

- Average survival for grade II tumours is 10 years and for grade III tumours 2–3 years.

Ependymoma

Definition
- CNS tumour composed of neoplastic ependymal cells arising from the ependymal-lined ventricular system or the spinal canal.
- Subdivided by degree of malignancy into 'classical' ependymomas (WHO grade II) and anaplastic ependymomas (WHO grade III).

Epidemiology
- Account for approximately 6% of intracranial gliomas.
- Occur at any age, more frequently in childhood and adolescence.
- In adults most arise in the spinal cord.
- In children most arise around the 4th ventricle.

Aetiology
- The majority of tumours are sporadic.
- Neurofibromatosis type 2 (NF2) is associated with the occurrence of spinal ependymomas

Pathogenesis
- Current data favours an origin from neural stem or progenitor cells, particularly region-specific radial glia.
- The most common genetic alterations involve chromosome 22.
- Genomic studies have shown a complex landscape of mutations the clinical significance of which is still being evaluated.

Presentation
- Symptoms depend on tumour location.
- Posterior fossa ependymomas often present with nausea, vomiting, and headache related to hydrocephalus due to obstruction of the 4th ventricle. Cerebellar symptoms may also be present. Spinal ependymomas present with motor and sensory disturbances depending on which tracts are involved.

Macroscopy
- Grey-red, lobulated, and usually well demarcated tumours.
- There is often a relationship to a ventricular cavity.
- Some ependymomas may spread widely throughout the CSF.

Histopathology
- Ependymomas are composed of cells with regular plump oval nuclei and fibrillary processes. The cells may form glandular structures (rosettes) and perivascular pseudorosettes in which the cell radially arranged around blood vessels.
- Anaplastic ependymomas (WHO grade III) show increased cellularity and significant mitotic activity. Necrosis and microvascular proliferation may also be present.

Prognosis
- Children with posterior fossa tumours have 5-year survival of about 50%. Outcome for adult patients with spinal tumours is better.

Meningioma

Definition

- Tumours from meningothelial (arachnoid cap) cells and attached to the inner surface of the dura mater.
- Majority are benign and correspond to WHO grade I.
- Certain histological subtypes are associated with less favourable outcome and correspond to WHO grade II (atypical) and very rarely grade III (anaplastic).

Epidemiology

- 13–25% of primary intracranial tumours and 25% of intraspinal tumours.
- Most occur in adults between the ages of 20 to 60.
- More common in females.

Aetiology

- The majority are sporadic tumours.
- Irradiation is a risk factor. There were a number of patients previously irradiated for tinea capitis (fungal scalp infection) who developed meningiomas. This treatment is no longer used.
- Radiation-induced meningiomas are more commonly multiple and show atypical or anaplastic morphology.
- Multiple meningiomas may occur in patients with neurofibromatosis 2.

Pathogenesis

- The most common molecular alterations in meningiomas are loss of chromosome 22q and mutations in the NF2 gene.
- As meningiomas increase in histological grade they may acquire loss of the short arm of chromosome 1, long arms of chromosomes 10 and 14 and 9p21 deletions.

Presentation

- Meningiomas are typically slow growing tumours and produce symptoms and signs by compression of adjacent structures. Deficits depend on the location of the tumour. Headaches and seizures are common symptoms more generally.

Macroscopy (Fig. 18.10)

- Most are smooth lobulated well circumscribed tumours with homogeneous cream beige cut surface. They are adherent to the dura mater and compress rather than invade the underlying brain.
- They may infiltrate the overlying skull or induce hyperostosis (thickening of the bone).

Histopathology

- Classical meningiomas are syncytial tumours composed of lobules and whorls of meningothelial cells. Calcified round concretions (psammoma bodies) may be present. However, the histology may vary considerably.

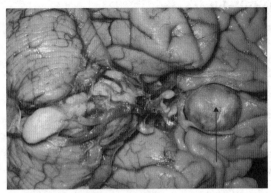

Fig. 18.10 Meningioma. this very well- circumscribed tumour (arrow) has the typical macroscopic appearance of a meningioma, a suspicion that was confirmed microscopically (see Plate 101).

Reproduced with permission from *Clinical Pathology* (Oxford Core texts), Carton, James, Daly, richard, and ramani, Pramila, Oxford University Press (2006).

- Atypical meningiomas (WHO grade II) typically show increased mitotic activity and a specific combination of other features (e.g. tumour cell necrosis, hypercellularity).
- Anaplastic meningiomas (WHO grade III) show significantly increased mitotic activity and severe pleomorphism. They may be barely recognizable as meningiomas.

Prognosis

- Benign meningiomas (the majority) have a low risk of recurrence following surgical resection.
- Atypical meningiomas have a higher rate of local recurrence and so may require radiotherapy following surgical excision.
- Anaplastic meningiomas are aggressive malignant tumours.

Medulloblastoma

Definition
• A primitive embryonal tumour of the cerebellum (WHO grade IV).

Epidemiology
• Most common malignant primary brain tumour in children, rare in adults (10–20% of primary paediatric brain tumours, less than 2% of brain tumours overall).

Aetiology
• Most are sporadic but rare examples are inherited (e.g. in patients with Gorlin's syndrome, *PTCH* mutations), Turcot's syndrome (*APC* mutations) and Li Fraumeni syndrome (*TP53* mutations).

Pathogenesis
• There are four molecular subgroups of medulloblastomas, each with significant clinical and pathological associations. Group 1 (WNT activation) with best clinical outcome, group 2 (SHH activation) with good/intermediate outcome and groups 3 with poor outcome and 4 with intermediate/poor outcome.
• Abnormalities affecting chromosome 17 are most common and are concentrated in medulloblastoma subgroups 3 and 4.
• *MYCC* and *MYCN* amplifications are linked with poor prognosis.
• Histogenesis is complex and may vary for the different subgroups. For Group 2 the cerebellar external granule cell layer has been postulated as the source of progenitor cells and for Group 1 dorsal brainstem progenitor cells.

Presentation
• Hydrocephalus (increased intracranial pressure, headache, vomiting). Cerebellar signs may be present.

Macroscopy
• Childhood medulloblastomas are typically located in the midline (vermis), rare adult tumours in the cerebellar hemispheres.
• Many are circumscribed, pink or grey, with areas of haemorrhage or necrosis. Texture may vary from soft to firm.
• There may be evidence of CSF dissemination.

Histopathology
• Highly cellular tumour composed of mitotically active small cells with hyperchromatic nuclei and scant cytoplasm ('small round blue cell tumour').

Prognosis
• Like all embryonal tumours the tumour grows rapidly and is fatal without treatment. The overall prognosis with modern therapy is favourable depending on tumour stage, subtype and extent of surgical resection (overall 5-year survival about 75%).

Primary central nervous system (CNS) lymphomas

Definition
- Primary extranodal lymphomas arising in the CNS.

Epidemiology
- Incidence has increased from around 1% to around 6% of primary intracranial neoplasms, mainly due to the AIDS epidemic.
- CNS involvement also occurs in 22% of post-transplant lymphomas, whereby about 55% are confined to the CNS.
- Typically occurs in two distinct groups: in **immunocompetent** individuals the peak incidence is from 50 to 70, in **immunocompromised** individuals it is typically seen at a younger age.

Aetiology
- Inherited or acquired immunodeficiency increases the risk of primary CNS lymphoma.
- Epstein-Barr virus plays a role in immunocompromised patients.

Pathogenesis
- Histogenetic origin in immunocompetent patients is a late germinal centre exit B cells (as evidenced by transcriptional profile).
- Epstein-Barr virus is expressed in virtually all AIDS and transplant-associated CNS lymphomas.

Presentation
- Symptoms may vary considerably and tumours may present with focal neurological deficits, neuropsychiatric symptoms, increased intracranial pressure and seizures.

Macroscopy
- Single or multiple masses in the cerebral hemispheres, often deep-seated and close of the ventricles. Lesions are typically ill-circumscribed, grey to yellow and fleshy. There may be haemorrhages and necrosis. There may be CSF involvement.

Histopathology
- More than 95% of primary CNS lymphomas are diffuse large B cell lymphomas composed of large atypical B lymphocytes. Tumour cells typically show an angiocentric pattern of arrangement.
- 2 Lymphocytes are highly susceptible to steroid-induced apoptosis. Steroids are commonly given to patients with brain tumours to help reduce oedema. Tissue diagnosis may be difficult in this situation as they tumour may have temporarily 'vanished'. Steroids are avoided pre-biopsy.

Prognosis
- Median survival of primary CNS lymphoma (diffuse large B cell lymphoma) of 2.5 to 5 years with radiotherapy and chemotherapy (especially methotrexate).

Cerebral metastases

Definition
- Tumours with origin outside the CNS which spread secondarily to the CNS via the haematogenous route. Rarely there may be direct invasion from adjacent tissues as opposed to metastatic disease.

Epidemiology
- Metastatic tumours are the most common CNS neoplasms.
- In autopsy studies CNS metastases are found in about 25% of patients who die of cancer.

Origin of CNS metastases
- Most common brain metastases in adults in descending order are from lung cancer (particularly small cell and adenocarcinoma), breast cancer, melanoma, renal cancer, and colon cancer.
- In children they arise from leukaemia, lymphoma, osteogenic sarcoma, rhabdomyosarcoma, and Ewing's sarcoma.

Pathogenesis
- Tumours typically spread to the CNS via the haematogenous route. Metastases tend to arise at the grey-white matter junction.
- Leptomeningeal, dural, and spinal epidural metastases may also occur.
- There may be isolated CSF involvement (malignant meningitis).

! Primary tumours may involve the CNS via 'remote' effects and there are a variety of paraneoplastic syndromes involving antibodies to tumour antigens which cross-react with normal CNS autoantigens).

Presentation
- Raised intracranial pressure or local effect of the tumour on the adjacent brain tissue.
- Patients may also present with seizures, infarcts, or intra-tumoural haemorrhage.

Macroscopy
- Typically well circumscribed rounded grey white or tan masses with variable necrosis and significant peritumoural oedema.
- Haemorrhage is often seen with choriocarcinoma, melanoma, and renal cell carcinoma.
- Melanoma may appear dark brown/black due to pigment content.

Histopathology
- Histology resembles the primary tumours from which they arise.
- Immunohistochemistry is used for metastases of unknown primary origin to aid with identification of the site of origin.

Prognosis
- Best outcome with surgical resection and/or radiotherapy is achieved in young patients with good performance status, single brain metastasis, and no extracranial metastases.

Multisystem diseases

Systemic lupus erythematosus

Definition
- A multisystem autoimmune disease characterized by autoantibody production against a number of nuclear and cytoplasmic autoantigens.

Epidemiology
- Incidence of 4 per 100 000 people per year.
- Most cases occur in women of childbearing age.
- More common in Africans and Asians.

Aetiology
- Current working theory is that defective phagocytosis of apoptotic bodies leads to priming of the immune system to intracellular self-antigens.

Pathogenesis
- Activation of autoreactive B and T cells leads to formation of immune complexes between autoantibodies and self-antigens.
- Immune complexes cause prolonged stimulation of interferon production by plasmacytoid dendritic cells in tissues.
- Chronic activation of the interferon system drives ongoing chronic inflammation and tissue damage in multiple organs systems.

Presentation
- Numerous possible manifestations, depending on sites of involvement.
- Fatigue, weight loss, and low-grade fever are common.
- Joint involvement causes arthralgia.
- Skin involvement causes scaly red lesions on sun-exposed sites.
- Pulmonary involvement causes pleural effusion, pneumonitis, and pulmonary fibrosis.
- Renal involvement causes glomerulonephritis (lupus nephritis), leading to CKD.
- Haematological involvement causes anaemia, lymphopenia, and thrombocytopenia.

Immunology
- >95% have anti-nuclear antibodies.
- 60% have anti-double-stranded DNA antibodies.
- 20–30% have anti-Smith antigen antibodies.
- 20–30% have antiphospholipid antibodies which cause a hypercoagulable state.

Histopathology
- Skin biopsies from involved skin show an interface dermatitis with vacuolar degeneration and apoptosis of basal keratinocytes.
- Renal biopsies from patients with renal disease show various type of immune complex glomerulonephritis.

Prognosis
- 15-year survival from diagnosis is 80%.
- Deaths are usually related to severe renal and lung involvement.

Systemic sclerosis

Definition
- A multisystem autoimmune disease in which fibrous tissue accumulates in multiple organs.

Epidemiology
- Rare disease with an annual incidence of 2–10 per million.
- Most cases arise in women aged 30–40y.

Aetiology
- Unknown.

Pathogenesis
- An abnormal immune response to an unidentified trigger results in production of cytokines such as IL-4 and TGF-β that stimulate collagen deposition by fibroblasts.

Presentation
- **Limited systemic sclerosis** (SS) usually starts with long-standing Raynaud's phenomenon. Then there is gradual tightening and thickening of the skin of the fingers, face, and neck. Calcium deposition is common, particularly in the finger pads. Small bowel involvement and pulmonary hypertension may occur as late complications after 10–15y.
- **Diffuse systemic sclerosis** presents more abruptly with widespread skin thickening, contractures, and skin ulcers. Visceral involvement occurs early with pulmonary fibrosis. An important complication is severe hypertension, leading to acute renal failure ('scleroderma renal crisis').

Immunology
- Anti-nuclear antibodies present in 65%.
- Anti-centromere antibodies present in 70–80% of limited SS.
- Anti-topoisomerase (Scl70) antibodies present in 40% of diffuse SS.

Prognosis
- No cure at present.
- Immunosuppressive regimes are used for organ involvement or progressive skin disease.
- Deaths are usually related to renal and lung disease.

Sarcoidosis

Definition
- A multisystem disease of unknown cause in which tissues are infiltrated by granulomas.

Epidemiology
- Prevalence of 10–20 per 100 000 population in the UK.
- Peak age of onset 20–40y.
- Those of African descent tend to show more severe disease.

Aetiology
- Unknown though mounting evidence indicates environmental and microbial antigens may trigger the disease.

Pathogenesis
- Antigen is presented to T cells via antigen-presenting cells resulting in activation and T helper (Th) 1 polarization.
- Th1 cells stimulate monocytes to form non-caseating granulomas in involved tissues.
- Proliferation of regulatory T cells elsewhere result in immunological anergy with T cell lymphopenia and reduced delayed-type hypersensitivity reactions.

Presentation
- Although any organ may be involved, the lungs and lymph nodes are the most common sites of disease.
- Presentation may be incidental on chest radiography or with symptoms such as cough or breathlessness or skin lesions.
- Acute sarcoidosis is a distinct form which presents suddenly with erythema nodosum, anterior uveitis, and cranial nerve VII palsy and has a good prognosis.

Histopathology
- Involved tissues contain non-necrotizing granulomas.
- The typical sarcoidal granuloma is well circumscribed with only minimal associated lymphoid inflammation (so-called 'naked' granulomas).
- Variable degrees of fibrosis may accompany the granulomas.
- No other explanation for the presence of granulomas can be found (e.g. pathogens, foreign material, tumour).

Prognosis
- Overall good prognosis with >70% of patients showing no significant disease on treatment.
- A minority develop long term disease which is difficult to treat leading to progressive lung fibrosis and respiratory failure.

Vasculitis

Definition

- A group of conditions in which inflammation and damage to blood vessels is the primary underlying pathology.

Polyarteritis nodosa (PAN)

- A systemic medium-vessel vasculitis, leading to areas of aneurysm formation and narrowing in involved vessels.
- A rare disease if diagnostic criteria are strictly applied.
- Main organs involved are the gastrointestinal (GI) tract (abdominal pain), nervous system (peripheral nerve palsies), and muscles (muscle aches).
- Imaging showing areas of vessel narrowing and aneurysm formation is highly suggestive. Biopsy proof of a necrotizing vasculitis is also helpful.

Granulomatosis with polyangiitis (GPA)

- A systemic ANCA-associated vasculitis characterized by dominant upper respiratory tract, lung, and renal involvement and cANCA positivity.
- Formally known as Wegener's granulomatosis.
- Presents with nasal symptoms, acute renal failure, and pulmonary symptoms.
- Renal biopsies show a focal segmental necrotizing glomerulonephritis with crescent formation (identical to microscopic polyangiitis).
- Lung biopsies show large 'geographical' areas of necrotizing granulomatous inflammation and a necrotizing vasculitis.
- Aggressive immunosuppression is needed to prevent mortality.

Microscopic polyangiitis (MPA)

- A systemic ANCA-associated vasculitis characterized by dominant renal and lung involvement and pANCA positivity.
- Most patients are adults with a median age of 55.
- Presents with acute renal failure and pulmonary symptoms.
- Renal biopsies show a focal segmental necrotizing glomerulonephritis with crescents (identical to Wegener's granulomatosis).
- Lung biopsies show marked alveolar haemorrhage and a necrotizing capillaritis within alveolar septae.
- Aggressive immunosuppression is needed to prevent mortality.

Eosinophilic granulomatosis with polyangiitis (EPA)

- A systemic vasculitis characterized by dominant lung and skin involvement, blood eosinophilia, and a history of asthma.
- Formally known as Churg–Strauss syndrome.
- Most patients are adults with a mean age of 40 at presentation.

Index

For the benefit of digital users, indexed terms that span two pages (e.g., 52–53) may, on occasion, appear on only one of those pages.
Tables and figures are indicated by *t* and *f* following the page number